Dr. Serge Rafal

Natural healing

HACHETTE
Illustrated

First published by Marabout, an imprint of Hachette-Livre, 43 Quai de Grenelle, Paris 75905, Cedex 15, France under the title *Médecines Douces*

This edition published 2003 by Hachette Illustrated UK, Octopus Publishing Group, 2–4 Heron Quays, London E14 4JP

ISBN: 1-8420-219-15

The information and recommendations given in this book are not intended to be a substitute for medical advice. Consult your doctor before acting on any recommendations given in this book. The authors and publisher disclaim any liability, loss, injury or damage incurred as a consequence, directly or indirectly, of the use and application of the contents of this book.

Translation supplied by First Edition Translations Ltd, Cambridge, in conjunction with Book Production Consultants plc, Cambridge.

Printed in

Table of contents

Foreword

This is a very valuable book for many reasons. Dr Rafal has written from the point of view of his own experience and there can be no better recommendation for practice than that. The book contains a wealth of information for both the layman and the expert and is one that every serious health seeker should own. Both traditional physicians and alternative practitioners alike will find it a rich source of information for both prevention and healing. There has been a huge increase in the popularity of complementary medicine in the past decade; the most popular therapies being herbal medicine, aromatherapy, homeopathy and acupuncture.

The book is written from the point of view of giving the reader a number of alternatives to choose from for their particular condition. At the same time, these options are underpinned with sound nutritional and supplemental recommendations. This is good naturopathic practice. One of the tenets in naturopathic medicine is that the person is treated and not the condition. Some people are going to respond better to homeopathy than they will to acupuncture, for example. We are all different, yet the basic raw materials that we need are the same. Here the reader can safely use the various modalities that suit them best. In addition, they can increase foods and supplements that provide the necessary vitamins and minerals that may be lacking for their particular condition. This is a truly holistic approach that not only serves to address the immediate or acute problem, but fosters a way to maintain our valuable health and alleviate chronic conditions.

Prevention is a word that is tantamount to natural healing and we are hearing more about this, as the idea that trying to fix something after it is broken is largely both ineffective and costly. We probably spend more time and money on our cars than we do on ourselves; expecting our bodies to keep 'running well without maintenance'. Our health care systems are buckling under the strain of having to 'fix' too many patients, many of whom could possibly have enhanced their treatment through augmenting complementary therapies.

In some health care systems, there is a growing demand by the public (as borne out by numerous surveys) for complementary therapies to be included and that they will be incorporated into the primary health care system. Indeed, some hospitals have set up complementary health centres to meet this demand and perhaps the future of complementary medicine will be in the primary health care systems.

Dr Rafal is one of a growing number of enlightened doctors working at the interface of both orthodox and holistic medicines. He is one of the pioneers of a system that in years to come will most likely be seen as the 'norm'. This integration, which is forging a different paradigm in medicine, can only greatly benefit the patient.

Stephen G. Langley,
The Hale Clinic, London.

Introduction

The aim of this book is a bold one, since I hope to be able to answer the many questions you might have concerning 'complementary therapies'.

I would like first of all to introduce you to them, to make you aware of their many advantages, before then explaining the best way to use them. This will then help you to ward off sickness and allow you to remain healthy, to stay in – or return to – peak physical and mental condition.

Finally, I hope to give you the means to take care of yourself using complementary medicines, by enabling you to manage and treat everyday problems, by offering you tips on easier ways to get well, and by guiding you towards the right choice for you and your family. I have chosen simple, effective instructions and protocols, and presented them in the order in which they should be used, with a view to sparing you the need for so many visits to a practitioner. Even if you do need to see a practitioner, this book can suggest some steps you might take before your appointment, and perhaps give you some ideas about any prescription given, should you wish to supplement it with any of my recommendations.

The advances and limits of modern medicine

The 20th century saw medicine make its greatest leap forward and take its place squarely in the modern scientific age. The average life expectancy has almost doubled in the Western world since 1900, and baby-boomers have now become grandparents, ushering in the 'grey power' generation. These wonderful improvements in longevity are partly the result of a reduction in infant mortality rates, but are also due to a better understanding of what causes disease (the risk factors), as well as much earlier diagnosis, and better management of the two illnesses which continue to plague us, cancers and cardiovascular diseases.

Although these conditions remain serious, and all too common, they are now much easier to detect thanks to better investigative tools (such as ultrasound, scans and magnetic resonance imaging) that have revolutionized both the way they are diagnosed and monitored and, to a lesser extent, their final outcome. Endoscopic instruments, for example, allow us to perform both preventive and therapeutic procedures at an earlier stage, avoiding the need for a major, possibly only palliative, operation.

In the field of pharmaceuticals, new medicines are now on the market which have changed the face of medical practice: the discovery of antibiotics in the 1940s means that our lives need no longer be cut short by infectious diseases. The antidepressants and tranquillizers developed in the 50s have allowed the anxious, the depressed, and those with real psychiatric conditions to leave the confinement of an asylum and lead almost normal lives at home. The anti-ulcer drugs in use since the 70s have pretty much eliminated our once-frequent recourse to surgery for stomach pain.

And yet...! For all its advances, modern medicine is far from being able to solve all health problems, and is especially unsatisfactory when faced with all the 'minor' illnesses or complaints which are not life-threatening, but which are literally poisoning people's lives. It is much too heavy-handed, for example, to deal with the everyday aches and pains or psychosomatic illnesses that make so many of us miserable.

So we GPs were not really prepared for the way complementary medicine, with its holistic, humane, and altogether less aggressive approach, caught on – nor for the growing trend of self-treatment. These two developments (which go hand in hand, since the second depends so much on the first) are now part of daily life for millions of people. It seems, then, not just a matter of interest, but of some importance, to clarify the role these therapeutic approaches play in a system of care that may complement, or in some cases replace, conventional treatment. How can they work for you?

A self-help guide for 'participants in their own health'

This practical guide, the synthesis of more than 25 years spent in the daily practice of complementary medicine, aims to be clear and simple, complete without being exhaustive. It is not designed to be a medical dictionary or encyclopedia, because I have deliberately chosen to deal with a limited, select number of conditions that respond especially well to complementary methods of treatment. But it is aimed at all those who care about their health, whether they already know and trust these therapies, or whether they would like to try out these safe, gentle treatments for the first time.

A plan of action

This book comprises two parts. The first aims to provide you with background information, a 'guide to the different methods', describing the essential techniques involved, classifying them and giving you the key to the best ways to use them. The second part is a practical guide to 'prevention and treatment', which will allow you to treat 80 symptoms or complaints that respond especially well to these therapies. The chapters are constructed in simple and consistent fashion: a brief list of the main symptoms, so that you can diagnose the problem; some general or dietary advice on how to stay healthy or build up your immune system; warnings to help you avoid some common mistakes; and above all the various, non-invasive treatments, presented to you in the order in which they should be used.

A word of warning

As with any self-help book, prudence, effectiveness, and simplicity are vital for the sake of both author and readers. This guide is for any reasonable person able to recognize a symptom and then to take the right approach, according to my recommendations. I have selected the contents so as to be able to advise you, to give you as much help as possible in preventing disease, and to offer you fast, effective solutions.

The ++ symbol in the text that follows is used to identify substances that have especially high concentrations (of trace elements or vitamins, for example), or especially strong symptoms.

How to use complementary medicine

Advice for all readers

This book offers you the most effective, gentle remedies for 80 everyday health problems. An accurate diagnosis must be made, and possibly even confirmed by further tests, for no self-treatment through complementary therapies can take place without it. I touch now on the limits of self-treatment, which must always be carried out with care, should bring noticeable results, must never exceed the stated dose or be continued beyond 48 hours – especially if there are no signs of improvement.

With homeopathic treatments there is no risk of overdose, but this is not the case with herbal therapies, especially when dealing with essential oils. These must never be used at higher doses than is recommended.

My choice of particular treatments and advice is a personal one, for although I could have prescribed other comparable products which act in similar ways, and produce the same effects, I have let myself be guided by my own experiences and habits. Certain brand-name products may be changed at any time, or taken off the market altogether. Your herbal medicine specialist or homeopath will be able to help you adjust the dosage or find an equivalent product.

A patent medicine is a preparation sold under a particular brand name, such as Berocca. Such names will always be indicated in this book by the ® sign, for example, Berocca®.

The doses I prescribe are for an adult of 'average' height, weight, and age, and are meant to be adapted in individual cases. Many of my treatments are intended for adults only, but if they are suitable for children I will say so and advise you of the appropriate dose to administer. Once again, homeopathic treatments can be safely given in the same way to everyone, whether to adults, children, pregnant women, or the elderly. Such is not the case with herbal remedies, and especially not with essential oils, which can be dangerous if not properly used, and which are therefore unsuitable, if not downright unsafe, for use in home remedies for infants and small children.

Advice for those who are new to complementary medicines

• Homeopathy may seem complicated to the uninitiated, as the treatments often come in the form of containers of granules or tablets with no instructions on them, just an obscure Latin name followed by a number and x (D) or c (according to whether it is a decimal or centesimal dilution). Thus, 'Hamamelis virginiana 6c' is a homeopathic preparation of witch hazel. The number 6 indicates the strength of dilution (in this example, the plant matter has undergone six successive dilutions at a ratio of 1:100), and 'c' stands for centesimal. Or alternatively, Hamamelis virginiana 6D has undergone six successive dilutions at a ratio of 1:10 and 'D' stands for decimal (the same as x). The first step in the process of homeopathic preparation is to develop a 'mother tincture' from the original substance by steeping animal, vegetable, or mineral products in water and alcohol, in order to extract their active properties. Successive dilutions or 'potentizations' result in the production of granules or tablets, which are the specific homeopathic form. These are composed of sucrose and lactose, impregnated with the active properties from the selected substance, and are taken as far away from mealtimes as possible. They are to be placed on or under the tongue, some of them dissolving almost immediately, whereas others are harder tablets that can be chewed. It is perfectly possible to mix homeopathic treatments with classical ('allopathic') medicines, as long as you do not take them at the same time.

• Phytotherapy or herbal medicine presents no particular complications or risks. The plant-based medications are prepared and packaged by a herbalist, mostly on special prescription, and generally come in the form of drops or capsules. The mother tincture, or preparation steeped in alcohol mentioned earlier, is easy to use. It is most often taken orally, having been diluted beforehand in half a glass of water according to the prescribed dose – commonly 1 teaspoon (5ml) three times daily either before or after meals depending on the condition.

– Aromatherapy's essential oils should be treated with caution, however. They should only be used if you know their effects, and when and how to take them
– Be very careful to adhere to the prescribed dose
– If you have any doubts, do not use them
– Do not use them over a prolonged period of time unless under strict medical supervision

For the sake of simplicity I have suggested taking essential oils with a little honey, but there are people who cannot tolerate them in this form, whether as a matter of taste or because of digestive difficulties. As an alternative, the oils can be prepared in an oral gel or in colloidal silica inside buffered capsules. To give you an example of the options, my recommendation to "take two drops of essential oil of cypress in a little honey, twice a day for ten days" could be substituted with: "obtain a preparation of one gram of essential oil in one hundred grams of oral gel", or alternatively with the suggestion to "ask for twenty buffered capsules each containing two drops of essential oil of mountain savory on colloidal silica, which you take for ten days, one capsule twice a day".

As a few general rules for using this book:

– Take prompt and informed action. It is a matter of the right diagnosis followed by the right decision, the right medicine at the right dose, taken at the right moment by the right patient, for the right amount of time

– Refrain from using any treatment that seems risky or vague, or which gives you cause for doubt

– Seek a conventional medical opinion if there seems to be no improvement

– Do not continue to treat yourself beyond a period of 24 hours, especially if you do not seem to be getting better (your health depends on it)

The cost of treatment

A portion of the cost of homeopathic preparations and herbal mother tinctures may be claimed back through some health insurance companies, provided it forms part of the consultation and provided the homeopath or herbalist belongs to an association recognized by the insurer.

1

Guide to the different methods

Introduction

Despite the extraordinary advances made by modern medicine, we have become attached to a different, vaguely old-fashioned approach – 'complementary medicine' – a social phenomenon of the 1980s. Alternatives to conventional treatment, particularly homeopathy, acupuncture, herbal therapy, osteopathy and chiropractic, are now very popular in the Western world. Many people use them in conjunction with conventional medicine, hence the term 'complementary', but others see them as a way of avoiding a visit to the GP.

Homeopathy is widely practised in the West. Three out of four Europeans are aware of it, and one in three uses it in four favourite areas: ENT, nervous problems, dermatology, and rheumatology. The homeopathy patient type is between 25 and 55 years old, politically involved and ecologically aware, a parent who is prepared to use this type of treatment for the children.

What should they be called?

There is, nevertheless, a problem in finding an acceptable name for a number of often disparate methods, whose only common feature is their rejection by conventional medicine. Many persist in using the term 'alternative medicine', because the underlying principle of most of the therapies is so different from that of conventional medicine.

The techniques of these 'alternatives' are more often seen as methods and treatments that complement conventional medicine than as entirely separate medical systems or remedies.

The essential characteristics of 'non-conventional treatments':

• they aim to strengthen natural defence reactions

• they depend on the notion of 'vital force'. (The term 'biological terrain' which is sometimes used refers more specifically to the biochemistry of the fluids in which the cells live. The cells cannot perform efficiently if the biological terrain is outside the healthy range)

• they are related to the concept of 'energy'

Vital Force

This apparently outdated notion, dear to the homeopath, constitutes the sum of inherited or acquired biological or immunological characteristics that help the organism defend itself against its aggressors, to tolerate or eliminate them.

The consideration of these factors, in which terrain therapy consists, is indispensable to an understanding of health and sickness.

A well-chosen, balanced diet, some rules for diet and hygiene, the restoration of intestinal balance, good stress management... all these undoubtedly help to strengthen defence reactions.

- they are primarily concerned with the whole suffering being, not the sick body alone
- they advocate a global physical, mental, and sometimes spiritual approach
- they are thought of as being 'alternative' because they suggest a non-aggressive therapeutic approach and maintain a privileged relationship with the patient
- they obtain results through procedures accepted (if at all) with some difficulty by conventional medicine

A series of different names...

For a long time the term 'parallel therapies' was the only one used. It embraces a hotchpotch of doctors and lay persons (medical counsellors, naturopaths, healers etc.). It cheerfully mixes proven methods supported by a long cultural past, some limited techniques that suddenly appear and just as quickly disappear, and still more dubious practices profiting from the jumble of ideas or from the limelight. The adjective 'parallel', implying that these therapies lie outside the medical system, has always pleased critics of such methods. In addition, the word is borrowed for controversial or critical articles on these methods.

The term 'different therapy' was once proposed as sounding milder than the above, but is no more used than 'new therapy', which is also scientifically incorrect. It would indeed be difficult to regard as 'new' ancient practices such as acupuncture, massage, and herbal medicine, or even homeopathy, which is two centuries old.

The term 'natural medicine' is much loved by 'naturopaths', and doctors are increasingly returning to this name that is liked and understood by the public. What comes from nature is certainly good for the health.

Natural healing

'Complementary medicine or therapy' and 'alternative medicine or therapy' are the terms most often known and used by the general public in Britain. Doctors like the term 'complementary' because it does not imply competition with conventional medicine.

In France, there is the term 'Médecines douces' or 'gentle medicine', which is the title of a magazine created in 1978, and which is overwhelmingly chosen by patients and preferred by numerous doctors, including the author. The adjective 'gentle' suggests two elements that are considered essential: a special relationship with the patient, and the use of therapeutic methods that are 'non-aggressive or mild'.

How many methods are there?

In addition to the principal, well-defined methods there is a profusion of 'minor' techniques that are derived from precedents or have been artificially created.

There are four 'gentle methods': acupuncture, homeopathy, herbal medicine, and manual therapies. Of the latter, osteopathy is the most well-known.

The list of alternatives is in fact much longer and, in addition to these four main techniques, there are at least 40 others. Here are some of them: acupressure, Alexander technique, anthroposophy, aromatherapy, auriculotherapy, biotherapy, cell therapy, qi gung, light therapy, etiopathy, electro-acupuncture, fascia therapy, Bach flower remedies, hydrotherapy, iridology, kinesiology, lithotherapy, macrobiotics, magnetotherapy, mesotherapy, Mézières method, music therapy, nature therapy, oligotherapy, organotherapy, ozone therapy, remedial massage, reflexology,

For adepts or adherents of complementary therapies in France, conventional medicine is described as 'hard', because it leaves less and less room for patient contact and because it resorts to heavily synthetic chemotherapy with numerous side effects. However, most practitioners or users of complementary therapies, while giving priority to their own methods, do not use them exclusively, but integrate them with modern medical methods.

Difficult classification

In classifying all these methods, their disparity raises issues that are more didactic than scientific.

At least in theory, most of them subscribe to a global concept, considering the patient in the context of his or her environment and personal history. The main methods pride themselves on a tradition by now ancient, on long experience that speaks for them and tries to provide scientific 'proof' of their efficacy.

The specific nature, reliability, and closely defined area of use of more contemporary methods such as mesotherapy and nutritional therapy have been rapidly established.

reiki, relaxation, shiatsu, sophrology, tai chi chuan, vegetarianism, vitamin therapy, yoga, zero balancing...

Sometimes some of these techniques are claimed to form part of a fairly large extended family, while hoping to be differentiated from it in order to be recognized.

How can the methods be classified?

It is possible to make a rough classification: it will certainly be artificial and simplistic, but indispensable when approaching an area that might well be likened to a great bazaar.

Methods based on the idea of energy: first comes acupuncture

Needles, hands, movements... allowing this ethereal flow to be channelled. Here we also find bioelectrical acupuncture and transcutaneous electro-stimulation, auriculotherapy, acupressure, and the body exercises of Chinese medicine.

Tai chi chuan is an energetic, physical, mental and spiritual method, but the dominating principle seems to be energetic. To many, auriculotherapy is a type of reflexology, but the use of needles brings it into this category. Transcutaneous electro-stimulation (bioelectrical acupuncture) is widely practised: it is a neurophysiological method that allows acupuncture to reach pain centres.

Methods using weak doses of medicines: first is homeopathy

Cell salts or Schuessler's salts are simple variants of homeopathy (6x or 12x potencies).

Natural healing

Methods based on plants: first is herbal medicine and its main branch, aromatherapy
The use of Bach flower remedies, highly prized in English-speaking countries, is not simple herbal medicine, for an essential overall spiritual approach is involved.

Manual methods: first is osteopathy
Included are chiropractic, etiopathy, bonesetting, fascia therapy, kinesiology, vertebrotherapy...

Certain techniques such as types of shiatsu can be included here since we have classed them among the methods involving energy.

Methods based on diet or diet supplements: first is oligotherapy
Macrobiotics, orthomolecular therapy, vegetarianism, and vitamin supplementation all find a place here.

Oligotherapy is a nutritional method, but could be classed with treatments using weak doses.

The use of vitamins is within the domain of conventional medicine, but many 'alternative' practitioners take a special interest in it.

Methods based on the elements (water, heat, cold, and earth) fall into the naturopathy category
Here we find clay, mud baths, light therapy, negative ions, and magnetotherapy.

Mental healing methods based on relaxation
Here we have music therapy, sophrology, yoga...

Reflex methods – by definition classified under reflexology
Here are neural therapy, palmar and plantar reflexology, sympathicotherapy, also mesotherapy.

Homeopathy is considered by some to be energy-based, since potentiation of the remedy is essential to its efficacy.
Catalytic trace element therapy can find a place alongside homeopathy, but since it is currently practised within the frame of nutritional therapy, it may be classed with methods involving diet supplementation. Some massage techniques are also tied up with energy. They produce improvements through the mobilization of this ethereal flow by the therapist's hands.

Thermotherapy and thalassotherapy are classic natural treatments, as are the physiotherapy used by kinesiotherapists and the phototherapy used by neurologists

Finally, we could have added some other diagnostic methods, such as iridology, which relies on the much-disputed claim that an illness leaves an indelible trace on the iris.

Some consider auriculotherapy to be a type of reflexology rather than an energy therapy. Mesotherapy, which involves the use of conventional medicines in very small doses, may well fall into this group.

Methods based on energy

In our bodies there exists a vital force that circulates and maintains physical and mental balance.

Energy therapy supports and influences this ethereal flux to maintain health or treat illness. Treatment consists of using the hands, needles, and precise movements to supply, reinforce, distribute, and channel this energy.

Acupuncture

Acupuncture was revealed to the whole world 40 years ago. To many, it still seems very mysterious, with an aura of magic.

Two ages, two worlds

Since its creation thousands of years ago, acupuncture has undergone fewer changes than any other therapeutic system. The splinters of stone have given way to bones, to bamboo, then to the metal needles we know today. This carefully worked out method, seemingly very simple, is an expression of the symbiosis between two worlds and two cultures. With a rich history and unparalleled longevity, it integrates perfectly with modern medicine.

From empiricism to scientific confirmation

Acupuncture, first used in the Yellow River valley, China, then throughout the Empire, then the whole continent of Asia, passed through a long period of development during which the mainstays of the method, the paths of the meridians and the positions and names of the points, and the rules for their use, all appeared. Its cultural significance was so great that bronze statues decorated with the acupuncture meridians were prized gifts during negotiations and peace treaties. The Ming dynasty (14th–15th centuries) marked the peak of Chinese influence in the whole of the Far East. King Louis XIV of France sent emissaries to bring back numerous documents on Chinese civilization and medicine. The special relationship between Italy and the 'Middle Empire' led to the introduction of acupuncture into Europe.

This short surge of interest was followed by a long eclipse lasting until the 19th century, when some attention was paid to it by prominent individuals, but not those in the scientific community, who judged it to be an esoteric, exotic practice. No man is a prophet in his own country: in 1929 it was even forbidden by the Nanking government... to be later rehabilitated by Mao during the Cultural Revolution.

Acupuncture attracted international attention in 1958, when for the first time it was substituted for general anaesthesia during a tonsillectomy. It became an object of curiosity and the point of departure for a multitude of studies by the scientific community in an attempt to penetrate its secrets and reproduce its effects. These researches gave it a scientific aura, and allowed its acceptance by conventional medicine.

The medicine of energy

The idea of energy is essential to an understanding of acupuncture and Chinese medicine. The latter embraces the concept of coherence between the laws of life, nature, and knowledge. The continuous rotation of the earth, its orbit around the

Throughout the Orient, health and the art of healing are based on the idea of a life force called 'prana' by the Hindus, 'Chi' by the Chinese, and 'Ki' by the Japanese. The term 'acupuncture' appeared in the 16th century and comes from the contraction of two Latin words, 'acus' (needle) and 'punctura' (prick). It was given the name by the Jesuits of the Society of Jesus on their return from a mission to China. Acupuncture consists in preventing or curing illnesses by means of needles placed in the skin. The points are chosen according to very precise rules.

Preventive medicine

In ancient China, a doctor was a sage who defined a way of life and an ethic. He was attached to a family in a preventive role and was paid as long as the family members remained healthy. He was concerned with food, supervised hygiene, gave massages, advised on physical exercise (tai chi chuan), organized treatments – frequently based on plants – and suggested and carried out acupuncture sessions.

sun, and relationship to the stars depends on the energy controlling the seasons, determining the climate, and influencing our bodies. Tao (the path, the way) symbolizes the essential, unique principle of beings and things, and the laws linking them with the universe and the cosmos.

In Taoist thought, the energy is unique and fundamental, present in each being as two opposing and complementary forces, in balanced proportions and indispensable to each other: Yin and Yang.

Good health is the result of a balance between the energy in us and the energy brought to us by the environment. Illness results if the energy is insufficient, blocked, badly balanced, or wrongly distributed. It is therefore necessary to watch over one's energy capital, one's supply of health.

Circulation along special paths

The energy stored or transformed in the body moves along special paths called meridians. The paths and the rhythm of this circulation are exact, but they cannot be seen or otherwise identified. They are like the aerial corridors used in aviation, in which aircraft pass along immutable but virtual routes. These meridians run at different depths, join the inside and the outside, above with below, left with right, and most fortunately cross the surface and are accessible to acupuncture needles.

Acupuncture consultation

Clearly, things have changed a great deal since those distant times when the court doctor had access only to the hands of his illustrious patient, the Empress, hidden behind a screen or a curtain, to make his diagnosis. This is the historic reason for the importance of the pulses in Chinese medicine. Consultation these days takes medical progress into account while preserving the features of the energetic approach.

Natural healing

As acupuncture can be separated from its place within Traditional Chinese Medicine (TCM) so as to stand alone as a therapy, its real power can be diluted to treating just symptomatically. A more holistic approach is usually undertaken which includes a number of diagnostic criteria, including both tongue and pulse diagnosis as well as observing and listening to the 'energy' of the patient. This gathered information will formulate the basis for the needle placement. Different doctors may work in different ways according to their training and some may use the five element approach which underpins TCM, namely the relationship of the patient, their environment and condition to the elements – water, fire, metal, wood and earth.

- The patient is stretched out on the back or the stomach, or sometimes is seated

- The placing of the needles, perhaps up to fifteen per session (depending on the treatment), so dreaded by those unfamiliar with acupuncture, causes little pain over most of the body, but can be slightly disagreeable on the extremities and the face. The needles, which are fine, solid, and very sharp, are swiftly inserted to a depth of a few millimetres. They may be left in place for up to twenty minutes, occasionally rotated, or sometimes connected to an electric stimulator to increase their effect

- At the start of treatment, weekly sessions are usual, but may be more frequent in the case of acute conditions such as shingles or for relieving the pain of sciatica

- As a general rule, five or six sessions are necessary to bring about an improvement or cure but may require many more for long-standing chronic conditions

Acupuncture is a discipline in full expansion. It has more than 5,000 registered practitioners in the UK and is perhaps the least controversial of the complementary therapies. Acupuncture is also carried out within the NHS (National Health Service) and has been taught in medical faculties since the early eighties...

Treatment consists of supplying energy, controlling its circulation, and channelling it. Sometimes it is a matter of disposing of an excess, sometimes of creating a shortage, sometimes of rebalancing.

Fear of communicable diseases (hepatitis, AIDS) has dictated the use of single-use steel needles. As a result, the gold or silver needles that were once used have been eliminated.

Acupuncture has no secondary effects, though there may be a temporary worsening of symptoms or transient tiredness. Thus, when we treat, for example, an athlete with hay fever, we avoid suggesting a session before an event or on the morning of a competition.

Mechanism

Two scientific hypotheses have been put forward to account for the efficacy of acupuncture.

• The implantation of needles creates competition between the nerve fibres concerned with touch and slower pain fibres: the former quickly convey messages to the brain, and the latter are inhibited. This is the 'gate control theory', so called because the brain gives priority to information on touch and closes the gate to pain messages

• The placing of needles in or on the skin causes the liberation within the central nervous system of neuro-modulatory substances – endorphins (endogenous morphines), which are involved in the control of the pain phenomenon

These two mechanisms probably do not explain all the effects of acupuncture, but have facilitated its introduction into most pain control centres.

Acupuncture indications

Acupuncture has four important targets:

• Pain:

– Rheumatology: neuralgia, back pain, lumbago, sciatica, stiff neck – which it can cure. Acute attacks of inflammatory rheumatism – which it can alleviate

– Trauma: strains, pulled muscles, sprains, tendinitis...

– Non-rheumatological: headaches and migraines, bladder pains (cystalgia) without urinary infection, sinusitis, shingles...

– It must be said that the symptomatic relief of these conditions through acupuncture is not the goal of the acupuncturist. The acupuncturist will be attempting to address the 'root' cause as well as attacking the 'branches'

• Autonomic nervous system problems:
– Anxiety states, feeling low or depressed, sleep problems, fatigue, overwork, spasmophilia
– Functional digestive problems (not associated with a precise cause): anorexia, bulimia, heartburn, constipation, diarrhoea, various digestive ailments... or gynaecological problems: dysmenorrhoea, premenstrual syndrome, hot flushes, circulatory problems...

• Allergy:
– Skin problems: from eczema to psoriasis...
– Asthma, allergic rhinitis, hay fever...

• Stopping smoking
– For some, acupuncture is a certain cure. It certainly helps correctly motivated patients

Bioelectrical acupuncture

Bioelectrical acupuncture reinforces the effects of acupuncture by means of current applied through the needles. This adjunct to conventional acupuncture began in China in 1934.

Indications
– Chronic pain
– Dealing with cellulitis (electrolipolysis)

Transcutaneous electro-stimulation

This was perfected by neurophysiologists working to understand the pain mechanism. It has developed in recent years thanks to the miniaturization of the equipment used for stimulation. It is mainly used in pain control centres, but some acupuncturists also use it.

Indications
– Residual pain after amputation
– The after-effects of shingles

The first anaesthesia using acupuncture had considerable worldwide impact. However, acupuncture anaesthesia is far less effective than modern Western methods. Delivery of babies under acupuncture has been offered in a few pregnancies and seems to relieve, but not suppress, back pains. Some Caesarean operations have been conducted under acupuncture, but the comfort it gave proved relative and it has been abandoned as an alternative to general or peridural anaesthesia.

If acupuncture does not cure all illnesses (and no modality can claim to cure all illnesses), its global approach means it can be offered to most patients, even those who are seriously ill, in combination with other treatments. Acupuncture does not cure cancer but can help the cancer patient.

A pharmacist in ancient Rome acquired fame through the miraculous gout cures he obtained by using electrical discharges from a torpedo fish: this was the first medical use of electricity.

Acupressure

This consists of applying pressure to the acupuncture points with the thumb. It is stimulating or calming depending on the technique used, and particularly useful for freeing up a pain or easing tension. It is sometimes used for patients who have a fear of needles or when treating some small children.

Auriculotherapy

Technique

Following diagnosis by questioning, then more specifically by using a blunt probe to locate painful points on the outer ear, the practitioner pricks these or massages them gently with a small instrument with a rounded point.

Auriculotherapists (those practising this technique) use:

– a simple acupuncture needle, carefully placed so as not to pierce the cartilage

– tiny, 'semi-permanent' press needles which are usually removed by the acupuncturist after about a week or so. This avoids any possible septic problems that might occur if they are left in for longer periods. However some people remove them themselves or find that they fall out of their own accord

Indications

– The same as those for acupuncture in general: the treatment of intractable pain or problems of the autonomic nervous system

– Particularly useful for stopping smoking or, under the right conditions, for following a diet

Some traditional Oriental methods

All of these are based on the circulation of energy.

Qi gung

Consists of exercises designed to develop the powers of concentration so as to be able to channel energy, the 'vital breath' – the life force – and use it at the right moment. Thus, a doctor trained in these methods can concentrate the energy in the palm of his hand and transmit it to a patient who needs it.

Shiatsu

This Japanese method of massage, relaxation and rebalance is the counterpart of Chinese acupressure. It is based on massage, rubbing, and stretching the pressure points or points found painful on examination. The treatment is applied in depth using the fingers, the palms… elbows, knees and feet… A session may last an hour. Regular practice may have a preventive role, since shiatsu regulates the circulation of energy, while taking the physical and existential globality of the being into account.

Tai chi chuan

Tai chi chuan was derived from the martial arts, but the aggressive gestures have been replaced with slow, circular movements akin to dancing or even choreography. It has a symbolic dimension, evoking victory in the suppleness of a snake facing the erratic movements of a bird. The aim is to externalize one's internal force or vital energy by channelling it. It allows mental concentration while using the body and encourages health, vitality, internal peace, and harmony with beings and things. Strongly rooted in Chinese culture, tai chi chuan has been practised in Europe since the borders of China were opened in the 1970s.

A method based on remedies in small doses

Despite being the subject of violent controversies ever since its creation in the 18th century, homeopathy stands at the forefront of complementary therapies. Many other methods (biotherapy, lithotherapy, organotherapy, etc.) are derived from it.

Two examples

– Coffee is a cardiovascular stimulant that hinders sleep. A patient who complains of palpitations and one who suffers from insomnia both have their conditions improved by taking diluted coffee (Coffea)

– A bee sting causes a red, burning oedema, relieved by a cold compress. A sunstroke victim with symptoms similar to those produced by a bee sting is relieved by prescribing a diluted bee preparation (Apis)

Homeopathy

This therapeutic method was advanced at the end of the 18th century by Samuel Hahnemann, regarded as the father of homeopathy, although the Swiss physician and alchemist Paracelsus (1493–1541) was instrumental in working with provings of homeopathic remedies. It consists in prescribing the substance that is experimentally capable of producing symptoms similar to those of the illness, after having enormously diluted and potentiated it; it thus creates a similar ('homeo') suffering ('pathos') – or homeopathy.

History

Samuel Hahnemann (1755–1843), a German doctor born in Saxony, was disappointed with indifferent results in his patients and began to give up his practice. He devoted himself to experimental research and made translations to earn his living.

He discovered a description of the properties of cinchona, a remedy recently introduced into Europe to combat 'marsh fever', or malaria, which then plagued the south of France. For several days in succession he took large doses of the bark, and soon felt the symptoms of the malaria attack normally treated with this substance. He realized that in a healthy person, cinchona is capable of producing symptoms identical to those that it can make disappear in a patient.

He brought the ancient Law of Similars described by Hippocrates, "like cures like", up to date and made it the basis for his method. He diluted remedies to avoid toxic reactions and to cause a minimal illness, capable of stimulating defence reactions without overcoming them. Homeopathy was born.

Out of step with the ideas of the time
The step taken by Hahnemann implied a fundamental criticism of medical methods of his time, since he decided to experiment with a substance before prescribing it. On the one hand he opted for the Law of Similars, setting himself against a medical profession that did not believe in it, and on the other he diluted his 'remedies' to a degree that apparently went beyond reason. He gave up his research into the cause of the illness, believing above all that the remedy must correspond to the ensemble of specific symptoms presented by the patient.

It is easy to imagine the difficulties he encountered, the determination of his adversaries to destroy him... all the more so since he alienated himself from the apothecaries by preparing and delivering his remedies to the patients himself.

A global treatment
Homeopathy is thus a therapy that treats the patient as a whole, not just the illness, deals with the physical body as well as the emotional, mental, and spiritual element. The patient's history of illnesses is assessed, and the treatment is not aimed solely at removing a troublesome symptom. The illness is not the cause, but the result of an imbalance that needs correction.

'Allopathy', a term used for conventional medicine, comes from the Greek words 'allos' (other) and 'pathos' (illness); it fights the symptoms, whereas homeopathy goes along with them.

By giving importance to physical and psychic signs, Hahnemann was one of the first to realize that the individual reacts with his body and spirit at the same time, and that the whole range of symptoms is more important than one symptom on its own. He was one of the forerunners of psychosomatics and the concept of global medicine.

The initial expansion of homeopathy followed the advance of Austria's armies; more specifically, its efficacy was proved in the face of fearful cholera epidemics. Its supporters began to preach its virtues: a Dr. Benoît Mure of Lyon left for Brazil and created some 22 dispensaries there, which explains the firm establishment of this method in South America. It was equally widely used in India under the influence of both the British and the French, because it constituted a cheap and effective preliminary treatment.
Dr. Frederick Quin (1799-1878) was a disciple of Hahnemann and introduced homeopathy to Great Britain in the late 1820s, founding the London Homeopathic Hospital.

The development of homeopathy
The number of homeopaths has grown enormously over the years, as has the public's demand for the treatment, despite the unfavourable opinion of the great majority of the medical profession. Homeopathy has not only stood the test of time, but has continued to develop, and the increasing numbers of patients are an indication of their satisfaction with the clinical results. It is much used by parents to treat their children, a good indication of its healthy status. The value of homeopathy has not been reduced or weakened by modern scientific discoveries. Currently the search is for further proof of the activity of high dilutions and its undisputed efficacy in human medicine.

Details of homeopathic consultation
Homeopathy, holistic human medicine, considers the patient as a unique, original reactional whole.

It not only takes into account the clinical signs that characterize the illness, but also strictly individual reactions in particular. Let us take an example:

– Two children with colds present common symptoms: fever, rhinitis, cough… but there are different additional symptoms: one has a high fever, is flushed and agitated, while the other has a slight temperature and is pale and very low

– These opposite types of behaviour indicate different ways of reacting and will not be treated with the same homeopathic remedy. Belladonna is indicated in the first case, Ferrum phosphoricum in the second

The consultation is thus highly individualized, searching for the patient's particular characteristics. This explains the sometimes disconcerting, unusual questions the homeopath is led to ask

Natural healing

The small details normally ignored in conventional medicine are given some weight: where? when? how? who?...

– Consultation is not a simple matter because there is no standard treatment. It takes accompanying signs and the reactional process into account, and can sometimes be lengthy, especially the first time

Highly diluted remedies
The homeopathic method rests on the need for dilutions that stimulate the body's defence mechanisms while avoiding violent reactions to toxic substances.

The extreme ('infinitesimal') dilutions used are a favourite target for the opponents of homeopathy, since after a dilution of 11c, going by the Avogadro constant in the laws of physics, no trace of the active principle can still remain.

This problem divides the medical profession and greatly intrigues and fascinates scientists. The mechanism of homeopathy could be explained by electromagnetism, since vigorous shaking or 'succussion' is essential to the efficacy of the homeopathic remedy.

The preparation of homeopathic remedies
Homeopathic preparations are remedies obtained by the so-called 'Hahneman' method of successive dilutions.

The homeopath obtains his raw materials from the three kingdoms of nature: animal, mineral, and vegetable.

Extracts of the natural ingredient are dissolved in a mixture of alcohol and water to form a 'mother tincture', which is the starting point for successive dilutions leading to the final remedy.

Consultation always has two aims

– One is the conventional medical consultation: questioning, observation, close examination, further examination as required, aimed at making as accurate a diagnosis as possible.

– The other is more specific: the search for the remedy, as studied by Hahnemann and listed in the 'materia medica', that corresponds as closely as possible to the reactive symptoms presented by the patient. Only the prescription of this remedy, homeopathically diluted, can bring about the cure.

No substance is homeopathic in itself; it is the method of preparation and prescription that makes it specific. Antibiotics or cortisone may become homeopathic if prepared as such, but clearly they will lose their initial properties and acquire others. Thus, patients being treated with cortisone may sometimes have it prescribed in homeopathic dilutions to lessen the almost inevitable undesirable effects of long-term treatment.

The mother tincture then undergoes successive dilutions according to either the decimal or the centesimal scale, denoted by 'x' and 'c' respectively, and is finally combined with lactose to form tablets, granules, or powder.

The number that follows the name of the remedy in Latin represents the number of 1/10 or 1/100 dilutions carried out to obtain it using the Hahnemann method: Nux vomica 4c is nux vomica to the 4th centesimal dilution and nux vomica 4x is nux vomica to the 4th decimal dilution.

The commonest standard dilutions are: mother tincture, 3x, 6x, 4c, 6c, 30c and 200c.

Forms of homeopathic remedies

– Various forms of homeopathic remedy are available. In addition to tablets, granules and powders, they can be prepared in other traditional forms: drops, ointments, creams, suppositories, etc.

Taking a homeopathic remedy

The granules are generally taken singly, in twos or fours, and placed under the tongue and sucked like sweets, between meals or refreshments

Touching homeopathic preparations with the fingers, taking coffee or strong mints concurrently or using mint-flavoured toothpaste is traditionally seen as undermining the energetic potential of the remedy due to its subtle energy nature.

The action of homeopathic remedies is not proportional to the quantity taken, but to the reaction sought from the body: it would be a mistake to imagine that ten granules have twice the activity of five, or that 7c is stronger than 5c.

Because of their extreme dilution, homeopathic remedies are neither toxic nor allergenic. If a child swallows a whole tubeful, there is no danger and no need to make an emergency call.

Prescribing rules

– More remedies are taken in acute conditions: after a shock, Arnica 6c may be prescribed every five minutes, four or five times in succession, then three or four times a day for two or three days

– In chronic illness the doses are taken at longer intervals: in asthma, Arsenicum album 30c is normally prescribed two or three times a week

– Higher dilutions are used for ailments with after-effects: after bereavement, Staphysagria is often prescribed at 200c, two or three times a week

– In acute illnesses, homeopathy is effective and rapidly so, provided it is prescribed at the appearance of the first symptoms; moreover, many paediatricians have taken it up. The results are certainly slower in more chronic illnesses that have developed over a number of years because the strengthening of the vital force is generally not a light matter to be dealt with instantly

Possible combinations

It is entirely feasible to combine homeopathy with the use of conventional medicines, a possibility clearly indicated by the term 'complementary therapies'. A patient with arterial hypertension may perfectly well benefit from homeopathic prophylaxis in the winter, and a complementary prescription of homeopathic remedies, vitamins, or trace elements is justifiable, even in a patient on antibiotics.

Indications for homeopathy

The field of activity of homeopathy is wider than imagined, covering the majority of everyday ill-

Note: homeopathy is not herbal medicine, even if some plants form the basis of certain homeopathic remedies; herbal medicine or phytotherapy will be described later. It is however true that plants are prescribed as mother tinctures, which are the starting point for homeopathic remedies, hence the confusion.

It is standard practice to prescribe the taking of remedies away from mealtimes: this still holds good but needs modification: granules taken ten minutes before or thirty minutes after a meal will be fully effective.

No value should be given to the saying "slight illness – homeopathy, serious illness – conventional medicine". Many people, even those with serious illnesses, turn to homeopathy for the first time when conventional medicine seems to have failed. While obviously cancer and AIDS cannot be treated with homeopathy, homeopaths frequently treat cancer or AIDS patients, because the method deals with patients, not diseases. It is a basic tenet of both naturopathy and homeopathy that the person is treated and not the disease. This understanding is also in Traditional Chinese Medicine and embraces the idea of 'wholeism': treating the mind, body and spirit as a total.

nesses, acute or chronic, functional, or sometimes due to injury, equally well in infants and the aged. Since it relies on the body's defensive potential, all that is needed for it to be fully effective is an unimpaired capacity for reaction.

• Autonomic nervous system problems constitute the major indication area:
– Anxiety states, depression, sleep problems, overwork, neurosis
– Functional digestive problems (precise cause unclear): anorexia, bulimia, heartburn, constipation, diarrhoea, and other difficulties with digestion... or gynaecological problems: dysmenorrhoea, premenstrual syndrome, hot flushes, circulatory problems...

• Infections in adults and children:
– Colds, sinusitis, sore throat, influenza, laryngitis, rhinopharyngitis, bronchitis, tracheitis, herpes...
– Its exceptional preventive role in winter ailments and recurrent urinary infection should be emphasized

• Allergy:
– Skin problems: from eczema to psoriasis...
– Asthma, allergic rhinitis, hay fever...

• Some painful conditions, especially:
– Arthritis
– Headache and migraine

• Veterinary practice: numerous veterinary surgeons have taken up homeopathy; here it is difficult to put a case for a solely psychological effect

• Some people say, or believe, that homeopathy has a slimming effect. This is not so; it simply helps with maintaining a diet, of which more later

It must be stressed right away that incorrect homeopathic instructions can be dangerous, especially if the patients are not informed or aware of a conventional medicine concealed among ten or twenty Latin names.

Methods based on plants

Even though advances in modern medicine had led to the general impression that plants would be returned to the apothecary's cupboard, or were only useful in making infusions to assist digestion or sleeping, they are back in favour. Day by day, as more and more consumers become aware of their usefulness, their appeal is on the increase.

Herbal therapy

Man used plants first to feed himself, then as a cure. Down through history, plants have been exploited for various purposes, and have been included in many more or less medical potions.

History

Ancient civilizations were witness to the growth of man's knowledge of medicinal plants. This knowledge was preserved and, as evidenced by numerous medicinal herb gardens, transmitted by medieval religious orders. The 15th century marked the beginning of the spread of knowledge of medicinal plants through herbariums. Culinary herbs, spices, ornamental plants, tea, cocoa, coffee, and tobacco were discovered and brought back by maritime expeditions to the Americas or the Indies.

At the end of the 19th century, treatment almost always involved the use the whole of the plant. The pharmacist was still an apothecary who prepared emulsions, infusions, decoctions, elixirs, liniments, macerations, ointments, tisanes (herbal teas), and topical remedies in his dispensary – sometimes nowadays a source of amuse-

Ancient civilizations and medicinal plants

The Chinese integrate plants into their traditional medicine along with acupuncture and diet.

Egyptian papyri show that the Egyptians were aware of the virtues of the poppy, from which morphine is extracted, and that they distributed energizing garlic to the workers building the pyramids.

In Rome, the Borgias became famous by exploiting the toxic properties of hemlock to perfection.

The Native Americans were aware of the antiseptic properties of certain fungi, which they applied to wounds; antibiotics have only been used extensively since the 1940s.

Whatever is quick and practical has consumer appeal. The public prefers tablets or capsules rather than decoctions. Nonetheless, the French in particular are very fond of tisanes, which they love to take in the evening to improve digestion or sleep.

ment or nostalgia. For some decades the herb trade was still a legally recognized profession.

The progress of medicine in the 20th century seemed finally to have put a brake on herbal medicine. But it has not turned out to be the case, and with some drugs, however extraordinary (antibiotics, tranquillizers etc.), the unwanted and sometimes dangerous side effects caused many patients to turn to less 'aggressive' treatments. This signalled the return in strength of 'gentle therapies', particularly the use of plants.

Large numbers of remedies are based on plants

The consumption of plants has tripled in the last 20 years. Sixty per cent of our medicines come directly or indirectly from the vegetable kingdom. The World Health Organization (WHO) has a list of some 20,000 plant names in 73 countries. Antibiotics are derived from fungi; atropine is used in eye lotion; digitalis is used to treat heart patients; rye ergot is still one of the main treatments for migraine; ginkgo biloba acts on the circulation; the horse chestnut, red vine, witch hazel, and blackcurrant are recognized venous tonics; melilot is used in making a synthetic anticoagulant; morphine controls pain; an extract of willow is used to prepare aspirin; derivatives of the periwinkle are anti-leukaemic.

All these uses demonstrate the therapeutic importance of plants.

Different plant preparations

Herbal medicine uses whole plants or one of their parts (leaves, flowers, stems, and roots...). After gathering, they are used fresh or dried, and subjected to various processes: drying, grinding, crushing, treatment with water or alcohol, glycol, or other solvents – all of which partially denature

Natural healing

them. As far as possible, the finished product handed to the patient should furnish the properties of the fresh plant in a stable form.

The herbalist provides plant remedies in solid or liquid form

– dry: powders (ten to twenty times more concentrated than an infusion) or dried extracts contained in capsules, sachets (infusions), in patent medicines, or made up as special preparations

– liquid: mother tinctures, liquid extracts, whole fresh plant suspensions…

Plant indications
Correctly handled by experienced practitioners, plants give remarkable results in most everyday illnesses.

• Autonomic nervous system problems
– Some plants to help with sleep: sweet woodruff, hawthorn, white horehound, poppy, hops, sweet marjoram, meadowsweet, orange blossom, passionflower, lime, valerian, verbena
– Some calming plants: angelica, hawthorn, camomile, California poppy, lettuce, bird's foot trefoil, passionflower, verbena
– some antidepressant plants: angelica, St. John's wort

• Digestive problems:
– Some plants that stimulate appetite: artichoke, fenugreek, gentian, bitter orange, dandelion…

– Some plants that stimulate gall-bladder action: artichoke, boldo, celandine, barberry, fumitory, dandelion, rosemary…

– Some plants that help the digestion: dill, anise, basil, caraway, blessed thistle, coriander, cumin, gentian, meadowsweet, mint, orange blossom, rosemary, savory, wild thyme, thyme, scented verbena…

Suspensions and mother tinctures

Fresh whole plants preserved as micro-suspensions in water and alcohol. These yield the therapeutic entirety of the plant with all its active principles. There are 14 of them in this form: artichoke, hawthorn, burdock, blackcurrant, bladderwrack, horse chestnut, melilot, lemon balm, nettle, passionflower, dandelion, horsetail, meadowsweet, and valerian.

Mother tinctures whose preparation involves a filtration stage lose all the active principles that are insoluble in alcohol: their action is therefore less complete than that of suspensions.

Plant quality

Currently, there are some 200,000 known species of plant. Of these, 20,000 are listed as therapeutic, 2,000 are well known, and 200 are used every day throughout the whole world in preparing pharmaceutical products that cover almost all common illnesses.

– Some antispasmodic plants: angelica, hawthorn, white horehound, celandine, cypress, bird's foot trefoil, melilot, meadowsweet, olive, marigold, valerian, and scented verbena

– Some laxative plants: barberry, linseed, mallow, psyllium, and tamarind… also aloes, buckthorn, cascara, rhubarb, sennapod, but be careful not to take too much of these

• Gynaecological problems:
– Some plants for the menopause: evening primrose, cypress, chasteberry, soya, and yam

• Circulatory problems:
– Some plants that act on the venous system: cypress, witch hazel, horse chestnut, red vine

– Some plants active against arterial hypertension: garlic, hawthorn, birch, mistletoe, olive

– Some diuretic plants: artichoke, berberis, birch, blackcurrant, cherry stem, fennel, pink sage, mouse-ear hawkweed, and dandelion

• Rheumatic illness:
– Some anti-inflammatory plants: devils' claw, horsetail, meadowsweet, white willow, and horseweed

• Infections:
– An anti-infective plant: echinacea
– Some plants that act on the airways: eucalyptus, ipecacuanha, marruba…
– Some plants that stimulate defence reactions: eleutherococcus, ginseng, kola, mate, quinine, tea…

• Skin problems: burdock, borage…

Aromatherapy

A branch of herbal therapy, this therapeutic method uses the essential oils of aromatic plants. Aromatherapy has many applications, but thanks to its bactericidal action, it is particularly effective in the treatment of infections.

Definition and main features

Since 1972 the term 'essential oil' has replaced the former 'essence' or 'aromatic essence'. Essential oils are steam-distilled plant extracts. They are volatile liquids, oily but not greasy (they do not stain paper) are less dense than water, and have very strong aromatic smells and flavours. They are insoluble in water, and soluble in alcohol and in fixed oils such as, for example, sweet almond. They are sensitive to air and light and therefore have special storage conditions.

The definition of essential oil differs appreciably depending on whether it has been prepared by a pharmacist, a botanist, a chemist, or a perfumer.

Plants and plant essential oils

Four hundred and twenty-two essential oils derived from plants or parts of plants are listed, but only about forty of them are used in aromatherapy.

Knowledge of the properties of the plants used in herbal therapy does not necessarily make it possible to deduce their properties in aromatherapy; this is of fundamental importance. One cannot assume that the properties of essential oils will be the same as those of the plants they are extracted from without the risk of making serious mistakes.

The main difficulty in the use of essential oils is that they are only moderately well tolerated; pharmacists are continually seeking improvement.

Not everything natural is necessarily harmless: you should definitely avoid any plant or mixture if you are not sure of its exact composition, provenance, quality, and relevant precautions.

Plants have enormous potential; many useful effects are still only partly recognized and are still to be defined. Plants are the oldest medicine; they are even more important today, and in all probability will remain so in the future.

Guide to the different methods

Essential oils have several advantages over plants:
– they are very effective
– they need little storage space
– they do not alter, so can be kept for a long time
– they are easily transported, easy to use, and require no complex infrastructure

Some essential oils are very expensive: some three to five tonnes of rose petals are needed to produce one litre of its essence. However, most of the essential oils that we will be recommending are very affordable.

A historical note

Some authors link the introduction of essential oils with ancient medicine, but this is incorrect: in those times they were used for embalming and for the preparation of perfumes, but only rarely actually as medicine. The arts of distillation and the use of essences are more recent, and date back to the invention of the alembic in the Middle Ages, some four centuries ago. It was the Arabs who were responsible for this discovery, and the alchemists perfected and spread distillation techniques. The first study that led to the use of essential oils in medicine – as antiseptics – was only carried out at the end of the 19th century.

Methods of administration

• Mainly in oral form:

For the sake of simplicity, we have recommended taking one or two drops of essential oil in a little honey one to three times a day, while realizing that the taste and smell of certain oils may cause digestive problems or make it impossible to continue treatment. In such cases, you can consult an aromatherapist who will be able to recommend a more acceptable mixture, or suggest a special preparation in the form of gastro-resistant capsules.

• The skin

Certain essential oils such as eucalyptus can be applied to the skin, but with sensitive skins there is a risk of allergy or irritation

• The respiratory tract

Inhalation methods and aerosols are rightly recommended because they are very effective. The stick inhaler is convenient for ENT infections

• Pessaries are used for gynaecological infections

Indications and limitations

• Infection is indisputably the major indication. Seven essential oils are used: Ceylon cinnamon, eucalyptus, cloves, Spanish oregano, mountain savory, tea tree, and thyme

• For the airways can be added cajeput, niaouli, and pine

• The stimulant essential oils are: coriander, ginger, mint, nutmeg, rosemary, and savory

• The sedative essential oils are: camomile, sweet marjoram, bitter orange, orange blossom, and verbena

• The digestive essential oils are: caraway, cumin, tarragon, and mint

• The antispasmodic, anti-neuralgic essential oils are: basil, cajeput, and camomile

• For dentistry: cloves

• The essential oil for circulation problems: cypress

• The essential oil for external treatment: lavender

The limits of aromatherapy are those imposed by the rigour and progress of modern medicine: there is absolutely no question of systematically replacing antibiotics with essential oils, but they can be very useful in handling some acute episodes or recurring infections (ENT, urinary etc....) that we practitioners of complementary medicine so often see in the course of consultation. However, in the hands of a skilled aromatherapist, many chronic ailments such as sciatica and migraine can also be relieved.

Two examples of treatment via the respiratory tract

■ Pour five drops of the essential oil onto a handkerchief and inhale it for two minutes, two or three times a day

■ Pour ten drops into a bowl of hot water, and breathe in over it for one or two minutes, two or three times a day. You can cover your head with a cloth to keep the heat in a little longer. This system is not ideal because, as we have seen, the essential oils are insoluble in water. Scientists are working to resolve this problem and provide more suitable presentations

Caution, danger

Without question essential oils are acutely toxic: self-medication should never take place without VERY clear advice. The haphazard use of essential oils in approximate doses may cause serious or even fatal accidents.

– You should never take essential oils without knowing their effects, indications, and method of use

– You should never take them if in doubt

– You must keep to the prescribed dosage

– You should never follow a prolonged course of treatment without authoritative advice

– Never use them on children

Manual methods

The range of these methods, in use since antiquity, has been gradually systematized, and in informed and trained hands is one of the most reliable medical techniques. The treatment mainly consists of massages and manipulative movements applied to the muscles, the vertebral column, or sometimes to more deeply seated organs.

Vertebral manipulation

This is defined as passive, forced, controlled, painless, mobilization taken to the limit of the possible movement of the joints. It is generally accompanied by a cracking noise, which is due to the sudden appearance of tiny bubbles within the joint fluid and never, as some patients imagine, to the movement of the vertebrae.

A little history

The history of manipulation overlaps that of medicine, since it was used by the Egyptians, the Greeks, the Romans... until the Middle Ages, when it was abandoned by doctors and left to barber-surgeons and bonesetters.

The 'renaissance' of manipulation took place at the end of the 19th century in the United States when, in the space of just a few years, two methods relying on very different concepts were outlined: chiropractic and osteopathy. The medical profession rediscovered spinal manipulation soon after the Second World War.

In Germany, Italy, Great Britain and America, manipulation by lay practitioners is permitted, but in France only doctors can carry out these medical procedures. However, although this legislation is clear, and was confirmed in the French parliament in 1995, many lay persons, most often kinesiotherapists, practise under the title of osteopath.

The three main methods
These may seem similar to the patient, but the thinking and theories behind them differ greatly.

Osteopathy

A system of medical thought as well as a therapeutic method, osteopathy was first described in 1873 by an American surgeon, Andrew Taylor Still. Nearly all current manipulative techniques are derived from it.

Blockage mechanism
To the osteopath, the illness creates blockages between the movement of normally mobile organs. Correction of this 'osteopathic lesion' restores the vascular and lymphatic circulation, together with correct joint mobility.

Associated problems
An osteopathic lesion develops as follows: a shock causes the primary lesion; pain and local muscle contraction ensue and may extend along a muscular chain; a secondary lesion may occur some distance away in the form of a residual pain or a functional imbalance; this process may take several months, or even years.

The osteopath must seek out and treat the primary lesion to obtain a medical result.

Consultation
This will show up the reduced mobility and muscular tension that osteopathic manipulative movements will later remove.

Manipulation brings about a marked improvement in most cases without it being possible to give a precise explanation: it works by a local mechanical 'unblocking' action. A blockage irritates a nerve and, unless it is quickly relieved, causes inflammation to spread to the surrounding tissues. The muscles protect themselves by contracting, which results in pain and the leaning posture associated with acute stiffness (torticollis, lumbago). Manipulation adjusts the spinal column and reduces the pain.

An accepted discipline

Osteopathy has been officially accepted in the United States since 1945, and is recognized by an advanced diploma.

Osteopaths in France are for the most part kinesiotherapists who have trained privately in France or abroad.

Osteopaths in Britain are professionally regulated and doctors cannot practise osteopathy unless they have completed the necessary requirements.

Cranial osteopathy consists of a very gentle manipulation by means of touching and adjusting the bones of the skull. Even some osteopaths question its theoretical basis.

Vertebrotherapy

This method, systematized in France by Dr. Robert Maigne, relies on strictly neuroanatomical factors. The spinal cord is located in the vertebral column; nerve roots emerge from it to connect with the organs and limbs. The nerves may be trapped or irritated, as in a 'minor intervertebral disruption', which can only be revealed by clinical examination. This blockage can produce symptoms in the related nerve area, as when a headache is produced if the cervical nerves are affected, or when intercostal or abdominal pain results from problems with the dorsal or lumbar nerves.

The examination seeks to identify this blockage, which cannot be seen on an X-ray. Manipulation suppresses the pain almost immediately by restoring the normal interplay of muscles and vertebrae.

Chiropractic

Described in 1894 by a Canadian hypnotist, David Palmer, who believed he had discovered the secret of illnesses. According to Palmer, they were all caused by vertebral misalignment, termed subluxation. He advanced this theory after having used manipulation to cure deafness in his caretaker and cardiovascular problems in several of his other patients. This method is widely practised in the United States, since there are more chiropractors (20,000) than osteopaths.

The indications for manipulation

– Mainly pain, be it cervical, dorsal, lumbar, or in the joints

– However, some thoracic or abdominal functional symptoms, nervous problems, headaches, vertigo, whistling or buzzing in the ear – caused by a 'vertebral blockage' – may be improved or cured by a manipulative movement

The dangers of manipulation
Manipulation is often criticized for being potentially dangerous, but it seems that in trained hands, the likelihood of a serious or even tragic accident is insignificant, bearing in mind the millions of manipulations carried out daily all over the world. Though they are very readily prescribed in rheumatology, anti-inflammatory agents have proved incomparably more dangerous.

Methods based on diet and/or dietary supplements

Diet holds a position of the utmost importance in our societies, whatever the culture, way of life, means, traditions. It is a vital factor in the prevention of illness as long as it is varied, balanced, carefully chosen, supplemented, and complemented.

The global approach in complementary therapy has always included careful consideration of diet in general and the status of minerals and vitamins in particular.

Oligotherapy (trace element therapy)

This continually developing method came into being during the first half of the 20th century. It relies on the prescription of trace elements, relatively inactive mineral substances present in tiny quantities, essential to life, not synthesized by the body, and therefore necessarily obtained from food sources. (The Greek 'oligos' means little, hence oligotherapy.)

The Mézières method

This method, described by the kinesiotherapist Françoise Mézières, combines the stretching of muscle chains with the maintenance of postures.

It aims to correct static problems and their consequences by restoring elasticity and lengthening the retracted muscle groups of the back and rear of the body.

It is used for both prophylaxis and the treatment of adolescents and adults with spinal problems.

Bodily awareness is not sufficiently well developed for this method to be beneficial for children under eight years of age.

Dietary deficiency, or rather, subclinical deficiency, common in industrialized countries, is most often due to:
– an insufficient food supply: malnutrition, vegetarian diet, too strict a diet (especially lacking protein)
– methods of cultivation (the use of many fertilizers, herbicides, pesticides...), of refinement, preserving, cooking...
– an increase in demands on the body: growth, overwork, pregnancy, sport, surgery for injuries, psychological stress, age...
– losses of the body's resources: dieting, extensive burns, heavy sweating...

Like vitamins, minerals take part in numerous chemical reactions, assisting tissue metabolism and stimulating defence mechanisms. Through a generally minute part of the diet, they contribute to the maintenance of health, which means they need to be present in balanced amounts.

The accumulation or diminution of trace elements disturbs bodily function, allowing illness to take a hold.

Scientists class the mineral elements that make up living beings into three large groups, according to their relative importance to the body. The first two of these alone represent 99 per cent of the human body:

- Elements making up living matter, present in substantial proportions: nitrogen, carbon, hydrogen, and oxygen
- Elements whose quantities in the body can be expressed in grams are classed as the so-called 'macro-elements': calcium, chlorine, magnesium, phosphorus, potassium, sodium, and sulphur. A daily intake of more than 100mg of each of these is required to maintain life
- Trace elements whose amounts vary between tens of milligrams for the more abundant (iron, zinc) down to a few milligrams or fractions thereof for the least abundant (chromium, selenium). These trace elements also include copper, fluorine, iodine, and manganese – to mention only the most important. They are present in food in small quantities, and the body needs only minute doses

An important role

About 30 elements are capable of playing a biological role in the body. Fifteen of these are considered essential: their lack causes functional signs of deficiency, which can be corrected by specific supplementation. However, they can be toxic in high doses. They include chromium, cobalt, copper, iron, fluorine, iodine, and zinc. Others such as aluminium, silver, lithium, and gold, are useful rather than essential.

Deficiency signs
Trace element deficiency not only manifests itself as a loss of fitness, with tiredness, susceptibility to stress, loss of concentration and intellectual capacity, changes in the skin, hair and nails, premature ageing, diminution of immune defences, increased risk of osteoporosis, but also leads to a serious increase in cardiovascular and cancer risks, the two great scourges of Western societies.

Three approaches
Oligotherapy encompasses some very different techniques or theoretical approaches:

• Traditional, or Ménétrier's reaction (catalytic) therapy employs small doses of trace elements to correct the 'vital force' dear to homeopaths

• Orthomolecular therapy, currently very much in fashion, consists in providing various dietary supplements or complements to treat and prevent deficiencies and their effects

• Finally, the use of trace elements in larger doses (within certain limits) to obtain beneficial activity not associated with their nutritional role

These different concepts of treatment with mineral elements do not make their use by practitioner and patient any simpler. The doses to be given and the combinations to be recommended are constantly changing, with considerable variations regarding physiological requirements. However, although 'catalytic' doses used to be sufficient, there now seems to be an overall tendency

A reference study has confirmed that many people, though apparently in good health, have lower than acceptable levels of minerals (and vitamins); this is not without its consequences. In descending order, magnesium, calcium, zinc, selenium, iron, and chromium are the minerals whose deficiency carries the greatest risk.

Common deficiencies

A balanced, varied diet normally supplies the body with all it needs for the building, functioning, and maintenance of good health.

In developed countries frank, serious deficiencies leading to a typical clinical picture are rarely seen.

On the other hand, moderate and subclinical deficiencies are much more frequent. The daily efficacy of such prescriptions for patient after patient provides plenty of evidence of this.

to use increased doses to take care of deficiencies and normal requirements at the same time. Moreover, it is quite legitimate to give a large dose of a mineral (to prevent or treat a deficiency) along with a catalytic dose (to strengthen the vital force) – a procedure currently in use with lithium, magnesium, manganese, copper...

The vitamins

The discovery of the first of the vitamins in 1910 brought about a revolution in medical thought. It showed that the absence of a substance could be responsible for an illness previously thought to be caused by a toxin (poisoning) or by bacteria (infection) in the body. The word 'vitamin' appeared in 1912, when the first amine recognised as vital was isolated (hence the name).

Many studies – rewarded by Nobel prizes – revealed the factors responsible for a number of diseases, and then their synthesis in the cure or prevention of deficiency-linked illness. The most recent research has led to a completely different way of understanding them and to their use against cardiovascular disease and cancer.

Definition and main properties

Vitamins seem to possess an almost magical quality, a supernatural power; they are synonymous with good health, growth and longevity. What is more:

– They are indispensable to life since they contribute to the production of blood cells, hormones, cerebral neurotransmitters... they provide energy, are absolutely essential to cell growth and organ function

– They are present in the body in small amounts

– They are organic chemical substances with no

energy value, to be considered as nutriment in the same way as are proteins, carbohydrates, fats, and minerals

– They are assimilated by the body during digestion

The 13 vitamins

Vitamin A (retinol), betacarotene (provitamin A), vitamin B1 (thiamine), vitamin B2 (riboflavin), vitamin B3 or PP (nicotinic acid, nicotinamide, niacin), vitamin B5 (pantothenic acid), vitamin B6 (pyridoxine), vitamin B8 or H (biotin), vitamin B9 (folic acid), vitamin B12 (cobalamin), vitamin C (ascorbic acid), vitamin D (ergocalciferol = D2, cholecalciferol = D3), vitamin E (tocopherol), vitamin K (phylloquinone).

A more complete role

Vitamins have a very wide range of activity since they take part in many, often very important, chemical reactions:

– They help us to fight infection better by improving the 'vital force'

– They neutralize toxic substances because of their antioxidant properties

– They encourage tissue repair since they are involved in the formation of some cell membranes

A new use that shows promise

For a long time, vitamins were used in small doses, solely to prevent or cure deficiency illnesses, but the attitude of the medical profession towards them has changed considerably over the last few years. Numerous studies have confirmed that larger doses are useful in delaying unavoidable processes such as ageing, in preventing the onset of cardiovascular disease, and in preventing the appearance of certain cancers, or improv-

The word 'vitamin' comes from the Latin 'vita' (life) and amine (a substance containing nitrogen), but contrary to what was once believed, they do not all contain nitrogen. However, the word remains.

We do not know how to synthesize most vitamins, thus we have to find them in our food or take them as a supplement. Each country has fixed the quantities for the RDA (recommended dietary allowances), designed to cover the needs of most (95 per cent) of the population.

The vitamin deficiencies, in descending order of frequency, are: carotenoids, vitamins E, D, C, B6, B9 (folic acid), B1, B12...then K, B3 and B8.

Micronutrients

In addition to the minerals and vitamins already mentioned, there are:

– Amino acids, involved in the make-up of proteins, an important source of energy, and the precursors of the neurotransmitters essential to cell function

– Essential fatty acids ensuring the integrity of biological membranes, the proper functioning of receptors, and also influencing platelet aggregation and inflammation

ing their prognosis. Thus they are now used more freely for prevention and cure, in the same way as conventional medicines.

Orthomolecular therapy

Originating in the United States about 25 years ago, this method seeks to optimize health, improve mental and physical performance, slow the effects of ageing, and avoid the risk of illness through the balanced supplementation of micronutrients: amino acids, minerals, vitamins, and essential fatty acids. When one of these is absent from food, or present in insufficient quantities, the body draws on its reserves. When these are dipped into, or exhausted, some symptoms of dysfunction appear, and an illness may develop. The treatment consists of adding useful or essential supplements or complements to the diet.

Methods based on nature's constituent elements

The very definition of a natural, alternative (complementary) medicine implies recourse to the 'elements' that make up our environment – air, earth, fire, and water.

So we come to hydrotherapy and thalassotherapy. However we will not expand on these since they form an integral part of conventional treatment, together with the treatments (heat, cold, electricity, ultrasound...) used by functional physiotherapists and kinesiotherapists, and some marginal methods such as magnetotherapy and light therapy.

Natural healing

Naturopathy

Since man's origins, all the world's civilizations have made use of nature for treatment or to remain healthy.

Hippocrates, the famous Greek physician, in announcing his "primum non nocere", which can be translated as "above all, do no harm", laid down the basis of natural medicine, harmless to the body it means to cure.

Naturopathy is a general means of providing help in most illnesses: it deals with the person as a whole, dictates a healthy lifestyle, makes use of simple rules of hygiene, gives plenty of dietary advice, recommends treatments based on plants or homeopathic remedies, and prescribes physical or mental care. Thus, at least in theory, naturopathy is the example which all complementary therapies must (or should) follow, since its sole aim is to help man to rediscover the healthy principles of life by using specific natural means.

Naturopathy is most often, but not exclusively, practised by non-medical persons. In the countryside one still refers to 'healers', meaning those who, in town, are called naturopaths or nature therapists. Countries such as England, America and Australia now have established naturopathic colleges which offer a four-year study programme leading to a diploma or degree in Naturopathic Medicine. The courses include in-depth orthodox studies in anatomy and physiology, symptomatology and diagnosis as well as pathology.

The once pejorative term 'natural medicine' is now becoming acceptable, and many practitioners of complementary therapy are recognized by the natural methods they use and readily combine with conventional medicine.

Hydrotherapy is probably one of the oldest treatments, popular with the ancient Greeks, the Romans, the Gauls... It underwent a long eclipse for many centuries, then reappeared in the 19th century. It is currently very popular with the public: every year some 600,000 people enjoy its benefits in some 105 centres in France alone, almost all of them located on or near ancient Roman baths. Thalassotherapy involves seawater and so is naturally included as a water cure.

Stress management

Many patients who suffer high stress levels neither need nor wish to be attended by psychiatrists or psychologists, nor do they want to take remedies. They are turning instead to increasingly popular stress management methods.

Qi gung, shiatsu and tai chi are the Oriental equivalents of Western psychological methods.

If few scientists question the influence of colour on our mood and behaviour, far fewer would accept the use of coloured light as therapy.

Relaxation methods

These methods are aimed at gaining improved control over body and mind. Relaxation in the medical sense does not mean resting and quietly listening to music or watching television. It involves breathing and mental exercises to make it easier to achieve calm and obtain release.

Relaxation methods are a real therapeutic tool, both prophylactic and curative.

Implementation
These methods call for a period of learning to secure the voluntary muscular and mental relaxation essential for awareness and better control of body and mind. Thus they allow the results of stress to be reduced, suppressed, and channelled, and the stressful situations of life to be tackled in a calm, determined and relaxed manner.

Three phases
Each of these methods passes through three phases:

– development of awareness of bodily sensations to (re-)establish harmony between the body and mind, and to obtain or reinforce self-confidence

– complete mastery of breathing in order to be able to empty the head, focus the attention, and increase self-control

– the incorporation of relaxation into daily life in situations of conflict, or when things are simply difficult

Two types of method
Relaxation techniques can be roughly divided into two groups:

– Passive methods using suggestion or release:

hypnosis, Schultz self-managed training, music therapy, and transcendental meditation

– Active methods necessitating physical movement: Jacobson's progressive relaxation, yoga

The importance of relaxation methods
They give the patient an active role in managing his condition or problem. They are important because of the speed with which they can effect changes, and the results they can produce, especially among those engaged in competitive sports. They provide an excellent alternative to the use of tranquillizers, which are too frequently prescribed and used, and they are an essential factor in success, in opening up, getting better, and being healthy. Their sole disadvantage is that they require effort, patience and time from patient and therapist alike.

The use of relaxation methods
– For most nervous problems, in conjunction with or instead of therapy

– In preparing for a scheduled event (athletes, artists…)

– Preventive treatment, feeling well and staying well

Reflex methods

Touching the body, pricking it with an instrument, injecting some 'miraculous' substance: all past civilizations have carried out these practices with initiatory, aesthetic or therapeutic aims. Any action affecting the skin, an extensive organ well supplied with nerves, is bound to trigger a profound reaction in the nervous system, the glands, and the organs: this forms the basis of methods of reflex therapy, under which we include mesotherapy.

Sophrology

Created in 1960 by a Colombian, A. Caycedo, sophrology is supposed to be both a philosophical and a therapeutic system, the science (logos) of a serene mind and a combination of Oriental and Western methods of relaxation.

Sophrology brings together mental techniques that can make a positive change in behaviour, with the aim of helping to build and maintain a balanced personality.

It has three main constituents:
– philosophy, based on another way of living, being, and thinking…
– therapy, useful in anxiety, neuroses, fears…
– prevention

Somatotopy is based more on empirical findings than on satisfactory scientific explanations. The connections between a point on the ear and the back, and the sole of the foot and the brain are far from being generally recognized.

The materials used vary greatly: massage with the hands or glass or metal rods, the use of needles, injections, magnets, tiny electric currents, soft laser rays, different heat sources... Those trying to stop smoking gladly accept the placement of temporary needles that are only kept in the ear for a week or so.

Reflex therapy

This term embraces diagnostic and/or therapeutic methods whose aim is to discover the body's dysfunction, then rebalance it by reflex or energetic means. In somatotopy, the body is represented by points on the ear, and other therapies use different organs such as the nose, the teeth, the iris, the tongue, the sole of the foot, the palm etc. for diagnosis. Starting with these links, it becomes possible to produce a reflex reaction at a distance in a precisely defined troubled area by massaging or needling certain points. The treatment is simple to carry out, and works quickly... most of the time.

Different methods

Here we find plantar, palmar, and dental reflexology, neural therapy, and sympatheticotherapy...

Reflexologists search for and locate spontaneously painful points by examining the palms, the soles of the feet, or the teeth. Stimulating these zones improves the symptoms or makes them disappear.

Neural therapy, a technique developed in Germany, and whose name comes from the Greek 'neuron', meaning nerve, consists of searching, locally or at a distance, for an irritant centre that may be causing the stubborn symptoms, and then treating it.

Sympathicotherapy is used to treat autonomic disorders such as asthma, also sterility and colitis, by stimulation or cauterization of the nasal mucosa. This re-balancing method, which was very fashionable for a time, is still in use, but more privately and selectively than before.

Mesotherapy

This method, developed about 50 years ago by a French doctor, Michel Pistor, is based on the carefully calculated injection of small doses of medicament. It is halfway between conventional and complementary therapy, seen as the gentlest conventional technique and the most conventional complementary technique.

Definition

Dr. Pistor himself defined his method very simply, in the clearest possible way: "A little, rarely, and in the right place." In fact, mesotherapy consists of using very small doses of conventional drugs (diluted anti-inflammatory agents, analgesics, relaxants, vasodilators, vitamins...) or of homeopathic remedies. These are injected intradermally or subcutaneously, into or near the area it is hoped to treat, by means of one or more fine needles.

Mechanism

This method of administering drugs changes their distribution in the body and increases and prolongs their activity. The skin acts as a reservoir, allowing the gradual diffusion of an injected drug. An intradermal injection spreads at a constant concentration for six hours, while an intravenous injection quickly reaches peak concentration in the blood and is almost completely eliminated in one hour.

Technique

The injection is given in very small amounts, using a syringe or an electronic injector. A papilla forms at each injection site. Some 50 of these mini-injections are carried out at each session. The papillae disappear after a few minutes or within two or three hours, depending on the products used. The doses used are generally between 1 and 5ml, but may be up to 20ml for cellulite.

Accidents

Mesotherapy is an effective, certain, safe method. If the technique is applied correctly, the only events seen are superficial haematomas, which are quickly resolved.

All mesotherapists use disposable needles, therefore the risk of transmitting infectious diseases (hepatitis, AIDS) is nil.

Occasionally some allergic reactions to the drugs used (anti-inflammatories, local anaesthetics) may be observed. This risk can be reduced or removed by using homeopathic injections.

Session frequency

The number of sessions depends on the condition... and on the practitioner:

– in acute conditions such as lumbago, the sessions will be close together and can take place every two or three days

– in more chronic conditions the sessions will be further apart – one every three weeks, or even every three or six months

– the frequency of sessions can be set by the patient, seeking consultation when the symptoms reappear or worsen

Indications

- Locomotor ailments, rheumatology, traumatology, sporting traumatology:
  – tendinitis, periarthritis
  – torticollis, lumbago
  – spasm, pulled muscles, strains
  – sprains and their sequelae
  – bouts of osteoarthritis...

- Circulatory problems:
  – arteritis
  – vein and capillary problems, vasomotor problems in the extremities
  – vertigo, whistling and buzzing in the ears...

- Infections:
  – prevention of recurrent ENT infections
  – sinusitis...

- Allergy:
  – asthma, above all
  – hay fever

- Dermatology:
  – hair falling out, with the inconvenience of unpleasant injection sessions
  – cellulite

Contra-indications

- Cuts on the skin where it is to be treated
- Febrile illness present
- Patient on anticoagulants
- Patient fearful or nervous
- Children
- Patient has weakened immunity
- Previous severe allergy

Diagnostic methods

One of the aims of every practitioner, whatever his method of treatment, is to arrive at a diagnosis.

A conventional doctor uses questioning, clinical examination, and additional tests. Like homeopaths, practitioners of complementary therapy who adopt a holistic approach will investigate patients' reactions or, like acupuncturists, the influence of the changing seasons on the appearance of symptoms. The medical profession finds these approaches easier to accept than some diagnostic means, such as those used in iridology, the Kirlian effect, or the mineral composition of the hair... The reliability and specificity of these methods are unconvincing.

You will have grasped the difficulties, limits, and dangers of classification: some methods may fall under one or more headings according to the way they are viewed and adopted. However, we hope this attempt will make your ideas clearer and allow you to understand the different approaches.

As explained in the introduction, this book is not exhaustive. It is based only on our own practice. Thus we have exercised a choice: in this 'guide to illnesses' you will find only the remedies in daily use in our practice.

The essential diagnostic phase

Complementary therapists do not distort medical practice, rather they enrich it, since contrary to what has long been supposed, they try to arrive at the most accurate diagnosis possible and will use modern means if necessary (biological examinations, X-rays etc), while adding their own special touches to refine, then adjust or supervise treatment.

2

Prevention and treatment

Nervous problems

Antidepressants and tranquillizers have revolutionized the treatment of nervous and psychiatric illness by allowing many patients who were confined to hospitals, hospices, and asylums to live an almost normal life. However, their excessive use has its drawbacks (numerous undesirable side effects and chiefly, the risk of habituation), and they should only be prescribed after mature reflection. Complementary therapies, with homeopathy and herbal treatment at their head, constitute a mild and effective alternative, worth trying first.

Anxiety states – Panic attacks – Phobias – Fright – Spasmophilia – Fatigue – Depression – Sleep disturbances and insomnia – Withdrawal from tranquillizers, antidepressants, and sleeping pills.

Anxiety states

These are frequent: as many as one person in five is affected in the West. Anxiety is a feeling of uneasiness in the face of a vaguely defined danger. Anxiety has no precise cause, occurs at any time and has some very disagreeable symptoms, from vague feelings of illness to acute panic attacks. It is often associated with a lump in the throat or knots in the stomach, a feeling of suffocation, trembling, palpitations, vertigo, sweating...

Useful advice

As soon as you feel tense, you should:
– keep an eye on the quantity and quality of your diet
– take some exercise, especially if this normally relaxes you
– engage in recreational activity
– arrange for periods of rest or recovery
– look after your most valuable ally, sleep

Two natural foods

Brewer's yeast

ORIGIN: a living substance specially prepared as a supplement, from a minute fungus that serves as a ferment in the preparation of beer. It is different from baker's yeast, and much better tolerated by the intestine.

COMPOSITION: yeast is an extraordinary dietary supplement containing little fat, salt, sugar, or calories, but is rich in proteins, essential amino acids, minerals (chromium, phosphorus, potassium, selenium...), and group B vitamins.

INDICATIONS: it is a sedative and improves and calms the nerves, as well as reducing the sensation of hunger and the need for sugar.

METHOD OF USE: you will find it in health food shops and pharmacies as tablets, capsules, flakes (be careful, it is very bitter). Take one dose three times a day.

Lecithin

ORIGIN: a water and fat-soluble phospholipid that dissolves and distributes fats. Made by the liver, it is present in high concentrations in the vital organs (brain, heart, liver, kidneys), and supplies the nerve cells with beneficial unsaturated fatty acids.

COMPOSITION AND PROPERTIES: because it is rich in phosphorus and amino acids, it encourages the development of the nervous system and also has a regulatory role. It is sedative, helps the memory, aids concentration, and assists sleep.

SOURCES: comes in the diet, and is found particularly in runny egg yolk, walnuts, soya, and sunflower, safflower or linseed oil.

Method of use: you will find it in health food shops, most often as an extract of soya. Take one teaspoonful twice a day.

Oligotherapy

Lithium, magnesium

Supplies of these two elements are obtained from a varied diet of good quality. You will find them mainly in cereals, chocolate, green vegetables, eggs, fish, meat, dried fruits…

• When there is a deficiency, which is frequent with these two elements, they can be supplied in the form of colloidal minerals such as Organic Minerals (Colloidals) which contains 70+ trace minerals
– Available in 946ml bottles
– Take 1–3 caps just before breakfast and/or evening meal
– Children 1 teaspoon daily for each 20lbs of body weight
Or Maximol (Ionized colloidals)
– Available in 500ml bottles
– Take ½ capful once or twice daily on an empty stomach
– One dose of magnesium to be taken three times a day, and one dose of lithium twice a day, for a few days or weeks
Or Lithium orotate (Vitamin Research Products) 120mg
– Available in containers of 120 capsules
– One capsule twice daily with meals

• You can also take higher doses of magnesium by using remedies such as Magasorb® (Lamberts) Containing 150mg of magnesium (as citrate)
– Available in containers of 60 and 180 tablets
– One to three tablets daily

• You can take Trispartate® (Thorne), which contains calcium, magnesium, and potassium
– Available in containers of 60 capsules
– One to three capsules three times daily

Vitamins useful in anxiety states

These are mainly **B group** vitamins: they have their own independent activity besides the absorption of magnesium. You will find them in the husks of cereals (wheatgerm, oat flakes) pulses (haricot beans, lentils, peas…), brewer's and baker's yeast, wholemeal bread, fish, and meat (especially poultry)…

Vitamin B1

• Thiamine (Lamberts): one tablet= 100mg
– Available in containers of 90 capsules
– One capsule to be taken each day

Vitamin B3

• NIASAFE® (Thorne) non-flushing: one tablet = 510mg of Niacin:
– Available in 60 or 180 vegetarian capsules
– One to three capsules daily

Vitamin B6

• Vitamin B6 (Lamberts): one tablet= 100mg:
– Available in containers of 100 tablets
– One tablet to be taken each day for adults, a quarter to half a tablet for a child

Folic Acid

• Folic Acid (Lamberts): one tablet = 400μg:
– Available in containers of 100 tablets
– One tablet to be taken each day

Vitamin B12

• Vitamin B12 BIO-B12® (Thorne): one capsule = 1000mcg B12, 800mcg Folic

acid, Zinc picolinate 15mg and Papain 75mg:
– Available in containers of 120 or 60 vegetarian capsules
– For adults, one capsule daily

• You can take Lamberts® B-100 complex, a mixture of vitamins B1, B2, B3, B5, B6, B12, folic acid, biotin,choline, inositol and PABA:
– Available in containers of 60 and 200 tablets
– One tablet to be taken each day

Homeopathy

Aconite, Ignatia
– Four granules of one of these remedies at 7c, to be sucked like sweets every 15 minutes, three or four times in succession until the symptoms improve

• You can take Nervoheel® (Heel) which contains Ignatia D4, Kalium Bromatum D4, Sepia D4, Acidum phosphoricum D4 and Zincum valerianum D4...
– Available in packs containing 50 or 250 tablets
– One tablet to be dissolved under the tongue three times daily

You can also add a constitutional remedy decided upon after consultation with your homeopath, which in this case will often be Argentum nitricum, Arsenicum album, Actaea racemosa...

Aconitum napellus

Vegetable origin: aconite, a plant from the mountains.
– Homeopathic remedy for nervous conditions with 'a fear of imminent death'
– Characteristic sign: extreme agitation

Ignatia amara

– Vegetable origin: a shrub, St Ignatius' bean
– A great remedy for nervous hypersensitivity
– Specific signs: the subject is contradictory, paradoxical, and even hysterical
– Rated as the homeopathic tranquillizer, it is too often used wrongly: the specific signs should definitely be present if it is to be prescribed

Herbal treatment

Hawthorn, passionflower
These plants can be prepared and made up by your herbalist as a mother tincture, as powder in capsules, as dried extracts...

POSSIBLE PRESCRIPTION: You can ask your herbalist to prepare a 60ml bottle of fresh whole-plant suspension of hawthorn or passionflower. Take a half-teaspoonful in a little water morning and night for a few days or according to the symptoms. For adults only.

SPECIAL NOTE: thanks to a method of cold stabilization, the suspension provides the full therapeutic effect naturally present in the whole plant.

Hawthorn

Hawthorn has been used since antiquity for many different purposes: it has been made into execution blocks as well as being taken to dissolve kidney or bladder stones. Its considerable cardiosedative properties were only recognized in the 19th century.

It regulates and slows the rhythm of the heart, and reduces awareness of distressing palpitations. It reduces nervousness and the signs of anxiety, in children as well as in adults, without producing drowsiness or memory loss.

• You can use Lamberts® Hawthorn 2500mg:
– Available in containers of 60 tablets
– One tablet daily for a minimum of 6 weeks

• You can also make an infusion with a dessertspoonful of flowers in a cup of boiling water

Plant essential oils

Lavender, sweet marjoram, bitter orange…
– Two drops of one of these essential oils to be taken in a little honey, twice a day

• You can also pour six drops of essential oil of lavender in your bath at night, for complete relaxation

Lavender

This is not just the aromatic plant that perfumes our wardrobes and repels insects; it is also very sedative and slightly antidepressant.

Sweet marjoram

This cousin to oregano has a stronger sedative action: the ancient Greeks planted it on the tombs of their next of kin to bring peace to their spirits.

Bitter orange

Native to China, bitter orange is used both as a food and as a medicinal plant. The essential oil of neroli, which is very sedative, is produced from the flowers. Petitgrain essential oil comes from the leaves and young shoots. Distillation produces the orange-flower water used by confectioners.

Acupuncture

Acupuncture has proved not merely useful but sometimes indispensable, thanks to its sedative action and ability to restore the equilibrium.

TREATMENT SCHEDULE: An initial weekly or twice-weekly treatment can be suggested in periods of great stress, followed by maintenance treatment once a month for several months.

Relaxation

Relaxation is essential in learning to take charge of the emotions and control muscular tension, and in reducing, channelling, and even suppressing the effects of stress.

Panic attacks

This medical term describes an acute, sudden, intense anxiety attack. Unpredictable and without a precise cause, it leads to a feeling of dread and an impression of impending death. It can last for a few minutes or hours and disappears gradually, leaving the patient worn out and terrified at the thought of another attack – which can happen at any time.

Panic attacks are twice as frequent in women as in men, and occur most often between the ages of 15 and 20. Questioning will often reveal a family history of the condition, which may indicate an unfortunate predisposition.

Homeopathy

Aconite

– Four granules at 7c, to be sucked like sweets every five minutes, and at longer intervals on improvement

Aconitum napellus

– Vegetable origin: aconite, a plant from the mountains
– Homeopathic remedy for panic attacks with 'a fear of imminent death'
– Characteristic sign: agitation

Opium

– Four granules at 15c to be sucked every 15 minutes, four or five times in succession, until there is some improvement

Opium

– Vegetable origin: the opium poppy
– Homeopathic remedy for extreme fright followed by strong emotions
– Characteristic sign: hypersensitivity, especially to sound

• You can use Lehning® Crataegus Complex 15, which contains Aconite 4x, Arsenicum album 4x and, naturally, mother tincture of Crataegus (hawthorn):
– Available in 30ml bottles of oral solution
– Fifteen drops to be taken in a little water, three or four times in succession, between meals

You should also definitely add a constitutional remedy, chosen through consultation with your homeopath. In this case it will often be Argentum nitricum, Arsenicum album, Ignatia...

Herbal treatment

Hawthorn, passionflower

These two plants can be prepared and made up by your herbalist, alone or in combination, as a mother tincture, powder in capsules, dried extracts...

POSSIBLE PRESCRIPTION: Ask your herbalist to prepare a 60ml bottle of fresh whole-plant suspension of hawthorn or passionflower. Take a half-teaspoonful in a little water morning and night for few days, depending on the symptoms. For adults only.

SPECIAL NOTE: Thanks to a method of cold stabilization, the suspension provides the full therapeutic effect naturally present in the whole plant.

Passionflower

A plant native to Brazil and Mexico: its name refers to Christ's Passion. Very effective in combating anxiety, signs of nervousness, and sleep problems.

Oligotherapy

Lithium

Supplies of most of the trace elements are normally provided in the diet, which should be varied and of good quality. When there is a deficiency, lithium can be taken as a supplement.

Dietary sources of lithium

There is little data on the presence of lithium in foods, but it is found in small amounts in cereals, lettuce, green vegetables, potatoes, meat, eggs, fish, drinking water, table salt…

• Lithium supplements: there are many brands and forms such as Organic Minerals (Colloidals) which contains 70+ trace minerals:
– Available in 946ml bottles
– Take 1–3 caps just before breakfast and/or evening meal
– Children 1 teaspoon daily for each 20lbs of body weight
Or Maximol (Ionized colloidals):
– Available in 500ml bottles
– Take ½ capful once or twice daily on an empty stomach
Lithium orotate (Vitamin Research Products) 120mg:
– Available in containers of 120 capsules
– One capsule twice daily with meals

Acupuncture

Acupuncture has proved not merely useful but sometimes indispensable, thanks to its sedative action and ability to restore the equilibrium.

– TREATMENT REGIME: An initial weekly or twice-weekly treatment can be suggested in periods of great stress, followed by maintenance treatment once a month for several months.

Relaxation methods

Relaxation is essential for learning to control the emotions and muscular tension, and reducing, channelling, and even suppressing the effects of stress.

Phobias

This term describes a tension, fear, or panic arising in a situation or during an activity that in itself usually presents little danger: the middle of a crowd, speaking in public, the sight or presence of an animal, a confined space (lift, cave), the edge of a void, or simply height, some means of transport (aeroplane, underground train …). Phobia affects as many as one in two people, and twice as many women as men. Half of them try to avoid the situation, one in seven make sure that they do, but only one in four have tried any treatment.

Homeopathy

Aconite, gelsemium

– Four granules of one of these two remedies at 7c to be sucked like sweets, two or three times in succession, depending on the symptoms

Natural healing

Aconitum napellus

– Vegetable origin: aconite, a mountain plant
– Homeopathic remedy for anxiety states with 'fear of imminent death'
– Characteristic sign: agitation

Gelsemium sempervirens

– Vegetable origin: jasmine, a climbing shrub with large, scented, white or yellow flowers
– Homeopathic remedy for fright, trembling
– Characteristic sign: a feeling that the legs are about to give way

• You can use Spascupreel® (Heel), which contains Gelsemium D6, Chamomilla D3, Passiflora D2...
– Available in containers of 50 or 250 tablets
– In general, one tablet dissolved under the tongue three times daily. In acute cases one tablet to be repeated every 15 minutes

You should also definitely add a constitutional remedy, chosen upon consultation with your homeopath; in this case it will often be Argentum nitricum, Arsenicum album, Ignatia.

Argentum nitricum

– Chemical origin: silver nitrate
– Homeopathic remedy for fear regarding what is about to happen
– Characteristic signs: patient agitated, in a hurry, anxious to finish before starting

Herbal treatment

Hawthorn, passionflower

These two plants can be prepared and made up by your herbalist, alone or in combination, as a mother tincture, powder in capsules, dried extracts...

• You can use a fresh whole-plant suspension: thanks to a method of cold stabilization, the suspension provides the full therapeutic effect naturally present in the whole plant
POSSIBLE PRESCRIPTION: Ask your herbalist to prepare a 60ml bottle of whole-plant suspension of hawthorn or passionflower. Take a half-teaspoonful in a little water, morning and night. For adults only.

• You can use Valerianaheel®, which contains mother tinctures of Crataegus, Valeriana, Chamomilla, Avena (oats)

For fear of flying

Ask your homeopathic pharmacy to prepare granules containing the following:
– Argentum nitricum 7c
– Arsenicum album 7c
– Gelsemium 7c
– Ignatia 7c

Four granules to be taken twice on the day before the flight, four granules in the morning, then, if needed, four granules on arrival at the airport, four on boarding the aircraft, four at takeoff...

Do not hesitate to repeat the doses.

and Lupulus (hops) combined with Hypericum (St. John's Wort) D1, Kalium bromatum D1:
– Available in drop bottles of 30 and 100ml
– In general, 15 drops 3 times daily, in the evening 25 drops. Single dose for infants and young children. Age 2–6 years, 5 drops; 6–12 years,10 drops

• You can use Passiflora complex (Bioforce), containing Passiflora and Oats:
– Available in drop bottles of 50ml
– 20 drops twice daily in a little water

Oligotherapy

Essentially magnesium

This trace element is normally supplied in the diet, which should be varied and of good quality. When there is a deficiency, which is frequent in the case of magnesium, it may be taken as a supplement.

Dietary sources of magnesium

Present in almost all foods, but unfortunately mainly in those that are rich in calories. Magnesium is found mainly in citrus fruits, bananas, whole cereals (oat flakes, bran...), cocoa and chocolate, shellfish (winkles, shrimps, oysters, clams...) and oily fish, snails, figs, hard cheeses, dried fruit and nuts (almonds, peanuts, hazelnuts, walnuts...), vegetables (spinach, dried haricot and green beans, split peas, soya...), wholemeal bread.

• Magnesium medications: there are many different brands and forms such as Organic Minerals (Colloidals) which contains 70+ trace minerals:
– Available in 946ml bottles
– Take 1–3 caps just before breakfast and/or evening meal
– Children 1 teaspoon daily for each 20lbs of body weight
Or Maximol (Ionized colloidals):
– Available in 500ml bottles
– Take ½ capful once or twice daily on an empty stomach

POSSIBLE PRESCRIPTION: One dose of magnesium to be taken twice a day for a few days or weeks.

• You can take higher doses of magnesium during the week preceding an event that you are worried about, using MagAsorb® (Lamberts) 150mg:
– Available in containers of 60 or 180 tablets
– One tablet one to three times daily

Relaxation

Relaxation is essential for learning to control the emotions and muscular tension, and reducing, channelling, and even suppressing the effects of stress.

After a few hours' work on the emotions with a qualified practitioner, certain techniques such as neurolinguistic programming (NLP) may eliminate a troublesome phobia.

Fright

A particular type of emotion that affects everyone at some point: students, sportsmen, artists, doctors... Fright has the symptoms of acute anxiety: knotted throat and stomach, a feeling of suffocation, trembling with quaking at the knees, sweating, a strong and rapid heartbeat, blushing with red ears, nausea and even vomiting.

All these signs are bad enough by themselves, but are slight compared with the dramatic psychological turmoil that can be brought on by an exam or a sports event.

Feverishness, difficulty in concentrating, sometimes with deep despair, feeling at a complete loss, incoherence – all these factors make success dubious and can also have lasting psychological effects.

Dietary advice

• Breakfast should be regular – consisting of protein, orange or other fruit juice, cereals – to avoid the well-known 'eleven o'clock low' due to hypoglycaemia

• Lunch and dinner should be easily digestible, and overgenerous helpings, which have a disastrous effect on alertness and concentration, avoided

Two natural foods that are useful against fright

Wheatgerm

ORIGIN AND COMPOSITION: Wheatgerm is a perfect food, the vegetable equivalent of the egg. It contains all the nutrients necessary for the growth of the plant. It is made up of the kernel, (three-quarters of the total weight) which yields flour when ground, and the husk (15 per cent of the total) which gives bran. Wheatgerm is obtained by soaking the grain in water and allowing it to germinate for two days. It contains all the constituents necessary for the plant's growth. It contains twice as much calcium, three times the magnesium and phosphorus, and many more vitamins, especially B and E, than wheat. It also contains vitamins A and C.

PROPERTIES: It helps to take care of nervous problems and is equally effective against fatigue and overwork.

METHOD OF USE: You will find it in health food shops as flakes that can be sprinkled on salads, yoghurt, or soft cheese. Take one or two teaspoonfuls a day.

Lecithin

ORIGIN: a water and fat-soluble phospholipid that dissolves and distributes fats. Made by the liver, it is present in high concentrations in the vital organs (brain, heart, liver, kidneys), and supplies the nerve cells with beneficial unsaturated fatty acids.

COMPOSITION AND PROPERTIES: because it is rich in phosphorus and amino acids, lecithin encourages the development of the nervous system and also plays a regulatory role. It is sedative, helps the memory, aids concentration, and assists sleep.

SOURCES: Lecithin is supplied by the diet, and is present mainly in runny egg yolk, walnuts, soya, and sunflower, safflower or linseed oil.

Method of use: You will find it in pharmacies and health food shops, most often as soya extract. One teaspoonful to be taken twice a day.

Acupuncture

Has a useful and much appreciated sedative and restabilizing action.

Treatment schedule: weekly or twice-weekly sessions, for the month preceding the event.

Relaxation methods

Relaxation is essential for learning to control the emotions and muscular tension, and reducing, channelling, and even suppressing the effects of stress.

Oligotherapy

Magnesium

This trace element is normally supplied in the diet, which should be varied and of good quality. When there is a deficiency, which is frequent in the case of magnesium, it may be taken as a supplement.

Dietary sources of magnesium

Present in almost all foods, but unfortunately particularly in those that are rich in calories. Magnesium is found mainly in citrus fruits, bananas, whole cereals (oat flakes, bran...), cocoa and chocolate, shellfish (winkles, shrimps, oysters, clams...) and oily fish, snails, figs, hard cheeses, dried fruit and nuts (almonds, peanuts, hazelnuts, walnuts...), vegetables (spinach, dried haricot and green beans, split peas, soya...), wholemeal bread.

• Magnesium is available in many different forms and brands such as Organic Minerals (Colloidals) which contains 70+ trace minerals:
– Available in 946ml bottles
– Take 1–3 caps just before breakfast and/or evening meal
– Children 1 teaspoon daily for each 20lbs of body weight
Or Maximol (Ionized colloidals):
– Available in 500ml bottles
– Take ½ capful once or twice daily on an empty stomach

POSSIBLE PRESCRIPTION: One dose of magnesium to be taken twice a day for a few days or weeks.

• You can take higher doses of magnesium during the week preceding a possibly frightening event, using MagAsorb® (Lamberts) 150mg:
– Available in containers of 60 or 180 tablets
– Take one to three tablets daily

• You can also use Phytisone® (Thorne), a combination of vitamins B1, B5, B6, C, and herbs liquorice root, red ginseng, Siberian ginseng and Ashwagandha
– Available in containers of 60 capsules
– One to two capsules twice daily

Natural healing

Homeopathy

Argentum nitricum, Gelsemium

– Four granules of one of these two remedies at 7c to be taken during the week preceding the event, to be sucked like sweets, two or three times a day between meals. Four granules to be taken on the day of an exam, possibly repeated on arrival at the examination centre, and even once more just before sitting it

Argentum nitricum

– Chemical origin: silver nitrate
– Homeopathic remedy for the fear regarding what is about to happen
– Characteristic signs: patient agitated, in a hurry, anxious to finish before starting

Gelsemium sempervirens

– Vegetable origin: the root of Virginia jasmine
– Homeopathic remedy for fright with trembling
– Specific sign: the legs feel as though they are about to give way

• You can use Spascupreel® (Heel), which contains Gelsemium D6, Chamomilla D3, Passiflora D2...
– Available in containers of 50 or 250 tablets
– In general, one tablet dissolved under the tongue three times daily. In acute cases one tablet to be repeated every 15 minutes

• You can also usefully add a constitutional remedy, chosen through consultation with your homeopath; in this case it will often be Argentum nitricum, Lycopodium, Pulsatilla

Herbal treatment

Hawthorn, passionflower

These two plants can be prepared and made up by your herbalist, alone or combined, as a mother tincture, powder in capsules, or dried extracts.

Possible prescription: Ask your herbalist to prepare 25 capsules of a mixture of dry extracts of hawthorn and passionflower, 150mg of each in a No.2 capsule (the particular size of the capsule that the herbalist uses). One capsule to be taken three times a day during the week before the appointed date, two capsules morning and night on the day before, and two capsules on the morning of the event.

Hawthorn

This delicate plant, with its beautiful white and pink flowers in bud, has been celebrated by many a poet. In former times its very hard wood was made into execution blocks.

Passionflower

The passionflower, a liana from Brazil and Mexico, owes its name to a Spanish Jesuit who saw elements of Christ's Passion in the shape of its flower.

• You can use a fresh whole-plant suspension: thanks to a method of cold stabilization, the suspension provides

For examination nerves

– Increase the supply of carbohydrates in the diet: fresh and dried vegetables (for phosphorus), bread, pastry, rice, potatoes, fruit...

– Make sure of a supply of foods rich in vitamin B1: cereal husk (wheatgerm and oat flakes), pulses (haricot beans, lentils, peas), brewer's and baker's yeast, wholemeal bread, fish, meat (especially poultry)

– Eat garlic and onion for their selenium, and cocoa, wheatgerm and coconut for vitamin E

– Coffee and tea are allowed because of their psycho-stimulant effects, but can cause insomnia if taken late in the day. At examination time sleep is the first thing to be threatened: losing sleep can bring about mental breakdown, so it should be protected at all costs

– Take care with alcohol and tobacco: they may superficially calm the nerves, but can affect the memory, and alcohol ultimately has a depressive effect

the full therapeutic effect naturally present in the whole plant

POSSIBLE PRESCRIPTION: You can ask your herbalist to prepare a 60ml bottle of fresh whole-plant suspension of hawthorn or passionflower. Half a teaspoonful to be taken in a little water, morning and night. For adults only.

• You can use Passiflora Complex (Bioforce): which contains passionflower and oats:
– Available in bottles of 50ml
– 20 drops twice daily in a little water

Spasmophilia

This term, which is only used in France, applies to various nervous symptoms suffered by six to ten million people in the country, without predisposing ethnic or social factors. Primarily, these patients (about 75%) come from an urban background. Most are in the 30–40 age group and four-fifths are women. They suffer muscular, mental, or sexual fatigue, sleep disorders, anxiety, and emotional disturbances, in that order of frequency.

The diagnosis is essentially clinical, based on questioning and examining the patient. There is one test, which if positive, is useful: the famous Chvostek sign. This is a contraction of the lip on one side when the cheekbone is tapped with a reflex hammer. Biological and paraclinical tests show few changes, the blood calcium level is normal, which is not the case with tetanus, and the magnesium level is diminished or normal. The electromyogram, thought for a long time to yield specific results, does not in fact do so.

The Germans use the word dystonia, the English say neurosis, and the Americans simply call it anxiety. Nonetheless it is a feature of society with many repercussions on personal, family, social, and professional lives, at a not inconsiderable cost to the health service and insurance companies.

Acupuncture

Acupuncture has proved not just useful but on occasion indispensable, thanks to its sedative action and ability to restore the equilibrium.

TREATMENT SCHEDULE: An initial weekly or twice-weekly treatment can be suggested in periods of great stress, followed by maintenance treatment once a month for some months.

Relaxation

Relaxation is essential for learning to control the emotions and muscular tension, and reducing, channelling, and even suppressing the effects of neurosis.

Two natural foods useful in neurosis

Wheatgerm

ORIGIN AND COMPOSITION: wheatgerm is a perfect food, the vegetable equivalent of the egg. It contains all the nutrients necessary for the growth of the plant. It is made up of the kernel, (three-quarters of the total weight) which yields flour when ground, and the husk (15 per cent of the total) which gives bran.

Wheatgerm is obtained by soaking the grain in water and allowing it to germinate for two days. It contains all the constituents necessary for the plant's growth. It contains twice as much calcium, three times the magnesium and phosphorus, and many more vitamins, especially B and E, than wheat itself. It also contains vitamins A and C.

PROPERTIES: It helps in dealing with nervous problems and is equally effective against fatigue and overwork.

METHOD OF USE: You will find it in health food shops as flakes that can be sprinkled on salads, yoghurt, or soft cheese. Take one or two teaspoonfuls a day.

Brewer's yeast

ORIGIN: a living substance, specially prepared as a supplement, from a minute fungus that serves as a ferment in the preparation of beer. It is different from baker's yeast, and much better tolerated by the intestine.

COMPOSITION: Yeast is an extraordinary dietary supplement containing little fat, salt, sugar, or calories, but rich in proteins, essential amino acids, minerals (chromium, phosphorus, potassium, selenium...), and group B vitamins.

INDICATIONS: It is a sedative and improves and calms the nervous state, as well as reducing the sensation of hunger and the need for sugar.

METHOD OF USE: You will find it in health food shops and pharmacies as tablets, capsules, flakes (take care, it is very bitter). One dose to be taken three times a day.

Oligotherapy

Magnesium is almost always lowered in people suffering from stress.

Copper, manganese

Phosphorus, involved in the contraction of muscles.

Supplies of the trace elements are normally provided in the diet, which should be varied and of good quality. When there is a deficiency, they can be taken as a supplement.

Dietary sources of magnesium

Present in almost all foods, but unfortunately particularly in those rich in calories. Magnesium is found mainly in citrus fruits, bananas, whole cereals (oat flakes, bran…), cocoa and chocolate, shellfish (winkles, shrimps, oysters, clams…) and oily fish, snails, figs, hard cheeses, dried fruit and nuts (almonds, peanuts, hazelnuts, walnuts…), vegetables (spinach, dried haricot and green beans, split peas, soya…), wholemeal bread.

Dietary sources of copper

Copper is present in small quantities nearly everywhere, except in milk, which contains very little. It is found especially in the liver ++ (calf, sheep), seafood (seaweed, lobsters, oysters, scallops, fish roe), almonds and nuts, certain vegetables (avocados, mushrooms), cereals (whole wheat, whole rice, soya), dried fruits, green vegetables, plums, cocoa, tea…

Dietary sources of manganese

Present primarily in vegetables, manganese is found mainly in whole cereals, chocolate, oily plants (almonds, walnuts, hazelnuts), wheatgerm, some condiments (cloves, ginger, thyme), vegetables (carrots, beetroot, chestnuts, haricot beans, peas, soya), coffee, tea… Manganese is scarce in or absent from food derived from animals (meat, fish, eggs) and fruit.

Dietary sources of phosphorus

Found primarily in dairy products ++ (100mg in a litre of milk) and also in bananas, whole cereals (cornflakes…), brewer's yeast, cocoa, chocolate, sparkling drinks, green and leafy vegetables (artichokes, asparagus, carrots, mushrooms, cabbage, parsley, soya…), dried vegetables (haricot beans, lentils, peas), dried fruit and nuts (almonds, peanuts, dates, figs, hazelnuts, walnuts…), eggs, fish++, potatoes, meat (especially poultry)…

• Copper, manganese and phosphorus medications are found in many different brands and forms such as Organic

Natural healing

Minerals (Colloidals) which contains 70+ trace minerals:
– Available in 946ml bottles
– Take 1–3 caps just before breakfast and/or evening meal
– Children 1 teaspoon daily for each 20lbs of body weight
Or Maximol (Ionized colloidals):
– Available in 500ml bottles
– Take ½ capful once or twice daily on an empty stomach

Magnesium supplements also come in many brands and forms such as these colloidals.

POSSIBLE PRESCRIPTION: One dose of magnesium to be taken twice a day for some weeks or even months.

Foods containing plenty of magnesium are also rich in calories, but it should be realized that a bar of dark chocolate (100g) provides fewer calories than a medium-sized portion of chips.

• If necessary, you can take a higher dose of potassium for some weeks, using Spartate® (Thorne) containing calcium 100mg, magnesium 90mg and potassium 30mg:
– Available in containers of 60 capsules
– Take one to three capsules three times daily

Calcium is often very useful in muscular hyperactivity (hyperkinesis)

Dietary sources of calcium

Essential supplies are provided by cheese and dairy products (1.2g per litre of milk, 200mg per litre of yoghurt) and various brands of mineral water, which as a rule should cover basic needs.

Calcium supplements: you can use homeopathic calcium such as Weleda® calcium salts:
– Available in packs containing two boxes of 50g oral powder
– One quarter-teaspoonful to be taken morning and night

Vitamins useful in neurosis

Mainly **group B** vitamins

Dietary sources of B vitamins

Mainly found in the husks of cereals (wheatgerm++, oat flakes), pulses (haricot beans, lentils, peas...), brewer's and baker's yeast, wholemeal bread, fish, meat (especially poultry)...

• You can take Lamberts® B-100 complex, a mixture of vitamins B1, B2, B3, B5, B6, B12, folic acid, biotin, choline, inositol and PABA:
– Available in containers of 60 and 200 tablets
– One tablet to be taken each day

Vitamin D is useful for fixing calcium.

Dietary sources of vitamin D

Found mainly in oily fish (halibut, cod++...), tinned sardines, egg yolk, meat (beef, chicken, veal, liver), cheeses, butter, milk, cereals, mushrooms...

• Vitamin D supplements: you can use Lamberts® chewable Calcium(400mg) with Vitamin D (2.5µg) and FOS:
– Available in containers of 60 tablets
– Children (from four years upwards): chew one tablet daily.
– Adults: chew 1–2 tablets daily

In sunlight the skin produces vitamin D. Supplements can be withheld during periods of exposure to sun in the summer.

Homeopathy

Ambra grisea, Nux moschata

– Four granules of one of these two remedies at 7c to be sucked like sweets once or twice a day for some weeks

Ambra grisea

– Animal origin: ambergris is a substance formed in the stomach of the sperm whale
– Homeopathic remedy for hypersensitive persons, overcome by anything – and nothing
– Characteristic sign: extreme shyness

Nux moschata

– Vegetable origin: nutmeg
– Homeopathic remedy for hypersensitivity with sudden, profound changes of mood
– Characteristic sign: a tendency to faint or have blackouts

You should also add a constitutional remedy chosen through consulting your homeopath; in this case it will often be Actaea racemosa, Ignatia, Lachesis...

Herbal treatment

Hawthorn, white horehound, passionflower...

• These three plants can be prepared and made up by your herbalist, alone or combined, as a mother tincture, powder in capsules, dried extracts...

Possible prescription: Ask your herbalist to prepare a 30ml bottle of a mother tincture of white horehound. Take 25 drops in a little water, two or three times a day, according to the symptoms.

White horehound

White, or stinking horehound, so named because it smells of musty cellars, will repel even animals. No restaurant would risk offering an infusion of it. It is sedative and helps with sleep.

• You can take hawthorn and passionflower in the form of a fresh whole-plant suspension, which provides the full therapeutic effect naturally present in the whole plant

Possible prescription: From your herbalist, obtain a bottle of 60ml fresh whole-plant suspension of one of these two remedies. Half a teaspoonful to be taken in a little water, morning and night for some days or weeks. For adults only.

• You can use Lamberts® Hawthorn 2500mg:

– Available in containers of 60 tablets
– One tablet daily for a minimum of six weeks

• You could also try lime, whose sedative properties are well known: ask your herbalist for a 60ml bottle of lime buds macerated in glycerine at 1x. Take 50 drops in a little water three times a day. The buds of some plants seem to possess greater activity than the adult plant itself; this is true of blackcurrant, lime, and a few others.

Sweet woodruff

Sweet woodruff is a scented, very sedative plant: it is used to perfume tobacco (Amsterdamer), and is considered by some to be the standard natural tranquillizer.

Plant essential oils

Sweet orange, petitgrain bitter orange

– Two drops of one of these oils to be taken in a little honey twice a day

Bitter orange

Bitter orange has been known in Europe since antiquity; the sweet orange, on the other hand, was not introduced into North Africa and Spain until the 15th century.

Fatigue

An everyday complaint; around four people in ten, mostly women, and mainly between 30 and 40, consider themselves to be suffering from fatigue. It can be defined as an abnormal lack of energy that renders the least physical or mental effort difficult.

In fact descriptions of fatigue are often vague and inaccurate, and may include signs of anxiety, difficulty in concentration, personality disorders, as well as problems with sleep. Fatigue accompanies a number of illnesses that need to be ruled out first (hepatitis, infectious mononucleosis…), but it is frequently psychological in origin, particularly in adolescents.

Popular anti-fatigue remedies contain vitamin C, which is better known for its anti-fatigue effects than for its antioxidant action.

General advice

Follow these simple but important rules:
– Take a little exercise, but not too much
– Arrange rest periods and take a siesta
– Engage in some distracting activity
– Try to relax
– Take care of your most valuable ally, sleep

Dietary advice

• You should choose cereals and dried fruits for their manganese and vitamin B, seafood for cobalt and vitamin B, brewer's yeast for vitamin B, and green vegetables and fresh fruit (kiwi, lemon, orange…) for vitamin C

- Use plenty of garlic, cinnamon, mint, ginger, and pollen, all of which have a long tradition as stimulants

Cinnamon

Native to India and Sri Lanka (formerly Ceylon), cinnamon grows in tropical regions. It is mainly grown as a spice, but nonetheless possesses medicinal properties, particularly as an antiseptic and stimulant. Cinnamon wine was once given out in hospitals to prevent the spread of infection.

Natural foods useful in fatigue

Royal jelly

ORIGIN AND COMPOSITION: The virtues of this precious form of honey, secreted by young worker bees during their second week of life, have been known since the 17th century. It is called 'royal' because it is given to queen bees and greatly prolongs their lives. Royal jelly is one of the foods richest in trace elements (calcium, copper, iron, phosphorus, potassium…), vitamins (A, B, C, D, and E), as well as some essential amino acids.

PROPERTIES: Royal jelly stimulates immunity and helps fight infection; it is recommended in extreme fatigue and in convalescence.

METHOD OF USE: if you are lucky enough to live near a beekeeper you may obtain it fresh. Take only a little at a time because, as you will have gathered, it is very concentrated. Otherwise you can buy sealed vials, airtight because it deteriorates easily. Take one vial at breakfast for a few days, at intervals of a few weeks.

Wheatgerm

ORIGIN AND COMPOSITION: Wheatgerm is a perfect food, the vegetable equivalent of the egg. It contains all the nutrients necessary for the growth of the plant. It is made up of the kernel, (three-quarters of the total weight) which yields flour when ground, and the husk (15 per cent of the total) which gives bran. Wheatgerm is obtained by soaking the grain in water and allowing it to germinate for two days. It contains all the constituents necessary for the growth of the plant. It contains twice as much calcium, three times the magnesium and phosphorus, and many more vitamins, especially B and E, than wheat itself. It also contains vitamins A and C.

PROPERTIES: It helps to take care of nervous problems and is also effective against fatigue and overwork.

METHOD OF USE: you will find it in health food shops as flakes that can be sprinkled on salads, yoghurt, or soft cheese. Take one or two teaspoonfuls a day.

Lucerne and **oats** are rich in minerals and vitamins A, B, D, and E, and in amino acids. They are both nutritive and stimulating.

- You can use Avena (Bioforce) tincture of oats:

– Available in 50ml bottles of oral drops
– Twenty drops to be taken in a little water two to three times daily

Acupuncture

Widely used and very useful in treating fatigue.

TREATMENT SCHEDULE: weekly sessions for a few weeks are helpful during periods of overwork.

Oligotherapy

Cobalt, copper, iron, magnesium, manganese

The provision of trace elements normally comes from the diet, which should be varied and of good quality, encouraging the intake of cereals, fresh or dried fruit, liver.

• When there is a deficiency, trace elements can be taken as supplements such as Organic Minerals (Colloidals) which contains 70+ trace minerals:
– Available in 946ml bottles
– Take 1–3 caps just before breakfast and/or evening meal
– Children 1 teaspoon daily for each 20lbs of body weight:
Or Maximol (Ionized colloidals):
– Available in 500ml bottles
– Take ½ capful once or twice daily on an empty stomach
Or Multi-Guard® (Lamberts), a mixture of trace elements (calcium, magnesium, phosphorus, selenium, zinc…) and vitamins (betacarotene, D, B, C, and E):
– Available in containers of 30 and 90 tablets
– One tablet to be taken each morning

Vitamin C is indispensable here.

Dietary sources of vitamin C

Vitamin C is mainly found in citrus fruits (lemon, orange, grapefruit…), green vegetables (celery, cabbage++, cress, sorrel, parsley, horseradish…), fruit, especially red fruit (strawberries, raspberries, redcurrants…), and others (blackcurrant++, kiwi++…), potatoes, leeks, tomatoes…

• Vitamin C supplements can be found in pharmacies in various forms and brands: Thorne vitamin C (500mg) with citrus bioflavonoids (75mg): one to two capsules three times daily; Lamberts® vitamin C one chewable tablet = 100mg: one to three tablets daily

• You can use Berocca® a mixture of vitamins B, C, calcium, and magnesium:
– Available in boxes of ten effervescent tablets
– One tablet to be taken in the morning for ten days

You can take natural vitamin C, which can be found in, for example, Weleda® sea buckthorn juice, or as Cynorrhodon-Acerola® 500 chewable tablets. A tablespoonful of sea buckthorn juice supplies about 30mg of vitamin C, and a tablet of the mixture of two fruits provides 500mg
– One tablespoonful to be taken each morning

Homeopathy

Kalium phosphoricum
Phosphoricum acidum
– Four granules of one of these two remedies at 5c to be sucked like sweets twice a day between meals for a few days

Kalium phosphoricum

– Chemical origin: dipotassium phosphate
– Homeopathic remedy for mental fatigue due to overwork
– Specific sign: muscular weakness

Phosphoricum acidum

– Chemical origin: phosphoric acid
– Homeopathic remedy for mental exhaustion
– Specific sign: relative absence of muscular weakness

You can use Phosphoric acid complex, which contains both substances at 3c.
– Available in tubes of 80 granules
– Four granules to be sucked like sweets, twice a day

Herbal treatment

Ginseng, eleutherococcus – and also **mint**
POSSIBLE PRESCRIPTION: Ask your herbalist to prepare 20 capsules of a mixture of dried extracts of ginseng and eleutherococcus, 150mg of each in a No.2 capsule (the particular size of the capsule that the herbalist will use). Take two capsules twice a day for about ten days.

Ginseng

When China began to open its doors to the world, it ensured the universal spread of ginseng, a mythical plant known and venerated there for four thousand years, and long reserved exclusively for the use of the emperor and the nobility. Above all, ginseng is famous for its fortifying and physical stimulant effects, strengthening natural defence mechanisms, as an aphrodisiac, anti-stress agent, antidepressant, regenerative...

Eleutherococcus

Eleutherococcus or Siberian ginseng is a plant of the ginseng and ivy family, but has its origins on the plains of Siberia, where it grows in abundance. It is widely used by people involved in sport because it increases resistance to physical and mental fatigue.

• You can also take Phytisone® (Thorne), a remedy based on ginseng, vitamins, herbs and trace elements:
– Available in containers of 60 capsules
– One to two capsules twice daily

• You can take one or two mint infusions

Plant essential oils

Nutmeg, rosemary, creeping thyme
– Two drops of one of these to be taken in a little honey, twice a day

• In the mornings you could also take one drop of essential oil of creeping thyme in 40 drops of oak macerated in glycerine 1x. Obtain a 30ml bottle of this from your herbalist

Nutmeg/rosemary/creeping thyme

Nutmeg was brought back to Europe in the 16th century by Portuguese sailors. It had the reputation of increasing sexual vigour, but care is needed because of its toxicity: eating just two nutmegs can result in lethal convulsions. Rosemary was once thought of as a miraculous plant, an ingredient in the waters of youth used by the Queen of Hungary. Creeping thyme, a heathland plant used by some to treat a lump in the throat, is basically antiseptic and energizing.

Oak

The oak is a common, very tall forest tree, once sacred to the druids and, because of its strength, much exploited for naval shipbuilding as well as for its medicinal properties. It relieves tiredness and possesses tonic, revitalizing, and immuno-stimulant properties. It is very useful during convalescence, even though its bark has long served as a cure for minor skin problems or sore throat.

Depression

A common illness that affects millions of people in the Western world. Two-thirds of cases are women. In the severe forms, in which there may be the wish to die, the diagnosis is obvious, but in the majority of less severe cases the symptoms can be mistaken for anxiety states or neurosis.

It is advisable to watch out for difficulty with concentration, behavioural problems (alternating between sadness and hyperactivity, apathy and excitement), slight or severe insomnia, difficulty in facing everyday life and the future, a persistent tiredness unrelieved by rest, and a partial or complete aversion to sex.

Depression is sometimes so insidious that it escapes the notice of the patient, the family, and medical staff, to the extent that about one-third of patients do not seek advice.

Depression calls for a marked degree of vigilance, since it is a serious illness that can lead to suicide attempts and deaths. Unfortunately, depression recurs in 50 to 80 per cent of cases.

Some important points

Depression affects around ten per cent of people, two women for every man (the latter are most likely to be delinquent or alcoholic). It tends to occur towards the age of 50 in men, and somewhat earlier in women. In the young it may follow the death of a parent. It affects the divorced more often than the married, and widowers more than widows. Women take twice as many psychotropic drugs as men, and attempt suicide three times as often.

Trigger factors in depression:
– loss of a loved one, a job, or objects (e.g. as in a burglary)
– family, personal, professional, or social conflict
– social isolation
– serious illness
– medicinal treatment (e.g. a slimming diet)
– after childbirth (post-partum depression is well known)
– menopause

Predisposing factors:
– family history++
– delicate personality

Some mistakes to avoid:
– do not tell the depressed person to "pull him/herself together"; he/she will be constantly trying to do this anyway
– do not ask the person to make an important decision; he/she is not capable
– do not advise the person to go on holiday; he/she will not necessarily improve
– do not try to persuade him/her that things will get better; it does not work
– do not attempt to dismiss irrational or paranoid notions; this requires massive patience or even more than that

Natural foods useful in depression

Pollen

ORIGIN AND COMPOSITION: Pollen consists of thousands of tiny grains, the male seed of flowers. It is collected by particular bees and distributed to feeding larvae in the hive. It contains many minerals (copper, iron, magnesium, potassium, silicon), amino acids (glutamic acid, methionine), and vitamins A, B, C, and E.

PROPERTIES: Pollen stimulates immunity and strengthens immune reactions, and is invaluable for restoring mental and muscular energy, re-establishing nervous equilibrium, fighting depression and fatigue, improving memory and mental performance.

METHOD OF USE: You can find it in health food shops, in capsules or sold loose from a jar. On retiring to bed, pour a teaspoonful of pollen into half a glass of water, cover it, let it stand overnight, and take the mixture in the morning at breakfast.

Brewer's yeast

ORIGIN AND COMPOSITION: a living substance, specially prepared as a supplement, from a minute fungus that serves as a ferment in the preparation of beer. It is different from baker's yeast, and much better tolerated by the intestine. Yeast is an extraordinary dietary supplement containing little fat, salt, sugar, or calories, but rich in proteins, essential amino acids, minerals (chromium, phosphorus, potassium, selenium...), and group B vitamins.

INDICATIONS: Brewer's yeast is a sedative and improves and calms the nervous state, as well as reducing the sensation of hunger and the need for sugar.

METHOD OF USE: You will find it in health food shops and pharmacies as tablets, capsules, flakes (take care, it is very bitter). One dose to be taken three times a day.

Chocolate

One of the foods that depressed persons eat most. Though from the nutritional point of view it may not be a good example of balance, (it is too rich in fat and sugar), chocolate is still very useful because it contains magnesium, calcium (when it is milk chocolate), and above all, precursors of the neurotransmitters involved in depression. But take care: one 100mg bar of chocolate provides more than 600 calories.

• You can also use Megavit® (Lamberts), a high potency combination of magnesium, group B vitamins, selenium, and vitamin E among others:
– Available in containers of 60 and 180 tablets
– One to two tablets to be taken daily

Acupuncture

Its balancing action is very useful, even indispensable in treating incipient depression. It may also help during withdrawal from antidepressant treatment.

TREATMENT SCHEDULE: weekly or twice-weekly sessions are effective in problems with mood, and tiredness. Acupuncture has a calming action and helps with sleep.

Light therapy

Light therapy has found its place as a service in many hospitals. It consists of exposing the depressed person to an intense light source for a few hours a day.

It is a good idea to encourage the patient to spend as much time as possible in broad daylight, or with all the lights on (fluorescent or halogen), and to take long walks in the sunshine. Of his own accord, the patient prefers to stay quiet, in darkness as gloomy as his thoughts.

Homeopathy

Sepia

– Four granules at 9c, to be sucked like sweets once or twice a day, between meals

Sepia

– Animal origin: cuttlefish ink
– A great homeopathic remedy for depression, deep despair
– Typical personality: apathetic woman, pessimistic, shuns society

You can use Lehning® Sepia Complex 20, which contains Sepia 4x, and Calcarea carbonica 3x.
– Available in boxes of 80 tablets
– Suck one tablet twice a day

Oligotherapy

Lithium

This trace element is normally supplied by the diet, which should be varied and of good quality.

When there is a deficiency, lithium can be taken as a supplement.

Dietary sources of lithium

There is little information on its presence in food, but it can be found in small quantities in cereals, lettuce, green vegetables, potatoes, meat, eggs, fish, mineral waters, table salt…

• Lithium supplements can be found as many different forms and brands, e.g.: Organic Minerals (Colloidals) which contains 70+ trace minerals:
– Available in 946ml bottles
– Take 1–3 caps just before breakfast and/or evening meal
– Children 1 teaspoon daily for each 20lbs of body weight
Or Maximol (Ionized colloidals)
– Available in 500ml bottles
– Take ½ capful once or twice daily on an empty stomach
Or Lithium orotate (Vitamin Research Products) 120mg:
– Available in containers of 120 capsules
– One capsule twice daily with meals
– One dose of lithium to be taken three times a day, for a few days

Vitamins useful in depression

Mainly in **group B**, especially **B1, B3, B5, B6, B12**

Dietary sources of B vitamins

You will find them mainly in whole cereals, brewer's yeast, wheatgerm, meat (liver), fish and seafood, vegetables (asparagus, mushrooms, Brussels sprouts, spinach, lentils), rice and wholemeal pastry…

• If you are looking for an energizing effect, take Berocca®, which contains group B vitamins, vitamin C, and also calcium and magnesium:
– Available in tubes of 10 or 20 effervescent tablets
– One tablet to be taken a day for 20 days

Depression and the aged

The aged are affected by depression partly because they stay inside at home too much, and do not expose themselves enough to light or sunlight.

Agitation or depression, especially in the aged, gives reason to suspect a deficiency in vitamin B9 and B12.

Herbal treatment

Angelica, St. John's wort

• These two plants can be prepared and made up by your herbalist as, for example, a mother tincture, powder in capsules, dried extracts…
POSSIBLE PRESCRIPTION: Ask your herbalist to make up 45 capsules each containing 200mg of dried angelica extract. Take one capsule three times a day for 15 days

Angelica

The fruit and roots of angelica are used in medicine. The roots are gathered in the autumn when they are particularly rich in the essential oil. Angelica is principally known for its digestive properties, as, for example in Benedictine liqueur, but recent studies have shown its value in depression.

• You can take Lamberts® St. John's Wort 1360mg (containing 500µg hypericin):
– Available in containers of 60 tablets
– One tablet to be taken twice a day for some weeks

• Or you can take St. John's wort (Bioforce) as a tincture:
– Available in bottles of 100ml
– One teaspoon in a little water with meals, two to three times daily

St.John's wort

This plant is called St. John's wort because it flowers in midsummer – St. John's day is 24 June. Once used to treat nervous problems and to dispel low spirits, it has been widely prescribed more recently for its antidepressant properties. The mother tincture contains small amounts of an active compound (hypericine), which makes an extract preferable.

Plant essential oils

Rosemary, for its energizing properties.
– Two drops to be taken in a little honey, twice a day

POSSIBLE PRESCRIPTION: Ask your herbalist to prepare a bottle with one gram of essential oil of rosemary and a bottle of 30ml of mother tincture of angelica. Place two drops of the essential oil in 30 drops of the mother tincture, add a little water and take it twice a day for two weeks.

Rosemary

This shrub can be recognized from afar by its fine appearance and strong aroma.
Rosemary leaves are rich in the essential oil and by tradition it fights fatigue, strengthens the memory, and activates the circulation, as well as improving morale and calming the nerves.

Sleep disturbances and insomnia

Characterized by a reduction in the length and quality of sleep, with serious effects on activities the following day. Insomnia, the severest form of sleep disturbance, is very widespread. Sleep, an extremely delicate function, is immediately affected by the smallest personal or professional setback, the slightest stress, anxiety, or depression.

Sleep occurs in successive passages of an hour and three-quarters or so, becoming shallower and less refreshing with the approach of the early hours. The first two cycles are much more refreshing than the two that follow. Sudden arousal by the telephone is much more traumatic when one has just gone to sleep than at the end of the cycle.

Those who keep watch or navigate alone know that just a little sleep can suffice, but only if the precise rules dictated by our rhythms are followed. In this respect we all differ: some need many hours of sleep, others, like Napoleon or Margaret Thatcher, for example, very little.

General advice

- Avoid a siesta
- Do not take tea or coffee after 5.00pm because they are too stimulating
- Do not dine too heavily or richly
- Choose lettuce, fish, lean meats, pastry, and rice, which improve sleep, and eat foods containing magnesium and lithium
- Do not take violent exercise before retiring to bed; instead a little exercise in the afternoon is recommended
- A glass of warm milk or an infusion with a little honey is the classic way to obtain a good night's sleep
- Always try to go to bed and get up at about the same times
- Do not go to bed unless you are sleepy
- Be careful about altitude (above 1,800 metres) if you are already a poor sleeper at sea level

Acupuncture

Almost indispensable because of its sedative action and ability to restore equilibrium.

Treatment schedule: four to eight sessions spread over a month are generally enough, especially if the insomnia is a relatively recent development. Then monthly maintenance treatment can take over.

Relaxation

Relaxation is essential if one is to learn to take charge of the emotions, control muscular tension, and to reduce, channel, and even suppress the effects of stress. Naturally, learning to relax can take some weeks, but it may then help with going to sleep or going back to sleep.

Homeopathy

Coffea

– Four granules at 9c, to be sucked like sweets a few minutes before retiring to bed

Coffea cruda

– Vegetable origin: coffee
– Homeopathic remedy for insomnia with a state of excitement – as after too much coffee

- You can use Valerianaheel®, which contains mother tinctures of Crataegus, Valeriana, Chamomilla, Avena (oats) and Lupulus (hops) combined with Hypericum (St. John's Wort) D1, Kalium bromatum D1

– Available in drop bottles of 30 and 100ml
– In general, 15 drops 3 times daily, in the evening 25 drops. Single dose for infants and young children: from age 2–6 years, 5 drops; from 6–12 years, 10 drops

Natural healing

Oligotherapy

Lithium, magnesium

Supplies of trace elements are normally provided by the diet, which should be varied and of good quality. When there is a deficiency, as there frequently is in this case, these elements may be taken as supplements.

Sources of lithium and magnesium

You will find them mainly in cereals, chocolate, green vegetables, eggs, fish, meat, and dried fruits.

• Lithium and magnesium preparations: Organic Minerals (Colloidals) which contains 70+ trace minerals:
– Available in 946ml bottles
– Take 1–3 caps just before breakfast and/or evening meal
– Children 1 teaspoon daily for each 20lbs of body weight
Or Maximol (Ionized colloidals)
– Available in 500ml bottles
– Take ½ capful once or twice daily on an empty stomach

Or Lithium orotate (Vitamin Research Products) 120mg:
– Available in containers of 120 capsules
– One capsule twice daily with meals

POSSIBLE PRESCRIPTION: one dose of magnesium during the day, one dose of lithium at bedtime.

• You can take Multi-Guard® (Lamberts), a mixture of trace elements (calcium, magnesium, phosphorus, selenium, zinc…) and vitamins (beta-carotene, D, B, C, and E)
– Available in containers of 30 and 90 tablets
– One tablet to be taken each morning

Herbal treatment

A number of well-known plants such as **lime, verbena**.

Others such as **sweet woodruff, white horehound, California poppy** are increasingly used.

Some of them, such as **hawthorn, passionflower, and valerian** have a tranquillizing effect, which makes them useful, if not actually indispensable.

These plants can be prepared by your herbalist, singly or in combination, as mother tincture, powder in capsules, dried extracts…

Sweet woodruff/Eschscholtzia

Sweet woodruff is added to silage to scent cows' milk, and is also used to freshen the air at home, to repel insects, and to give a fruity aroma to "Amsterdamer" pipe tobacco. Eschscholtzia or California poppy is antispasmodic, analgesic, and sedative.

• For hawthorn, passionflower, and valerian, you can use a fresh whole-plant suspension which, thanks to a method of cold stabilization, provides the full therapeutic effect naturally present in the whole plant

POSSIBLE PRESCRIPTION: obtain from your herbalist a 60ml bottle of fresh whole-plant suspension of one of these three plants. Take a half-teaspoonful in a little water at bedtime.

Lime

The pale yellow flowers of the lime tree, whose pleasant and characteristic scent is familiar to all, are antispasmodic, sedative, and mildly laxative in action.

- You can ask your herbalist to prepare a 60ml bottle of lime buds macerated in glycerine at 1x. Take 50 drops in a small sedative infusion at bedtime
- Those who like infusions can buy the plants in speciality shops or from herbal suppliers. Allow one dessertspoonful of plant for a cup of boiling water and leave it to infuse for ten minutes

Plant essential oils

Lavender, sweet marjoram, petitgrain bitter orange

– Two drops of one of them to be taken in a little honey at bedtime

Petitgrain bitter orange

Petitgrain bitter orange is one of the constituents of the bitter orange leaf, whereas neroli, which is used to make 'orange-flower water', is prepared from the flowers.

Withdrawal from tranquillizers, antidepressants, and sleeping pills

Most people who choose complementary remedies do so to avoid the use of 'heavier' medications. An increasing number of patients coming for treatment do so because they begin to take mood-altering drugs or sleeping pills as a temporary measure, and then find they have trouble stopping them.

Withdrawal is a delicate phase calling for much patience and active cooperation from the patient, because these very effective drugs cause real physical and psychological dependence. Conventional drugs cannot be suddenly withdrawn; rather they can be substituted, then progressively replaced by gentler therapy. A suitable period for successful withdrawal from, for example, a soporific drug (hypnotic) and its replacement, is about two months.

Acupuncture

Acupuncture heads the list because its powerful sedative action and ability to restore the equilibrium make it invaluable.

Treatment schedule: Weekly or twice-weekly sessions are necessary from the start of withdrawal. Generally the intervals should be increased as soon as possible. The maintenance treatment can extend over several months. In the right conditions, for complete withdrawal from all medication, a series of 12 to 15 sessions is not unusual.

Auriculotherapy

This technique, related to the one above, involves placing tiny needles the size of a pinhead in the external ear. They are left in place at the end of the session and are usually removed after a week or so. Sometimes they fall out themselves. The advantage over a normal acupuncture session is that these temporary needles provide longer-lasting beneficial stimulation.

Relaxation

Relaxation is essential for learning to control the emotions and muscular tension, and reducing, channelling and even suppressing the effects of stress. Naturally, a few weeks' practice are necessary to permit withdrawal under the best conditions.

Oligotherapy

Lithium when withdrawing from antidepressant treatment; **magnesium** if stopping tranquillizing treatment.

Supplies of these two trace elements are normally provided by the diet, which should be varied and of good quality. When there is a deficiency, they may be taken as supplements.

Dietary sources of lithium

There is little data on the presence of lithium in foods, but it is found in small amounts in cereals, lettuce, green vegetables, potatoes, meat, eggs, fish, drinking water, and table salt.

Dietary sources of magnesium

Present in almost all foods, but unfortunately particularly in those rich in calories. Magnesium is found mainly in citrus fruits, bananas, whole cereals (oat flakes, bran), cocoa and chocolate, shellfish (winkles, shrimps, oysters, clams) and oily fish, snails, figs, hard cheeses, dried fruit and nuts (almonds, peanuts, hazelnuts, walnuts), vegetables (spinach, dried haricot and green beans, split peas, soya), wholemeal bread.

• Lithium and magnesium medications: there are many different forms and brands: Organic Minerals (Colloidals) which contains 70+ trace minerals
– Available in 946ml bottles
– Take 1–3 caps just before breakfast and/or evening meal
– Children 1 teaspoon daily for each 20lbs of body weight
Or Maximol (Ionized colloidals):
– Available in 500ml bottles
– Take ½ capful once or twice daily on an empty stomach

Or Lithium orotate (Vitamin Research Products) 120mg
– Available in containers of 120 capsules
– One capsule twice daily with meals

POSSIBLE PRESCRIPTION: One dose of magnesium to be taken in the morning and at midday, and one dose of lithium in the evening for a few days or weeks.

• You can also use Megavit® (Lamberts), a high potency combination of

magnesium, group B vitamins, selenium, and vitamin E among others:
– Available in containers of 60 and 180 tablets
– One to two tablets to be taken daily

Vitamins useful during withdrawal

Mainly vitamins in group B, particularly B1, B3, B5, B6, B9, and B12.

Dietary sources of group B vitamins

You will find them mainly in whole cereals, brewer's yeast, wheatgerm, meat (liver), fish and seafood, vegetables (asparagus, mushrooms, Brussels sprouts, spinach, lentils), rice and wholemeal pastry…

• You can take Lamberts® B-100 complex, a mixture of vitamins B1, B2, B3, B5, B6, B12, folic acid, biotin, choline, inositol and PABA:
– Available in containers of 60 and 200 tablets
– One tablet to be taken each day

Homeopathy

Almost always used at some stage or other of withdrawal. Strictly speaking there is no homeopathic tranquillizer or hypnotic; it is therefore *essential* to consult a homeopath to establish the constitutional treatment that most closely matches the patient's personality.

A number of remedies stand out, among them **Arsenicum album, Natrum muriaticum, Nux vomica**…

Arsenicum album

– Chemical origin: arsenic anhydride
– Homeopathic remedy for anxiety with fear of death
– Symptoms and typical personality: alternating agitation and depression in a person who is meticulous and extremely fussy

Natrum muriaticum

– Chemical origin: sea salt
– Homeopathic remedy for the psychic problems of adolescence
– Characteristic personality: solitary, moody, irritable, made worse by comforting

Nux vomica

– Vegetable origin: the seeds of the tree Strychnos nux-vomica
– Homeopathic remedy for the hyperactive patient who takes stimulants
– Characteristic signs: physically and mentally hypersensitive, quick-tempered, aggressive

– These 'constitutional remedies' are often prescribed at 7c, four granules to be sucked once a day

• You can take Lehning® Gelsemium Complex 70, which contains Arsenicum album 3x, Nux vomica 3x, and, naturally, Gelsemium 3x:
– Available in 30ml bottles of oral drops
– Fifteen drops in a little water four times a day

Herbal treatment

Numerous sedative plants can be used: **hawthorn, white horehound, camomile, poppy, melilot, lemon balm, passionflower, lime, valerian**...

These can be made up by your herbalist either singly or in combination as mother tincture, powder in capsules, dried extracts.

POSSIBLE PRESCRIPTION: hawthorn, melilot, lemon balm, passionflower, and valerian can be obtained as fresh whole-plant suspensions. Ask for one of them to be made up into a 60ml bottle of fresh whole-plant suspension. Half a teaspoonful to be taken in a little water once or twice a day for a few weeks.

• You can use Valerianaheel®, which contains mother tinctures of Crataegus, Valeriana, Chamomilla, Avena (oats) and Lupulus (hops) combined with Hypericum (St. John's Wort) D1, Kalium bromatum D1

– Available in drop bottles of 30 and 100ml

– In general, 15 drops 3 times daily, in the evening 25 drops. Single dose for infants and young children: from age 2–6 years, 5 drops; from 6–12 years, 10 drops

Plant essential oils

Lavender, sweet marjoram, and petitgrain bitter orange are sedatives.

– One drop of essential oil of one of these to be taken in a little honey, three times a day

POSSIBLE PRESCRIPTION: Ask your herbalist to prepare a 30ml bottle of lime buds macerated in glycerine at 1x. Pour two drops of the first into thirty drops of the second, add a little water, and take this mixture at bedtime.

Infectious diseases

There are those who regard homeopathy and other alternative or complementary therapies as outdated, but these methods remain effective and quick in treating infectious complaints; this is one of their main raisons d'être. In each of the following chapters you can use them as initial treatment, switching quickly to another, particularly antibiotics, if improvement is slow to appear. The efficacy of complementary remedies depends essentially on the choice of products, the illness, the patient's reactive capacity, how early treatment is started, and the choice of dose. This may be summarized by the formula: "the right remedy for the right illness, in the right patient, at the right time, in the right dose". If a complementary treatment is carried out properly, the use of antibiotics, which are prescribed far too much in the Western world, can often be avoided.

The start of infection

Though complementary remedies are naturally very specific, the very start of infection calls for a relatively straightforward prescription, to be refined when the first individual symptoms appear. These should then be prevented or minimized by the rapid use of appropriate treatment.

Standard anti-infective treatment

To be started as quickly as possible at the first abnormal symptom:

• Start with Aconitum-Homaccord® (Heel) which contains Aconitum D2, D19, D30, D200, Eucalyptus D2, D10, D30 and Ipecacuanha D2, D10, D30, D200:
– Available in drop bottles containing 30 and 100ml
– Generally 10 drops to be taken three times daily. Initially 10 drops every 15 minutes

• Add copper as a trace element with silver and gold in colloidal form

• Six tablets of Pyrogenium 5c, once a day in a single dose, for a few days

• Twenty drops of Lehning® L52 in a little water, three or four times a day, if the patient already has a temperature

• Vitamin C: one gram a day for adults, 0.5g for children, for a fortnight

Aconitum napellus

– Vegetable origin: the plant aconite, also known as wolf's bane because the poison it contains was once used in hunting
– Homeopathic remedy for infections that are sudden in onset

Pyrogenium

– Animal origin: prepared from putrefied beef
– Homeopathic remedy for the prevention or treatment of serious infection

• To this standard treatment composed of three homeopathic remedies, one to three trace elements, and a vitamin, the homeopath may add remedies that are specific to each illness and fundamental for each personality

Dietary advice

Essential:

• Stop all heavy, greasy foods, particularly dairy products, fried food, and dishes with sauces

• Drink plenty

• Choose foods rich in vitamin C and copper

• Supplement your diet with wheatgerm and brewer's yeast, which are rich in group B vitamins and trace elements

• Take royal jelly

• Eat plenty of garlic and onion

• Make free use of herbs and spices

such as thyme, cinnamon and oregano, known for their anti-infective properties

Garlic/Onion

Native to Central Asia, garlic has been cultivated for centuries. The Egyptians, Greeks, Romans, and the Gauls ate large amounts, mainly for its invigorating and antiseptic qualities. The onion originated in Asia too: it has been an excellent food throughout history, a symbol of health, longevity, and indeed, eternity. In the Renaissance, its smell came to be considered offensive, and only the peasantry continued to use it.

Some foods rich in vitamin C

Citrus fruits (lemon, orange, grapefruit), green vegetables (celery, green cabbage++, cress, spinach, sorrel, parsley, horseradish), fruit, especially red fruit (strawberries, raspberries, redcurrants), and also other types (pineapple, blackcurrants++, guava, kiwi++), potatoes, green peppers, tomatoes…

Some remedies based on vitamin C.

• Synergisti-C (Thorne) which contains 650mg ascorbic acid, 400mg Echinacea angustifolia, 100mg Baptisia tinctoria and 100mg hesperidin:
– Available in containers of 60 capsules
– Take one to two capsules twice daily

• Biocare vitamin C (citrus free) 500mg containing magnesium ascorbate and bilberry:
– Available in containers of 180 veg capsules
– Take one to two capsules daily

• Lamberts®. Rutin +C +bioflavonoids (containing vitamin C 500mg, citrus bioflavonoids 100mg, rutin 50mg and hesperidin complex 30mg):
– Available in containers of 90 capsules
– Take one to two capsules daily

• You can take natural Vitamin C in chewable form – Lamberts® Vitamin C 100mg:
– Sold in containers of 90 tablets
– One to three tablets daily

Sea buckthorn/Dog rose/Barbados cherry

The sea buckthorn, a shrub with ornamental foliage and fruit, is very rich in natural vitamin C. This is also the case with the Barbados cherry from the West Indies, and the dog rose.

Some foods rich in copper

Seaweed, almonds, avocado, cocoa, cereals (especially whole wheat and whole rice), mushrooms, shellfish, oysters, crustaceans, calf and sheep liver++, dried fruit, nuts, fish roe, plums, tea…

Royal jelly

ORIGIN AND COMPOSITION: The virtues of this luxurious honey, secreted by young worker bees during their second week of life, have been known since the 17th century. It prolongs the life of the hive queen. Royal jelly is one of the foods richest in trace elements and group B vitamins. It contains the three antioxidant vitamins (A, C and E), and vitamin

D, as well as calcium, copper, iron, phosphorus, potassium ... and some essential amino acids, which impart general invigorating properties as well as stimulating immunity.

Method of use: if you are lucky enough to live near a beekeeper you may obtain it fresh. Take only a little at a time because, as you will have gathered, it is very concentrated. You can buy sealed vials, airtight because the jelly deteriorates easily. Take one vial at breakfast for a few days, at intervals of a few weeks.

Two plants to combat infection

Anti-infective **Echinacea**, very stimulating **ginseng**.

PRESCRIPTION: Ask your herbalist to prepare a 30ml bottle of a mother tincture of each of these two plants: take 25 drops of the first in a little water three times a day, 25 drops of the second, twice a day.

Although it may seem to taste very alcoholic, the mother tincture contains very little alcohol: 100 drops are equivalent to about a centimetre of wine in the bottom of a glass.

Echinacea

Echinacea or coneflower is very effective against snakebite, stubborn wounds, fevers... it comes to us from Native American tribes, who were using it long before the arrival of antibiotics.

Ginseng

By opening China's doors to the world, it ensured the universal spread of ginseng, a mythical plant known and venerated for 4,000 years and, because of its value in prolonging life, long the exclusive reserve of the emperor and nobility.

- You can use Echinaforce (Bioforce), a tincture of Echinacea purpurea:
  - Available in 50ml and 100ml bottles of oral drops
  - Fifteen drops to be taken in a little water, three times a day by adults, seven drops three times a day by children (6–12 years old)
- And Lamberts® Korean ginseng 600mg:
  - Sold in containers of 60 capsules
  - Take one to two capsules daily

About vaccines

The French scientist, Louis Pasteur, was famous for his rabies vaccine. We are reminded daily of the importance of this discovery, since vaccination is one of the most certain, most economical ways of preventing illnesses. The principle is no longer in dispute... even if some doctors have their own opinions on the importance, efficacy, and harmlessness of some vaccines.

Essential oils to combat infection

Spanish oregano, mountain thyme, common thyme…

Prescription: Obtain a 2ml bottle of one of these essential oils from your pharmacist or health-food store; take three drops in a little honey, two or three times a day.

Oregano

Oregano prefers to grow on chalky soils on the coast. The flowers have digestive properties and its essential oil is an antiseptic.

Thyme

Thyme is best known for its aromatic qualities, and is greatly appreciated by bees. The essential oil is a powerful anti-infective agent.

Winter savory

The Latin name for savory, *Satureia montana* is linked to the word satyr, strongly suggesting psychic and physical stimulation.

Warning, essential oils can be dangerous

– You should not take them unless you are fully aware of their effects, indications, and method of use

– You must adhere strictly to the prescribed dose

– If in doubt, do not take them

– Avoid prolonged treatment without expert advice

– Never give them to children

Fever

We talk of fever when the rectal temperature is more than 37.3° C (99.1° F) in the morning, 37.8° C (100° F) in the evening. The temperature should be taken at rest, over several minutes, at some time before or after meals. Fever is mostly due to an infectious process, and is often the main symptom, but sometimes it may also indicate another illness. It may be accompanied by shivering, sweating, headache, occasionally agitation, pain in the joints or muscles, skin eruptions… all signs that will narrow and clarify the diagnosis.

A rise in body temperature, a fever, is a natural defence reaction. It helps resist infection by killing the bacteria responsible or impeding their reproduction with body heat. When you have an infection, very often the first reaction is to take aspirin or paracetamol to lower the body temperature, and you will soon feel better, for a while… but you are suppressing your best means of natural defence. As long as the temperature is not too high and you are not running the risk of convulsions, you should try to resist this temptation, however legitimate it may seem.

Standard anti-infective treatment

To be started as quickly as possible at the first abnormal symptom.

• Start with Aconitum-Homaccord®(Heel) which contains Aconitum D2, D10, D30, D200, Eucalyptus D4, D10, D30 and Ipecacuanha D2, D10, D30, D200:
– available in drop bottles containing 30 and 100ml
– Generally 10 drops three times daily. Initially 10 drops every 15 minutes

• Add copper as a trace element with silver or gold in colloidal form

• Six tablets of Pyrogenium 5c once a day in a single dose for a few days

• Twenty drops of Lehning® L52 in a little water, three or four times per day

• Vitamin C: one gram per day for adults, 0.5 gram for children, for a fortnight

Some foods rich in vitamin C

Citrus fruits (lemon, orange, grapefruit), green vegetables (celery, green cabbage++, cress, spinach, sorrel, parsley, horseradish), fruit, particularly red fruit (strawberries, raspberries, redcurrants), and also others (pineapple, blackcurrant++, guava, kiwi++), potatoes, green peppers, tomatoes...

Some foods rich in copper

Seaweed, almonds, avocado, cocoa, cereals (especially whole wheat and whole rice), mushrooms, shellfish, oysters, crustaceans, calf and sheep liver ++, dried fruits, green vegetables, nuts, fish roe, plums, tea...

Silver

Silver, which has no known function in the body, has a general bactericidal and local antiseptic action (silver nitrate) which explains its use as an anti-infective.

• You can also use silver liquid SILV-LQ (Vitamin Research Products) 400ppm:
– Available in bottles of 4 fluid ounces
– Mix half a teaspoon with 1 ounce of water, rinse in mouth for 15 seconds before swallowing

• To this standard treatment composed of three homeopathic remedies, one to three trace elements, and a vitamin, the homeopath may add remedies that are specific to each illness and fundamental to each personality.

Dietary advice

To be strictly followed:

• Stop all heavy, fatty food, particularly dairy products, fried food, and dishes with sauces

• Drink plenty

• Choose foods rich in vitamin C and copper

• Supplement your diet with wheatgerm and brewer's yeast, which are rich in vitamins and trace elements

• Eat plenty of garlic and onion

• Eat herbs such as thyme, cinnamon, and oregano, known for their anti-infective action

Garlic / Onion

Garlic has been cultivated for millennia and has long been taken for its stimulant and antiseptic qualities. Throughout history the onion has been a food beyond compare, a symbol of longevity, even eternity. These two foods played a large part in combating the great epidemics of the Middle Ages.

• You can take Garlic-Chili Flax seed oil (Jarrow) to improve resistance to infection:
– Sold in 12 fl.oz bottles
– Take one to three teaspoons daily (may be used as salad dressing)

• You can take natural vitamin C in, for example, Weleda® Argousier (sea buckthorn) juice:
– Available in 200ml bottles
– One tablespoonful to be taken in the morning, providing about 30mg of the vitamin

Specific homeopathic treatment for fever

Aconite, Belladonna, Ferrum phosphoricum
– Four tablets of one or more of these remedies at 5c, to be sucked like sweets between meals, three or four times a day

Aconitum napellus

Vegetable in origin: the plant aconite was also called wolf's bane because the poison it contains was formerly used in hunting.

A homeopathic remedy for use in infections that are sudden in onset.

Belladonna

Vegetable in origin: the leaves and fresh flowers of belladonna, deadly nightshade.

A homeopathic remedy for infections with high fever, agitation, and intense thirst.

Ferrum phosphoricum

– Chemical in origin: iron phosphate
– Homeopathic remedy for slight fever with a very weakened state

How to choose between these remedies

It is usual to start with aconite, followed by belladonna or ferrum phosphoricum. The difference is that clinical reaction to the latter is slower and less pronounced than the reactions to aconite and belladonna.

• You can take Traumeel®,(Heel) which contains Aconite D3 and Belladonna D4, among other ingredients:

– Available in containers of 50 or 250 tablets
– In general, one tablet to be dissolved under the tongue three times daily...

Herbal treatment

Anti-infective **Echinacea**, very stimulating **ginseng**.

PRESCRIPTION: Ask your herbalist to prepare a 30ml bottle of a mother tincture of each of these two plants; take 25 drops of the first in a little water, three times a day, and 25 drops twice a day of the second.

Echinacea

Echinacea is a plant native to North America, where it was widely used by Native American tribes for its antiseptic properties.

• You can use Echinaforce (Bioforce), a tincture of Echinacea purpurea:
– Available in 50ml and 100ml bottles of oral drops
– Fifteen drops to be taken in a little water, three times a day by adults, seven drops three times a day by children (6–12 years old)...

You may also take infusions of **thyme**, and of **lime** and **camomile** flowers.

Lime

The flowers of the lime tree, best known for their sedative action, have always been widely used in illnesses involving a chill: the infusion can be sweetened with a little honey.

Influenza

Primarily a winter infection, influenza epidemics, viral in origin, affect millions of people every year. Influenza is most often benign, but sometimes leads to serious complications, mainly in the elderly and frail. After a short, apparently symptom-free incubation period of from 12 to 48 hours, it takes hold rapidly. Airborne droplets containing the virus from the saliva and the breath make it highly contagious during this initial phase.

The diagnosis is arrived at on the basis of an infectious period, a flare-up at the start with the temperature raised to 39–40°C, accompanied by intense fatigue, aching all over, muscle and joint pain, and even ear, nose, and throat signs as seen in any ENT infection.

Incubation is the time that elapses between the moment of infection and the appearance of the first symptoms of the illness.

Homeopathic prophylaxis

Aimed at preventing the illness from appearing or at reducing its harshness. There are three commonly prescribed remedies:

Influenzinum: Prepared from a strain of the current year's anti-influenza vaccine.

Aviaire: Prepared from chicken tuberculin.

Yersin serum: Prepared from plague serum.

PRESCRIPTION EXAMPLE:
– Influenzinum 7c, four tablets on Monday and Thursday
– Avaire 7c, four tablets on Tuesday and Friday
– Yersin 7c, four tablets on Wednesday and Saturday
Taken from September to January.

Natural prophylactic food

Cider vinegar: its virtues were discovered by an American veterinary surgeon who noticed that the rotten apples he added to his livestock's feed protected them from winter infections.

– Add a small teaspoonful of natural vinegar (of known origin) to half a glass of water, to be drunk before breakfast. Take a calcium supplement to avoid mineral deficiency

Standard anti-infective treatment

At the start of a bout of influenza. To be instituted as quickly as possible after the first abnormal symptoms appear.

• Start with Aconitum-Homaccord® (Heel) which contains Aconitum D2, D10, D30, D200, Eucalyptus D4, D10, D30 and Ipecacuanha D2, D10, D30, D200:
– available in drop bottles containing 30 and 100ml
– Generally 10 drops three times daily. Initially 10 drops every 15 minutes

• Add copper as a trace element with silver and gold in colloidal form

• Six tablets of Pyrogenium once a day, in a single dose, for a few days

• Twenty drops of Lehning ® L52 in a little water, three or four times a day, if there is fever

• Vitamin C: one gram per day in adults, 0.5g per day in children, for a fortnight

• You can take natural vitamin C in Weleda Hippophan®:
– Sold in 200ml bottles
– One tablespoonful taken in the morning provides about 25mg of the vitamin

Some foods rich in vitamin C

Citrus fruits (lemon, orange, grapefruit); green vegetables (celery, green cabbage++, cress, spinach, sorrel, parsley, horseradish); fruit, particularly red fruit (strawberries, raspberries, redcurrants), but also others (pineapple, blackcurrants++, guava, kiwi++); potatoes, green peppers, tomatoes...

Some foods rich in copper

Seaweed, almonds, avocado, cocoa, cereals (especially whole wheat and whole rice), mushrooms, shellfish, oysters, crustaceans, calf and sheep liver++, dried fruits, green vegetables, nuts, fish roe, plums, tea...

Gold

In the Middle Ages gold was considered a panacea that healed almost everything. Innumerable medical properties were attributed to it, and it was widely used for all illnesses. It "cured" gout, smallpox, plague, leprosy, strengthened the heart, and even revived the dead... It sank into oblivion as a treatment for some decades, but was rehabilitated during the 19th century, thanks to its efficacy against syphilis and other venereal diseases; then it became an accepted treatment, and still is today, because of its role in stimulating immunological defences.

• You can take Oscillococcinum® which is not a vaccine in the strict sense of the term, but a remarkable initial treatment composed of filtered, autolysed Barbary duck liver and heart:
– Available in boxes of three or six doses (generally tablet form)
– One dose to be taken at the first shivers, and once or twice again on the first day, and possibly the following day

• Or you may take Gripp-Heel® (Heel) which contains Aconite D4, Bryonia D4, Eupatorium D3, Lachesis D12 and Phosphorus D5:
– Sold in containers of 50 and 250 tablets
– In general, 1 tablet to be dissolved under the tongue 3–5 times daily. In acute disorders 1 tablet every 15 minutes (over a period lasting up to 2 hours)

Since influenza is a viral infection, antibiotics, which act only against bacteria, are useless, yet they are frequently prescribed.

• This treatment, combined with the dietary advice given in the section 'The start of infection', brings about improvement or cure in a good number of cases, but it is wise to add the following specific homeopathic remedies, as well as the basic remedy chosen by your homeopath

Homeopathy

Eupatorium, Gelsemium
– Four tablets of one of these remedies at 5c, to be sucked like sweets, between meals, three to four times a day

Eupatorium perfoliatum

– Vegetable origin: comfrey, a herbaceous plant with tall stems and pink flowers
– The homeopathic remedy for intense aching
– Specific sign: an agitated state

Gelsemium sempervirens

– Vegetable origin: jasmine, a climbing shrub with large scented yellow or white flowers
– Homeopathic remedy for infectious illnesses with extreme fatigue and shivering
– Specific sign: prostration

• You can take Lehning® Gelsemium Complex 70, which includes Aconite 2x, Belladonna 3x, and Gelsemium 3x...
– Sold in 30ml bottles of oral drops
– Fifteen drops to be taken in water, three times a day by adults, eight drops three times a day by children

Two plants to combat influenza

Anti-infective **Echinacea**, very stimulating **ginseng**.

Prescription: Ask your herbalist to prepare 30ml bottles of the mother tincture of each of these two plants. Take 25 drops of the first, in water, three times a day, and 25 drops of the second, twice a day.

Echinacea

Echinacea is a plant native to North America, where it was widely used by native tribes for its antiseptic properties.

• You can use Echinaforce (Bioforce), a tincture of Echinacea purpurea:
– Available in 50ml and 100ml bottles of oral drops
– Fifteen drops to be taken in a little water, three times a day by adults, seven drops three times a day by children (6-12 years old).

Three essential oils to combat influenza

Ceylon cinnamon, Melaleuca (tea tree), **Ravensara aromatica**

Prescription: Obtain a 2ml bottle of the essential oil of one of these plants from your pharmacist, health-food shop or herbalist. Take three drops in a little honey, twice a day.

Cinnamon

Cinnamon bark has been used since the dawn of time for its tonic and stimulant properties. Until recently, cinnamon wine was given out in hospitals and hospices in some countries to combat the spread of disease.

Melaleuca/Niaouli

The leaves of the tea tree (Melaleuca), originally an Australian tree, have considerable antiseptic properties, thanks to their essential oil. Naiouli, which belongs to this family, is extremely effective against most infections.

• You can use Comvitar Propolis and Honey Elixir which contains tea tree oil, Irish moss, peppermint oil, honey and propolis:
– Available in bottles of 200ml
– Adults two teaspoons per day. Children one teaspoon per day

• If you prefer a good toddy, here is a recipe: one drop of essential oil of cinnamon, three drops of essential oil of orange, one drop of essential oil of Spanish oregano, one drop of essential oil of thyme, some honey, the juice of a lemon, and hot water.

Colds and rhino-pharyngitis

The majority of people in the Western world catch a common cold at least once a year. This ailment, a viral infection of the nasal mucosa and air passages, is transmitted from one person to another by minute airborne droplets from the saliva and the breath.

The well-known symptoms of the cold are a thick, fairly clear, nasal discharge, but the nose can sometimes be blocked.

Rhinopharyngitis, inflammation of the nose and throat at the same time, is usually viral or bacterial in origin, but can sometimes be due to allergy; it is very contagious and frequent in crèches and amongst groups.

It also involves a running nose, but with a temperature, which can be high, a sore throat, and a cough set off by the nasal discharge.

To oversimplify, one could say that babies have simple colds, children suffer from rhinopharyngitis, and adolescents from tonsillitis.

Preventive measures

These are important and easily put into practice:

• If possible, take the child out of the crèche

• Hygienic precautions: wash hands frequently, and show children how to blow their noses

• Reduce the heating and forbid smoking in the bedroom

• Humidify the atmosphere with a humidifier: add eucalyptus

• Look for an infectious person in the family circle

• Eliminate any allergic factor

Standard anti-infective treatment

At the beginning of any cold – to be started as quickly as possible at the first abnormal symptom:

• Start with Aconitum-Homaccord® (Heel) which contains Aconitum D2, D10, D30, D200, Eucalyptus D4, D10, D30 and Ipecacuanha D2, D10, D30, D200:
– available in drop bottles containing 30 and 100ml
– Generally 10 drops three times daily. Initially 10 drops every 15 minutes

• Add copper as a trace element with silver or gold in colloidal form

• Six tablets of Pyrogenium 5c, once a day in a single dose, for a few days

• Twenty drops of Lehning® L52 in a little water, three or four times per day

• Vitamin C: one gram per day for adults, 0.5g for children, for a fortnight

Some foods rich in vitamin C

Citrus fruits (lemon, orange, grapefruit), green vegetables (celery, green cabbage++, cress, spinach, sorrel, parsley, horseradish), fruit, particularly red fruit (strawberries, raspberries, redcurrants), but also others (pineapple, blackcurrants++, guava, kiwi++), potatoes, green peppers, tomatoes...

Local treatment

• You can use Rhinodoron (Weleda) nasal spray which contains an isotonic salt solution of sodium and potassium chloride in pure distilled water with aloe vera.
– Available in glass bottles of 20ml as a spray

• You can use Euphorbium composition Nasal Spray S (Heel):
– Available as a 20ml atomizer
– Spray 1–2 shots into each nostril 3–5 times daily. For children under 6 years, 1 shot 3–4 times daily

This treatment, along with the dietary advice given in the section 'The start of infection' will bring about improvement or cure in a good number of cases.

Homeopathy

Allium cepa, Hepar sulfur

– Four tablets of one of these two remedies at 5c to be sucked like sweets three or four times a day, between meals

Allium cepa

– Vegetable origin: the common onion used in cooking
– A homeopathic remedy for a running, irritated nose

– The symptoms of a patient with a cold are identical to the effects of peeling an onion: the eyes and nose smart and begin to run, there is violent sneezing. You can prescribe Allium cepa to alleviate the symptoms: this is the very principle of homeopathy

Hepar sulfur

– Chemical origin: a mixture of sulphur and oyster shell
– Homeopathic remedy for infections with suppuration
– Characteristic sign: irritation caused by the smallest current of air

• You can use Naso-Heel® (Heel) which contains Kalium bichromicum D5, Phosphorus D6, Arum maculatum D4
– Available in drop bottles of 30ml and 100ml
– In general, 10 drops three times daily; in acute disorders, initially 10 drops every 15 minutes

• It is also necessary to add a basic remedy chosen after consulting a homeopath: often Calcarea phosphorica, Pulsatilla, Silicea...

Oligotherapy

Essentially with **copper**, but also **zinc**. Trace elements are normally supplied by the diet, which should be varied and of good quality. When there is a deficiency, the elements can be taken as preparations.

Dietary sources of copper

Copper is present in small quantities nearly everywhere, except in milk, which contains very little.

It is found especially in liver++ (calf, sheep), seafood (seaweed, lobsters, oysters, scallops, fish roe), almonds and nuts, certain vegetables (avocados, mushrooms), cereals (whole wheat, whole rice, soya), dried fruits, green vegetables, plums, cocoa, tea…

Dietary sources of zinc

Zinc is widespread in seafood: oysters++, other shellfish, and fish. However it is also found in meat, egg yolk, cereals, wholemeal bread, brewer's yeast, nuts, some vegetables (broccoli, mushrooms, spinach, haricot beans)…

• Copper and zinc preparations: there are various brands and presentations: colloidal minerals such as Organic Minerals (Colloidals) which contains 70+ trace minerals:
– Available in 946ml bottles
– Take 1–3 caps just before breakfast and/or evening meal
– Children 1 teaspoon daily for each 20lbs of body weight

Or Maximol (Ionized colloidals):
– Available in 500ml bottles
– Take ½ capful once or twice daily on an empty stomach

Herbal treatment

Anti-infective **Echinacea**, very stimulating **ginseng**.

– Ask your herbalist to prepare 30ml bottles of the mother tincture of each of these plants, and take 25 drops three times a day of the first and 25 drops twice a day of the second

• You can use Echinaforce (Bioforce), a tincture of Echinacea purpurea:
– Available in 50ml and 100ml bottles of oral drops
– Fifteen drops to be taken in a little water, three times a day by adults, seven drops three times a day by children (6–12 years old).

Some plant essential oils

Niaouli, mountain savory, and **common thyme**, for their anti-infective properties.

Mint, nutmeg, rosemary, for their stimulant properties.

– Two drops of one of these to be taken in a teaspoonful of honey, twice a day by adults

For children, you can choose between **eucalyptus radiata, niaioli**, and **thyme linalol**.

– One drop of one of these to be taken in a teaspoonful of honey, twice a day

Eucalyptus

Australian in origin, the eucalyptus is a very large ornamental tree that can reach tens of metres in height, and has long been used by the Aborigines to combat infections and fevers. It was introduced into Europe in the 19th century, not for medical purposes but for geographic and agricultural reasons: its great roots, which absorb large quantities of water and deter the growth of neighbouring plants, have made it possible to dry up marshy areas, mainly in the south of France and in southern Europe. Its characteristic pleasant smell kept insects away and drove malaria towards Africa. Its long leaves are sometimes distilled fresh to obtain the essential oil, and sometimes dried for the preparation of remedies. Among the 600 existing species of eucalyptus, the *globulus* variety is almost exclusively used in medicine.

Sore throat, tonsillitis

Tonsillitis is a common illness today, rare before the age of three, which is diagnosed from three signs: fever, pain on swallowing and the appearance of the tonsils on examination. It is bacterial or viral in origin, and sometimes has serious complications, particularly acute rheumatism in the joints with an attendant risk of problems involving the heart (murmurs) or the kidneys (acute glomerulo-nephritis); these are rare in the West, but unhappily still common in Third World countries.

Standard anti-infective treatment

To be started as quickly as possible at the first abnormal symptom.

• Start with Aconitum-Homaccord® (Heel) which contains Aconitum D2, D10, D30, D200, Eucalyptus D4, D10, D30 and Ipecacuanha D2, D10, D30, D200:
– available in drop bottles containing 30 and 100ml
– Generally 10 drops three times daily. Initially 10 drops every 15 minutes

• Add copper as a trace element with silver or gold in colloidal form

• Six tablets of Pyrogenium 5c once a day in a single dose for a few days

• Twenty drops of Lehning® L52 in a little water, three or four times a day

• Vitamin C: one gram a day for adults, 0.5 gram for children, for a fortnight

• You can use natural Vitamin C in, for example, Lamberts® Vitamin C with Bioflavonoids 500mg:
– Sold in containers of 100 tablets
– One to six tablets daily

Some foods rich in vitamin C

Citrus fruits (lemon, orange, grapefruit), green vegetables (celery, green cabbage++, cress, spinach, sorrel, parsley, horseradish), fruit, particularly red fruit (strawberries, raspberries, redcurrants), and also others (pineapple, blackcurrant++, guava, kiwi++), potatoes, green peppers, tomatoes...

Can a sore throat be treated without antibiotics?

Yes, since it is viral in three-quarters of cases, but the symptoms should disappear within the first 24 hours: you always have some hours to try an complementary treatment first, then move quickly to antibiotics if the condition does not improve or if you have any worries.

Local treatment

Propolis is useful, as a spray or in the form of tablets to be sucked.

• You can use Comvitar propolis tincture:
– Available in bottles of 25ml
– 6 to 10 drops to be taken in water, three times daily

• Or you can take Comvtar propolis lozenges:
– Available in packs of 12 lozenges
– Take up to 5 lozenges per day

Propolis

Propolis is a reddish gum collected by bees from chestnut and willow buds, which they use in the hive to block gaps and fix the wax.

• This treatment, along with the dietary advice given in the section 'The start of infection' will bring about improvement or cure in a good number of cases

Homeopathy

Belladonna, Mercurius corrosivus

– Four 5c tablets of either, to be sucked like sweets, three or four times a day, between meals

Belladonna

– Vegetable origin: the leaves and fresh flowers of deadly nightshade, also called belladonna
– The homeopathic remedy for an inflamed, painful throat
– Two specific signs: the patient has a raised temperature and easily becomes agitated

Mercurius corrosivus

– Chemical origin: mercuric chloride or corrosive sublimate
– The homeopathic remedy for spots or for throat ulcers
– Characteristic sign: burning pain
– Mercuric chloride, once used as a local antiseptic, is now used as a fungicide for the treatment of plants and flowers

• You can use Mercurius-Heel® (Heel) which contains Hepar sulfur D8, Mercurius solubilis D10, Belladonna D4, Phytolacca D4 and Echinacea angustifolia D3 among others:
– Sold in containers of 50 and 250 tablets.
– In general, one tablet to be dissolved under the tongue three times daily between meals. In acute conditions, initially one tablet every 15 minutes

• If the condition recurs you should add

the basic remedy decided upon after consulting your homeopath: in this case it will often be Calcarea carbonica or phosphorica

Calcarea carbonica

– Animal and mineral origin: calcium carbonate extracted from oyster shells
– Homeopathic remedy for recurrent ENT infections in overweight patients

Calcarea phosphorica

– Chemical origin: tricalcium phosphate
– The homeopathic remedy for recurrent ENT infections in tall, thin patients
– A characteristic sign: extreme tendency to tiredness

Herbal treatment

Echinacea for its anti-infective properties.

Echinacea

Echinacea is a plant native to North America, where it was widely used by native tribes for its antiseptic properties.

• You can use Echinaforce (Bioforce), a tincture of Echinacea purpurea:
– Available in 50ml and 100ml bottles of oral drops
– Fifteen drops to be taken in a little water, three times a day by adults, seven drops three times a day by children (6-12 years old)

Pokeweed (Phytolacca), **marigold** (Calendula), for their local action.

PRESCRIPTION: Ask your homeopathic pharmacy to prepare a 30ml bottle of mother tincture of one of these plants, and pour ten drops into half a glass of moderately warm (not hot) water, or into a camomile infusion. Gargle with this three times a day

Phytolacca

The root of pokeweed, a plant originating in North America, used by the Native Americans to treat wounds and skin problems. It is effective against the pain of sore throat, and in infection.

Marigold

Marigold, or *Calendula officinalis*, is better known for its ornamental qualities than its very real medical properties: it is a good antiseptic and healing agent.

• If you have no remedy or plants to hand, you can gargle with warm water to which has been added a spoonful of honey and the juice of a lemon

Some plant essential oils

Rosewood, mountain savory, and **common thyme**, for their anti-infective properties.

Mint, nutmeg, and **rosemary**, for their vitalizing properties.

– For adults, two drops of one of these to be taken in a spoonful of honey, twice a day

Rosemary

The essential oil of rosemary is one of the main ingredients of eau de Cologne.

Eucalyptus radiata, clove, thyme linalol may be used in children.

DOSAGE: One drop of one of them to be taken in a spoonful of honey, twice a day.

• You can make or ask to be made the following mixture: two drops of essential oil of clary sage and one drop of lavender in a bowl of hot water to which is added a spoonful of honey. Use it to gargle three or four times a day

Clary sage

Clary sage is a hardy, sticky, aromatic plant that is found growing alongside the arid roads of the South of France. Its action, mainly antispasmodic, is gentler than that of the essential oil of common sage, which is more toxic (risk of convulsions).

Laryngitis, tracheitis, bronchitis

An anatomical reminder: the larynx and its vocal chords are situated at the entrance to the trachea, which divides into two bronchi that carry the air we breathe into the lungs.

Viral or bacterial infection, or sometimes allergy, can originate at one of these three levels, leading to laryngitis, tracheitis or bronchitis, all of which entail irritation of the airways, with a roughening or change in the voice, pain or discomfort in the throat, cough, and sometimes fever.

Standard anti-infective treatment

At the first signs of a cough – to be started as quickly as possible at the first abnormal symptom.

• Start with Aconitum-Homaccord® (Heel) which contains Aconitum D2, D10, D30, D200, Eucalyptus D4, D10, D30 and Ipecacuanha D2, D10, D30, D200:

– Available in drop bottles containing 30 and 100ml

– Generally 10 drops three times daily. Initially 10 drops every 15 minutes

• Add copper as a trace element with silver or gold in colloidal form

• Six tablets of Pyrogenium 5c once a day in a single dose for a few days

• Twenty drops of Lehning® L52 in a little water, three or four times a day, if there is fever

• Vitamin C: one gram a day for adults, 0.5 gram for children, for a fortnight

• This treatment combined with the dietary advice given in the section 'The start of infection' will bring about improvement or cure in a good number of cases

Homeopathy

Arum triphyllum, Bryonia, Coccus cacti

– Four tablets of one of these three remedies at 5c to be sucked like sweets between meals every two hours at the beginning, then at greater intervals on improvement

Arum triphyllum

– Vegetable origin: the fresh root of the Indian turnip, a wild, hardy North American plant
– The homeopathic remedy for inflammation of the mucosa with the appearance of raw lesions, often prescribed for singers and public speakers
– Specific sign: the tone of the voice constantly changes

Bryonia alba

– Vegetable origin: the fresh root of white bryony
– The homeopathic remedy for dry cough aggravated by the slightest movement
– Two characteristic signs: improved by rest and by high atmospheric pressure

Coccus cacti

– Animal origin: the cochineal insect, an aphid
– The homeopathic remedy for laryngeal inflammation with abundant secretion of thick, runny mucus
– Two characteristic signs: the cough is worsened by heat, improved in a cold room

• You can use Mercurius-Heel® (Heel), which contains Hepar sulfur D8, Mercurius solubilis D10, Belladonna D4, Phytolacca D4 and Echinacea angustifolia D3 among others:
– Sold in containers of 50 and 250 tablets.
– In general, one tablet to be dissolved under the tongue three times daily between meals. In acute conditions, initially one tablet every 15 minutes

• Also Droperteel® (Heel) which contains Drosera D4, Lachesis D12, Carbo vegetabilis D12, Coccus cacti D4 and Kalium carbonicum D12.
– Available in containers of 50 and 250 tablets
– One tablet to be dissolved under the tongue three times daily. In acute disorders initially one tablet every 15 minutes

• If the illness recurs, you should also add the basic remedy decided upon after consulting your homeopath: in this case it will often be Pulsatilla, Silicea, Sulfur iodatum...

Silicea

– Mineral origin: silica, once extracted from quartz or flint
– One of the homeopathic remedies for persistent infections
– This remedy is best for a thin, tired, patient, deficient in essential minerals and sensitive to the cold
– Silica, the main component of most rocks, confers and preserves the vigour of plants that absorb it through their stems – and reinforces human defences equally well

Three plants for the airways

Eucalyptus, white horehound, plantain

PRESCRIPTION: Ask your herbalist to prepare a 30ml bottle of a mother tincture of one of these three plants; take 25 drops in a little water, three times a day.

Plantain

The plantain is a highly paradoxical plant: it is useful for its anti-infective, anti-tussive and anti-allergic properties, but its pollen is often responsible for allergic rhinitis.

White horehound

White horehound has been used since antiquity for coughs and respiratory problems and before the advent of antibiotics, it was used in the treatment of tuberculosis.

• You can add coneflower for its anti-infective properties, using Lehning® which contains Echinacea 1x...
– Available in 30ml bottles of oral drops
– Fifteen drops to be taken in a little water, three times a day by adults, eight drops three times a day by children

Essential oils for the airways

Eucalyptus

– Two drops of this essence to be taken twice a day in a little honey

Eucalyptus

Australian in origin, eucalyptus was introduced last century into the South of France and other parts of southern Europe in order to drain the marshy regions and drive away insects. Its leaves contain eucalyptol, widely used in pharmacy for its action on the lungs.

Guayacum

Lignum vitae, the hard, dense, resinous wood of the African jasmine, a shrub native to Central America and the Antilles: anti-inflammatory and anti-rheumatic.

Peppermint

The essential oil of peppermint (*Mentha piperita*) is delicate and effective; it contains large amounts of menthol, its antibacterial active principle.

Cough

A protective reflex aimed at clearing the bronchi of mucus or other foreign matter that may obstruct the respiratory system.

A dry cough is most often allergic in origin, and a loose cough resulting in the expulsion of secretions generally indicates that the lungs are irritated, but this is not a firm rule: the flow of mucus may come from the nose or the sinuses, causing irritation... and giving rise to a cough with phlegm. Acid reflux into the oesophagus, the tube through which food passes from the mouth to the stomach, may be responsible for a purely reflex cough. This should be considered when suggesting appropriate treatment, for the condition is digestive rather than pulmonary.

Caution: Never neglect a cough.

Homeopathy

Symptom identification is important: distinguish a dry from a loose cough.

Three remedies for a dry cough
Bryonia, Drosera, Ipeca
– Four tablets of one of these three remedies at 5c to be sucked every hour at the start, then at longer intervals as improvement occurs

Bryonia alba

– Vegetable origin: fresh bryony root
– Homeopathic remedy for dry cough aggravated by the smallest movement and by warmth
– Two characteristic signs: improvement with rest and high atmospheric pressure

Drosera rotundifolia

– Vegetable origin: *Drosera rotundifolia* or sundew
– The homeopathic remedy for a dry, hacking, barking, cough
– Characteristic sign: the cough causes rib pains, which the patient relieves by pressing the arms against the chest

Ipecacuanha

– Vegetable origin: ipecacuanha, a Brazilian shrub
– Homeopathic remedy for a choking cough accompanied by nausea and vomiting
– Two characteristic signs: improved with rest, worsened by movement

A remedy for turning a dry cough into a loose cough
Hepar sulfur
– Chemical origin: a mixture of sulphur and oyster-shell chalk
– Homeopathic remedy for infections with suppuration
– Two characteristic signs: hoarse or barking cough improved by warmth, worsened by the slightest draught

Two remedies for a loose cough
Antimonium tartaricum, Coccus cacti
– Four tablets of one of them at 5c to be sucked like sweets, every two hours at the start, then at longer intervals as improvement occurs
– Chemical origin: antimony and potassium tartrate
– The homeopathic remedy for severe hacking cough with plentiful secretion of thick mucus expelled with difficulty
– Normally reserved for severe, resistant or stubborn cases

Coccus cacti

– Animal origin: the cochineal insect
– The homeopathic remedy for inflammation of the larynx with abundant secretion of thick, runny mucus
– Characteristic signs: here the cough presents as short, intense fits, worsened by warmth and improved in a cold room

• You can take Tartephedreel® (Heel)

which contains Lobelia inflata D4, Ephedra vulgaris D3, and Belladonna D4 among others....
– Sold in drop bottles containing 30 and 100ml
– In general, 10 drops 3 times daily. In acute disorders initially ten drops repeated every 15 minutes

• Also Droperteel® (Heel) which contains Drosera D4, Coccus cacti D4, Carbo vegetabilis D12 and Kalium carbonicum D12:
– Available in containers of 50 and 250 tablets
– One tablet to be dissolved under the tongue three times daily. In acute disorders, initially one tablet every 15 minutes

• If the illness recurs, you can also add the basic remedy chosen by your homeopath: in this case, it will often be Pulsatilla, Silicea, Tuberculinium...

Herbal treatment

Eucalyptus, white horehound
PRESCRIPTION: You can ask your herbalist to prepare 21 capsules, each containing 200mg of powder of each of these plants. Take one capsule three times a day for a week

• You can choose Drosinula (Bioforce), containing Drosera, Spruce extract and Ivy extract:
– Available in 100ml bottles
– 1–2 teaspoons to be taken 3–4 times a day. Children (6–12) take 1 teaspoonful 2–4 times daily

• Or you can take Ivy-Thyme Complex (Bioforce), a:tincture combination of Thyme, Ground Ivy and White Horehound:
– Available in bottles of 50ml
– Adults 15 drops 2–3 times daily. Children (2–12 years old) 1 drop per year of age, 2–3 times daily

Drosera

Drosera (sundew) is a carnivorous plant found in peat bogs, used in the preparation of remedies of the same name.

A mustard poultice

This counter-irritation treatment consists of applying a poultice or plaster of mustard powder. Through different processes (poultice, cautery, scarification, cupping), counter-irritation draws a flow of blood towards an organ or a region of the body, to combat congestion.

Plant essential oils

Essentially **Eucalyptus**.
– Two drops to be taken, twice a day, in a little honey

Eucalyptus

Eucalyptus is a large tree with pointed aromatic leaves, native to Australia. The leaves contain an essential oil which gives the plant considerable anti-infective properties (for the respiratory passages and urinary ducts).

• If you have a cough, make this little cocktail: take a glass of warm water, mix in two tablespoons of honey, add two drops of essential oil of cypress, five drops of essential oil of *Eucalyptus radiata*, four drops of essential oil of lavender, and six drops of essential oil of Scots pine. Take one teaspoonful every two hours.

• Ask your herbalist to make up the following preparation: six drops of essential oil of *Eucalyptus radiata*, three drops of essential oil of lavender, two drops of essential oil of Scots pine, one drop of essential oil of thyme linalol, suspended in 90 per cent alcohol. Two or three times a day pour several drops into a little warm water and inhale over it for two minutes.

Otitis

Otitis is a frequent and serious condition, responsible for millions of prescriptions a year, two-thirds of which are for children under three years of age. It often starts as a cold, a sore throat, or any infectious condition.

The symptoms consist of severe pain, a fever that may reach 39.5° C, a feeling of deafness, and purulent or mucous discharge from the ear. Sometimes there is a singing in the ears, especially in adults, and vomiting in children.

Most cases are resolved without complications, the most serious being meningitis, which is fortunately rare. The hearing is rarely affected for long – provided that treatment is started promptly and continued for long enough.

Caution: an ear infection should never be taken lightly. It is very important that the need for tapping or for antibiotic treatment is not missed.

Standard anti-infective treatment

To be started as quickly as possible at the first abnormal symptom:

• Start with Aconitum-Homaccord® (Heel),which contains Aconitum D2, D10, D30, D200, Eucalyptus D4, D10, D30 and Ipecacuanha D2, D10, D30, D200:
– Available in drop bottles containing 30 and 100ml
– 10 drops to be taken three times daily. Initially ten drops every 15 minutes

• Add copper as a trace element with silver and gold in colloidal form

• Six tablets of Pyrogenium 5c, once a day, in a single dose, for a few days

• Twenty drops of Lehning® L52 in a little water, three or four times a day if the patient already has a temperature

• Vitamin C: one gram a day for adults, 0.5 gram for children, for a fortnight

• To this standard treatment composed of three homeopathic remedies, one to

Natural healing

three trace elements, and a vitamin, the homeopath may add remedies that are specific to each illness and fundamental for each personality

Dietary advice

To be strictly followed:

• Stop all heavy greasy foods, particularly dairy products, fried food, and dishes with sauces

• Drink plenty

• Choose foods rich in vitamin C and copper

• Supplement your diet with wheatgerm and brewer's yeast, which are rich in group B vitamins and trace elements

• Eat plenty of garlic and onion

• Make free use of condiments such as thyme, cinnamon and oregano, known for their anti-infective action

A natural food

Wheatgerm

ORIGIN AND COMPOSITION: obtained by soaking the grain in water and allowing it to germinate for two days. This is the living part of the plant, incorporating all the constituents necessary for its growth, with twice the amount of calcium, three times the magnesium and phosphorus, and much more vitamin B and E than wheat. It also contains vitamins A and C. This concentration of minerals and vitamins makes it effective against infections.

Use: Wheatgerm is sold in pharmacies and health food shops in the form of flakes to be sprinkled on salads, yoghurt, or soft white cheese. Take two teaspoonfuls a day. You can also use the oil, sold in bottles or as capsules.

Homeopathy

Capsicum

– Four tablets at 5c, to be sucked like sweets, between meals, three or four times a day

Capsicum annuum

– Vegetable origin: capsicum peppers
– Homeopathic remedy for the start of otitis, particularly if the condition evokes a sensation of baking heat
– Two characteristic signs: improved by warmth, worsened by cold or by touching

You can add **Chamomilla** for children.
– Four tablets at 7c to be sucked like sweets three times a day

Chamomilla

– Vegetable origin: German camomile
– Homeopathic remedy for the symptoms of teething
– Specific signs: unbearable pain, accompanied by irritability and extreme agitation, lessened by rocking or carrying the child

• You can use Traumeel® (Heel), which contains Belladonna D4, mercurius solubilis D8, Hepar sulfur D8, Chamomilla D3 and Bellis perennis D2 among others:
– Sold in containers of 50 or 250 tablets

– In general, one tablet to be dissolved under the tongue three times daily..

Oligotherapy

Essentially **copper** or a **copper/gold/silver** combination.

Dietary sources of copper

Copper is present in small quantities nearly everywhere, except in milk, which contains very little.

It is found especially in liver++ (calf, sheep), seafood (lobsters, oysters, scallops, fish roe) and seaweed, almonds and nuts, certain vegetables (avocados, mushrooms), cereals (whole wheat, whole rice, soya), dried fruits, green vegetables, plums, cocoa, tea…

• Copper remedies: found in various forms and brands, e.g.: colloidal minerals such as Organic Minerals (Colloidals) which contains 70+ trace minerals:
– Available in 946ml bottles
– Take 1–3 caps just before breakfast and/or evening meal
– Children 1 teaspoon daily for each 20lbs of body weight
Or Maximol (Ionized colloidals):
– Available in 500ml bottles
– Take ½ capful once or twice daily on an empty stomach

• You can use a copper/gold/silver mixture: (Colloidal minerals)

• You can also use silver liquid SILV-LQ (Vitamin Research Products) 400ppm:
– available in bottles of 4 fluid ozs
– Mix half a teaspoon with one ounce of water, rinse in mouth for 15 seconds before swallowing

Silver

Silver, which has no known effect on the body, has a general bactericidal and local antiseptic action (as silver nitrate) which determines its use as an anti-infective agent.

Herbal treatment

Anti-infective **Echinacea**, very stimulating **ginseng**.

– Ask your herbalist to prepare 30ml bottles of the mother tincture of each of these two plants: take 25 drops of the first in a little water, three times a day, 25 drops of the second, twice a day

Echinacea

The coneflower is very effective against snakebite, stubborn wounds, fevers… It comes to us from Native American tribes who were using it long before the arrival of antibiotics.
• You can use Echinaforce (Bioforce), a tincture of Echinacea purpurea:
– Available in 50ml and 100ml bottles of oral drops
– Fifteen drops to be taken in a little water, three times a day by adults, seven drops three times a day by children (6–12 years old)

Plant essential oils

Ceylon cinnamon, *Eucalyptus radiata*, cloves, *Melaleuca alternifolia*, niaouli, Spanish oregano, mountain savory, and

common thyme for their anti-infective activity.

– Two drops of one of these to be taken in a spoonful of honey, twice a day

Cloves

Cloves are the buds of the clove, a very tall, exotic tree. They are used for anaesthesia in dentistry, and for flavour in some dishes (sauerkraut, for example).

• You can have the following mixture made up for local use: 0.25g essential oil of lavender, 0.25g essential oil of cloves, 10g glycerine, suspended in enough oil of sweet almonds to make up a 30ml bottle. Place five drops in the ear two or three times a day.

Sinusitis

This term means acute or chronic inflammation of the sinuses, the deep, air-filled cavities in the facial bones, lined with a tissue similar to the nasal mucosa. The sinuses give resonance to the voice and provide added protection to the eyes, nose and brain.

Nine times out of ten sinusitis starts as a cold, causing congestion of the mucosa, most often affecting the maxillary sinus, as shown by X-ray or better by using a scanner. It presents as a continuous, pulsing, piercing pain on one side, which worsens when the patient leans forward or coughs. The pain is often accompanied by a discharge or a blocked nose, and sometimes fever. Sinusitis occurs most frequently in the winter.

A moderately severe episode may last two or three weeks, but the infection may become chronic with frequent relapses. The treatment should deal simultaneously with the infection, the inflammation and the congestion. It aims to relieve the pain, eliminate the germ responsible, allow improved draining of the sinuses, prevent complications and avoid relapses.

Sinusitis is too frequently diagnosed in children

This condition is rare before the age of five or seven, because only the ethmoid sinuses are present at birth (the frontal sinuses have not yet formed, and the maxillary sinuses are only very slightly developed). The differences between child and adult become indistinct after the age of 12.

Standard anti-infective treatment

At the start of the first symptoms of sinusitis – to be initiated as quickly as possible at the first abnormal symptom.

• Start with Aconitum-Homaccord®, (Heel) which contains Aconitum D2, D10, D30, D200, Eucalyptus D4, D10, D30 and Ipecacuanha D2, D10, D30, D200:

– Available in drop bottles containing 30 and 100ml
– ten drops to be taken three times daily. Initially ten drops every 15 minutes

• Add copper as a trace element with silver or gold in colloidal form

• Six tablets of Pyrogenium 5c once a day in a single dose for a few days

• Twenty drops of Lehning® L52 in a little water, three or four times a day

• Vitamin C: one gram a day for adults, 0.5 gram for children, for a fortnight

– This treatment, combined with the dietary advice given in the section 'The start of infection', brings improvement or cure in a good number of cases

Acupuncture

Vital, particularly when pain predominates. Combined with effective homeopathic treatment, it is one of the best treatments for discharge in sinusitis.

– Four or five twice-weekly sessions will be needed to start with, with longer intervals on improvement. A maintenance treatment of one session every three weeks can be carried out during critical periods

Homeopathy

Hepar sulfur, Hydrastis, and **Kalium bichromicum**

– Four tablets of one of these three remedies at 5c to be sucked like sweets three or four times a day, between meals, for a few days

Hepar sulfur

– Chemical origin: a mixture of sulphur and oyster chalk
– Homeopathic treatment for infections with suppuration
– Two characteristics: improved with warmth, worsened with cold

Hydrastis canadensis

– Vegetable origin: the roots of golden seal, a plant long used by the Native Americans
– Homeopathic remedy for discharges of thick, still yellow, viscous mucus

Kalium bichromicum

– Chemical origin: potassium bichromate
– Homeopathic remedy for suppuration with thick, sticky, foul, green mucus

• You can use Euphorbium composition S (Heel), which contains Euphorbium D3, Hepar sulfur D10 and Sinusitis nosode D13 among others:
– Sold in drop bottles containing 30 and 100ml
– In general, ten drops three times daily. In acute disorders, initially ten drops every 15 minutes followed by a reduction to ten drops six times daily

You should also add the basic remedy decided upon after consulting your homeopath: in this case, it will often be Calcarea carbonica, Calcarea phosphorica, Sulfur.

Natural healing

Sulfur

– Mineral origin: sulphur
– Homeopathic remedy for resistant and recurrent mucosal infections

Herbal treatment

Echinacea: anti-infective.

Eleutherococcus and **ginseng** – both very stimulating.

PRESCRIPTION: Ask your herbalist to prepare 30ml bottles of the mother tincture of each of these two plants. Take 25 drops three times a day of the first, and 25 drops twice a day of the second

Eleutherococcus and Echinacea

Eleutherococcus or devil's shrub is a plant of the ginseng and ivy family, but originates from the plains of Siberia where it grows in abundance. It owes its fame to athletes from the countries of the former Soviet Union and Asia who use it because it increases resistance to physical and mental fatigue. Echinacea originates from North America, and was used by the Native American tribes for its anti-infective properties.

• You can use Echinaforce (Bioforce), a tincture of Echinacea purpurea:
– Available in 50ml and 100ml bottles of oral drops
– Fifteen drops to be taken in a little water, three times a day by adults, seven drops three times a day by children (6–12 years old).

Plant essential oils

Niaouli, mountain savory, common thyme for their anti-infective properties.

Mint, nutmeg, rosemary for their stimulant properties.
– For adults, two drops of one of them to be taken in a spoonful of honey, twice a day

Mint

Mint, whose effectiveness is due to the menthol in its essential oil, is tonic, antiseptic, analgesic and digestive. It is thus one of the ingredients of stimulating drinks, as well as of Tiger Balm.

Niaouli

Niaouli, the New Caledonian paperbark tree (*Melaleuca leucadendron*) possesses properties close to those of the Cajput tree (*Melaleuca quinquenervia*), and the tea tree (*Melaleuca alternifolia*). They are all in the same family.

Nutmeg

Portuguese sailors brought nutmeg to Europe in the 16th century. It is a general and sexual stimulant, but can easily be toxic, thus caution is advised.

Eucalyptus, cloves, thyme linalol can be used in children.

– One drop of one of these to be taken in a spoonful of honey, twice a day

Thyme

An infusion of thyme used for its medicinal properties can easily be drunk instead of a cup of tea or coffee. There are various varieties of thyme, each of which contains a different essential oil. These essential oils are powerful, aggressive or toxic to different degrees.

Cloves

The essential oil of cloves is antiseptic, calming, and antispasmodic; the dried buds we use as a spice are virtually regarded as a panacea in the whole of Southeast Asia.

Two childhood illnesses

Whooping cough

A bacterial infectious disease (caused by Bordetella pertussis bacteria) epidemic, and highly contagious for two months, necessitating caution in those close to the patient. Whooping cough mainly affects children, but can be seen at any age: thanks to vaccination it is rare in the Western world. The incubation period varies, lasting from one to three weeks, then the illness starts like a common cold, soon accompanied by noisy breathing and fits of spasmodic coughing on exhalation. The repeated fits are suffocating, produce thick phlegm, and often cause vomiting as the patient attempts to cough. This disease is serious in infants and older persons because there is a risk of pulmonary and cerebral complications. Once cured, the patient is immune for life.

Standard anti-infective treatment

To be started as quickly as possible at the first abnormal symptom:

• Start with Aconitum-Homaccord®, (Heel), which contains Aconitum D2, D10, D30, D200, Eucalyptus D4, D10, D30 and Ipecacuanha D2, D10, D30, D200:
– Available in drop bottles containing 30 and 100ml
– Ten drops to be taken three times daily. Initially ten drops every 15 minutes

• Add copper as a trace element with silver and gold in colloidal form

• Six tablets of Pyrogenium 5c, once a day, in a single dose, for a few days

• Twenty drops of Lehning® L52 in a little water, three or four times a day, if the patient already has a temperature

• Vitamin C: one gram a day in adults, 0.5 gram in children, for a fortnight

• To this standard treatment composed of three homeopathic remedies, one to three trace elements, and a vitamin, the homeopath may add remedies that are specific to each illness and fundamental for each personality

Dietary advice

To be strictly followed:

- Stop all heavy, greasy foods, particularly dairy products, fried food, and dishes with sauces
- Give the child plenty to drink
- Choose foods rich in vitamin C and copper
- Supplement the diet with wheatgerm and brewer's yeast, which are rich in group B vitamins and trace elements
- Give the patient plenty of garlic and onion, known for their anti-infective action

Homeopathy

Aconite, Belladonna, Ferrum phosphoricum against fever.

– Four tablets of one of these remedies at 5c to be sucked like sweets between meals, three or four times a day

Aconitum napellus

– Vegetable origin: aconite, also known as wolf's-bane because the poison it contains was once used in hunting

– Homeopathic remedy for infections that are sudden in onset

Belladonna

– Vegetable origin: the leaves and fresh flowers of belladonna, deadly nightshade

– Homeopathic remedy for infectious conditions with high fever, agitation and intense thirst

Ferrum phosphoricum

– Chemical origin: iron phosphate.

– Homeopathic remedy for slight fever in a very weak patient.

Drosera, Coccus cacti to work against the cough.

– Four tablets of one of these two remedies at 5c to be sucked three or four times a day between meals

Drosera

Vegetable origin: *Drosera rotundifolia*, or sundew

– Homeopathic remedy for dry, hacking cough

– Characteristic sign: the cough causes pain in the ribs, which the patient relieves by pressing the arms against the chest

Coccus cacti

– Animal origin: the cochineal insect

– Homeopathic remedy for laryngeal inflammation with abundant thick, runny mucus

– Two characteristic signs: short but intense coughing fits, worsened by warmth, improved in a cold room

- You can use Drosera-Homaccord® (Heel) which contains Drosera and Cuprum aceticum in various D potencies:

– Available in drop bottles containing 30 and 100ml

– In general ten drops three times daily. In acute cases initially ten drops every 15 minutes

Oligotherapy

Essentially **Copper** or a **copper/gold/silver** combination.

Trace elements are normally supplied by the diet, which should be varied and of good quality. When there is a deficiency, they can be given as preparations.

Dietary sources of copper

Copper is present in small quantities nearly everywhere, except in milk, which contains very little. It is found especially in liver++ (calf, sheep), seafood (lobsters, oysters, scallops, fish roe) and seaweed, almonds and nuts, certain vegetables (avocados, mushrooms), cereals (whole wheat, whole rice, soya), dried fruits, green vegetables, plums, cocoa, tea...

• Copper and zinc preparations: there are various brands and presentations: colloidal minerals such as Organic Minerals (Colloidals) which contains 70+ trace minerals:
– Available in 946ml bottles
– Take 1–3 caps just before breakfast and/or evening meal
– Children 1 teaspoon daily for each 20lbs of body weight
Or Maximol (Ionized colloidals):
– Available in 500ml bottles
– Take ½ capful once or twice daily on an empty stomach

Herbal treatment

Echinacea an excellent anti-infective.
– Ask your herbalist to prepare a 30ml bottle of mother tincture of the plant. In an older child, give 15 drops in a little water twice a day for a few days
– You can use Echinacea complex (Bioforce) tincture which contains Echinacea purpurea:
– Available in 50ml bottles of oral drops
– Adults fifteen drops in a little water, three times daily . Children 6–12 years old – eight drops to be taken in a little water, three times a day. Children 2–5 years old – four drops in a little water, three times daily.

Plant essential oils

Eucalyptus, niaouli, thyme linalol may be used in children. Their main activity is antibacterial.
– One drop of one of them to be taken in a spoonful of honey, twice a day

Niaouli

New Caledonian niaouli (*Melaleuca viridifolia*) has properties similar to the Cajput tree (*Melaleuca leucadendron*) and the tea tree (*Melaleuca alternifolia*).

Mumps

A communicable viral infection affecting the parotid glands located under the jaw. Mumps is epidemic, and extremely contagious via droplets from the nose and saliva, but is almost always benign in children. After puberty it can be more serious for males, since it may affect the testicles and cause sterility.

Incubation takes two or three weeks. The illness is accompanied by fever and painful, if not unbearable, swelling of the glands, which is fortunately short-lived, disappearing towards the tenth day. The entire course of the illness is about three weeks from the first symptom to recovery. In the West, children account for about 80 per cent of cases of mumps.

Standard anti-infective treatment

To be started as quickly as possible at the first abnormal symptom:

• Start with Aconitum-Homaccord® (Heel), which contains Aconitum D2, D10, D30, D200, Eucalyptus D4, D10, D30 and Ipecacuanha D2, D10, D30, D200:
– Available in drop bottles containing 30 and 100ml
10 drops to be taken three times daily. Initially ten drops every 15 minutes

• Add copper as a trace element with silver and gold in colloidal form

• Six tablets of Pyrogenium 5c to be taken in a single dose, once a day for a few days

• Twenty drops of Lehning® L52 to be taken in a little water, three or four times a day, if the patient already has a temperature

• Vitamin C: 0.5 gram for children, each day for 15 days

• To this standard treatment composed of three homeopathic remedies, one to three trace elements, and a vitamin, the homeopath may add remedies that are specific to each illness and fundamental for each personality

Dietary advice

To be strictly followed:

• Stop all heavy, greasy foods, particularly dairy products, fried food, and dishes with sauces

• Give the child plenty to drink

• Choose foods rich in vitamin C and copper

• Supplement the diet with wheatgerm and brewer's yeast, which are rich in group B vitamins and trace elements

• Give the patient plenty of garlic and onion, known for their anti-infective action

Homeopathy

Bryonia, Mercurius solubilis
– Four tablets of one of these two remedies at 5c to be sucked like sweets, three or four times a day, between meals

Bryonia alba

– Vegetable origin: fresh bryony root
– Homeopathic remedy for inflammation worsened by the least movement or by warmth
– Two characteristic signs: improvement with rest and pressure

Mercurius solubilis

– Chemical origin: Mercury and ammonium nitrates
– Homeopathic remedy for acute and chronic inflammation with a tendency to suppurate
– Characteristic sign: profuse, evil-smelling saliva.

• You can use Traumeel® (Heel), which contains Belladonna D4, mercurius solubilis D8, Hepar sulfur D8, Chamomilla D3 and Bellis perennis D2 among others:
– Sold in containers of 50 or 250 tablets
– In general, one tablet to be dissolved under the tongue three times daily

• It is almost essential to add the basic remedy or remedies for convalescence decided upon after consulting the homeopath: in this case, they will often be Calcarea phosphorica, Pulsatilla, Sulfur iodatum...

Oligotherapy

Essentially **copper**, or **copper/gold/silver**

• The combination can be found in many brands and presentations: colloidal minerals such as Organic Minerals (Colloidals) which contains 70+ trace minerals:
– Available in 946ml bottles
– Take 1–3 caps just before breakfast and/or evening meal
– Children 1 teaspoon daily for each 20lbs of body weight
Or Maximol (Ionized colloidals):
– Available in 500ml bottles
– Take ½ capful once or twice daily on an empty stomach

Herbal treatment

Echinacea an excellent anti-infective agent.

Eleutherococcus and **ginseng**, very good general tonics for adults.

– Prescription: Ask for a 30ml bottle of a mother tincture of one of these plants to be prepared. Take 25 drops (for an adult) in a little water, twice a day for 3 weeks.

• For children you can use Echinacea complex (Bioforce) tincture which contains Echinacea purpurea...
– Available in 50ml bottles of oral drops
– Eight drops to be taken in a little water, three times a day. (6–12 years old) or four drops in a little water, three times daily (2–5 years old)

Plant essential oils

Eucalyptus, naiouli, thyme linalol can be given to children. Their main property is anti-infective.
– One drop of one of them to be taken in a spoonful of honey, twice a day
– A possible prescription for an adult would be a mixture made up of 0.01

gram essential oil of eucalyptus and 0.01 gram essential oil of thyme linalol, in a colloidal silica excipient, for a No.1 capsule (this is the capsule size that the herbalist would use for the ingredients). Take one capsule twice a day for 10 days

Thyme

There are many varieties of thyme, each of which contains a different essential oil (thymol, carvacrol, cineol, and linalol…), powerful, aggressive, or toxic to different degrees.

Three childhood eruptive illnesses

Measles

A contagious viral infection, epidemic, and more common in winter, measles spreads via airborne droplets from the nose and saliva. It mainly affects children, but adults are not entirely spared.

The incubation period is from one to two weeks, then the illness starts with what appears to be a feverish cold.

The first sign may be conjunctivitis with bloodshot eyes, but Koplik's spots are characteristic. These white spots with a pink areola appear inside the cheeks and allow reliable diagnosis.

The rash appears on the fourth or fifth day, first on the scalp and temples, spreading to the neck and the rest of the body. The raised spots disappear more quickly than their brown pigmentation, which can persist for a while. The illness lasts about ten days, during which the patient should be isolated.

Measles can be complicated by pulmonary problems or by severe encephalitis. A prescription for antibiotics should be readily available. This is a serious illness, responsible for a million and half deaths per year throughout the world. Vaccination is recommended.

Standard anti-infective treatment

To be started as quickly as possible at the first abnormal symptom:

• Start with Aconitum-Homaccord® (Heel), which contains Aconitum D2, D10, D30, D200, Eucalyptus D4, D10, D30 and Ipecacuanha D2, D10, D30, D200:
– Available in drop bottles containing 30 and 100ml
– ten drops to be taken three times daily. Initially ten drops every 15 minutes

• Add copper as a trace element with silver and gold in colloidal form

• Six tablets of Pyrogenium 5c, once a day, in a single dose, for a few days

• Twenty drops of Lehning® L52 in a little water, three or four times a day, if the patient already has a temperature

• Vitamin C: one gram a day for adults, 0.5 gram for children, for a fortnight

• To this standard treatment composed of three homeopathic remedies, one to three trace elements, and a vitamin, the homeopath may add remedies that are specific to each illness and fundamental for each personality

Dietary advice

To be strictly followed:

• Stop all heavy, greasy foods, particularly dairy products, fried food, and dishes with sauces

• Give the child plenty to drink

• Choose foods rich in vitamin C and copper

• Supplement the diet with wheatgerm and brewer's yeast, which are rich in group B vitamins and trace elements

• Give the patient plenty of garlic and onion, known for their anti-infective action

Some foods rich in vitamin C

Citrus fruits (lemon, orange, grapefruit), green vegetables (celery, green cabbage++, cress, spinach, sorrel, parsley, horseradish), fruit, especially red fruit (strawberries, raspberries, redcurrants), and others (pineapple, blackcurrants++, guava, kiwi++), potatoes, green peppers, tomatoes...

Homeopathy

Sulfur to encourage eruption.
– Six tablets at 7c to be sucked like sweets once a day, between meals

Sulfur

– Mineral origin: sulphur
– One of the main homeopathic remedies for skin ailments
– Sulfur may cause a transient worsening of the symptoms: if this happens, it is essential to consult your homeopath

Pulsatilla
– Four tablets at 7c to be sucked like sweets, two or three times a day between meals

Pulsatilla

– Vegetable origin: the pulsatilla anemone
– Homeopathic remedy for rashes of small red spots (maculo-papules) which disappear with finger pressure and are not found in healthy areas
– Characteristic sign: a desire for fresh air and the outdoors

Allium cepa if the watering of the eyes is not a problem. If it is, **Euphrasia**.

– Four tablets at 5c of one of these two remedies to be sucked like sweets, three or four times a day between meals

Allium cepa

– Vegetable origin: the common onion, used in cooking
– Homeopathic remedy for irritant nasal discharge
– The patient's symptoms are identical to those caused by peeling an onion

Natural healing

Euphrasia

– Vegetable origin: eyebright, or ophthalmic herb (*Euphrasia officinalis*)
– Homeopathic remedy almost solely used for the eyes
– Characteristic symptom: watering of the eyes is irritant, the nasal discharge is not.

• You can use Engystol® (Heel), which contains sulfur D4, D10, and Vincetoxicum hirundinaria D6, D10, D30:
– Available in containers of 50 and 250 tablets
– One tablet to be dissolved under the tongue one to three times daily

Oligotherapy

Essentially **copper** or a **copper/gold/silver** combination.

• Copper remedies: found as various presentations and brands, e.g. colloidal minerals such as Organic Minerals (Colloidals) which contains 70+ trace minerals:
– Available in 946ml bottles
– Take 1–3 caps just before breakfast and/or evening meal
– Children 1 teaspoon daily for each 20lbs of body weight
Or Maximol (Ionized colloidals):
– Available in 500ml bottles
– Take ½ capful once or twice daily on an empty stomach
One dose four times on the first day, three times on the second day, then twice a day for two weeks

Some foods rich in copper

Seaweed, almonds, avocado, cocoa, cereals (especially whole wheat and whole rice), mushrooms, shellfish, oysters, crustaceans, calf and sheep liver++, dried fruit, nuts, fish roe, plums, tea...

Herbal treatment

Echinacea, an excellent anti-infective agent.

Eleutherococcus and **ginseng**, very good general tonics for adults.

Prescription: Ask for a 30ml bottle of a mother tincture of one of these plants to be prepared. Take 25 drops (for an adult) in a little water, twice a day for up to 3 weeks.

Echinacea

Echinacea, the coneflower, a plant originating in North America, is widely used by native tribes for its anti-infective properties.

Eleutherococcus

Eleutherococcus is a plant of the ginseng and ivy family, but is native to the plains of Siberia where it grows in abundance. It increases resistance to fatigue.

• For children you can use Echinacea complex (Bioforce) tincture which contains Echinacea purpurea...
– Available in 50ml bottles of oral drops

– Eight drops to be taken in a little water, three times a day (6–12 years old) or four drops in a little water, three times daily (2–5 years old)

Plant essential oils

Eucalyptus, naiouli, thyme linalol can be given to children. Their main property is anti-infective.

One drop of one of them to be taken in a spoonful of honey, twice a day.

Cloves

The dried buds of the clove tree are used for flavouring some dishes. Their anti-infective and stimulant properties are unquestionable, and for this reason cloves are widely used throughout Asia.

Rubella or German measles

An infectious, eruptive, epidemic disease of viral origin, seen mainly in the spring and the winter.

It is highly contagious, spreading via airborne droplets from the nose and from saliva. Incubation takes from fifteen days to three weeks. Rubella is diagnosed from three signs: fever, a light rash appearing mainly on the face and neck, then on the rest of the body, and swellings behind the ears and near the nape.

The course of the illness is generally benign and lasts about a week, often unnoticed. This is a common illness without serious repercussions except at the start of pregnancy, when it can cause abortion or serious malformation (auditory, cardiac, and ocular) or mental deficiency in the future baby. Vaccination is advisable before pregnancy for women who have not had the disease in their childhood.

Standard anti-infective treatment

To be started as quickly as possible at the first abnormal symptom:

- Start with Aconitum-Homaccord® (Heel), which contains Aconitum D2, D10, D30, D200, Eucalyptus D4, D10, D30 and Ipecacuanha D2, D10, D30, D200:
– Available in drop bottles containing 30 and 100ml
– Ten drops to be taken three times daily. Initially ten drops every 15 minutes

- Add copper as a trace element with silver and gold in colloidal form

- Six tablets of Pyrogenium 5c, once a day, in a single dose, for a few days

- Twenty drops of Lehning® L52 in a little water, three or four times a day, if the patient already has a temperature

- Vitamin C: one gram a day in adults, 0.5 gram in children, for a fortnight

- To this standard treatment composed of three homeopathic remedies, one to three trace elements, and a vitamin, the homeopath may add remedies that are specific to each illness and fundamental for each personality

Dietary advice

To be strictly followed:

- Stop all heavy, greasy foods, particularly dairy products, fried food, and dishes with sauces
- Give the child plenty to drink
- Choose foods rich in vitamin C and copper
- Supplement the diet with wheatgerm and brewer's yeast, rich in group B vitamins and trace elements
- Give the patient plenty of garlic and onion, known for their anti-infective action

Some foods rich in vitamin C

Citrus fruits (lemon, orange, grapefruit), green vegetables (celery, green cabbage++, cress, spinach, sorrel, parsley, horseradish), fruit, especially red fruit (strawberries, raspberries, redcurrants), and others (pineapple, blackcurrants++, guava, kiwi++), potatoes, green peppers, tomatoes...

A natural food

Brewer's yeast

– A living substance prepared from a microscopic fungus that acts as the ferment for beer. As a food it contains little fat, little sugar, and few calories. It is different from baker's yeast, and much better tolerated by the intestine. It contains group B vitamins, minerals (chromium, phosphorus, potassium, and selenium...) and essential amino acids;
– Brewer's yeast reinforces immunity, has anti-infective properties, and restores the intestinal flora;
– You will find it in health food shops and pharmacies as tablets, capsules or flakes (take care, it is very bitter).

Homeopathy

Sulfur to encourage eruption.
– Six tablets at 7c to be sucked once a day between meals

Pulsatilla
– Four tablets at 7c to be sucked like sweets, two or three times a day between meals
– You might want to ask your homeopathic pharmacy to prepare the following mixture: Gelsemium 7c, Kalium phosphoricum 5c, Pulsatilla 7c, Sulfur iodatum 7c. Take (or give) four tablets twice a day for a fortnight

Sulfur iodatum

– Chemical origin: sulphur iodide
– Homeopathic remedy for the effects of rashes
– Its action is milder than that of sulfur

Oligotherapy

Essentially **copper** or **copper/gold/silver** combination.

- The combination can be found in many brands and presentations: colloidal minerals such as Organic Minerals

(Colloidals) which contains 70+ trace minerals:
– Available in 946ml bottles
– Take 1–3 caps just before breakfast and/or evening meal
– Children 1 teaspoon daily for each 20lbs of body weight
Or Maximol (Ionized colloidals):
– Available in 500ml bottles
– Take ½ capful once or twice daily on an empty stomach then twice a day for two weeks

Some foods rich in copper

Seaweed, almonds, avocado, cocoa, cereals (especially whole wheat and whole rice), mushrooms, shellfish, oysters, crustaceans, calf and sheep liver++, dried fruit, nuts, fish roe, plums, tea...

Herbal treatment

Echinacea, an excellent anti-infective.

Eleutherococcus and **ginseng**, very good general tonics for adults.

Prescription: Ask for a 30ml bottle of a mother tincture of one of these plants to be prepared, or a mixture of both. Take 25 drops (for an adult) in a little water, twice a day for several weeks

• You can use Echinaforce (Bioforce), a tincture of Echinacea purpurea:
– Available in 50ml and 100ml bottles of oral drops
– Fifteen drops to be taken in a little water, three times a day by adults, seven drops three times a day by children (6–12 years old).

Plant essential oils

Eucalyptus, naiouli, thyme linalol can be given to children. Their main property is anti-infective.
– One drop of one of them to be taken in a spoonful of honey, twice a day

• You can use Lehning® Gouttes aux essences®:
– A preparation containing cinnamon, cloves, lavender, mint, thyme...
– Available in 45ml and 90ml bottles
– Twenty drops to be taken four times a day (adult dose), five to ten drops three times a day (children's dose), diluted in a small drink

Chickenpox

An infectious, eruptive, illness, viral in origin, epidemic, and very contagious via airborne droplets from the nose and saliva. Chickenpox occurs mainly in the winter and spring, and affects children more readily than adults.

After an incubation period averaging 15 days, an itchy rash appears, consisting of small maculae, which soon turn into more prominent papules, then into vesicles filled with liquid. These leave scabs, which mark the end of the contagious period. This takes over four days, but the process is repeated in successive overlapping waves for a fortnight.

The course of the illness is generally benign, but scratching must be avoided because the scars may be permanent. The illness confers immunity for life.

Standard anti-infective treatment

To be started as quickly as possible at the first abnormal symptom:

• Start with Aconitum-Homaccord® (Heel), which contains Aconitum D2, D10, D30, D200, Eucalyptus D4, D10, D30 and Ipecacuanha D2, D10, D30, D200:
– Available in drop bottles containing 30 and 100ml
– Ten drops to be taken three times daily. Initially ten drops every 15 minutes

• Add copper silver and gold found in Organic Minerals (Colloidals) which contains 70+ trace minerals:
– Available in 946ml bottles
– Take 1–3 caps just before breakfast and/or evening meal
– Children 1 teaspoon daily for each 20lbs of body weight
Or Maximol (Ionized colloidals):
– Available in 500ml bottles
– Take ½ capful once or twice daily on an empty stomach

• Six tablets of Pyrogenium 5c, once a day, in a single dose, for a few days

• Twenty drops of Lehning® L52 in a little water, four times a day, if the patient already has a temperature

• Vitamin C: one gram a day in adults, 0.5 gram in children, for a fortnight

• To this standard treatment composed of three homeopathic remedies, one to three trace elements, and a vitamin, the homeopath may add remedies that are specific to each illness and fundamental for each personality

Dietary advice

To be strictly followed:

• Stop all heavy, greasy foods, particularly dairy products, fried food, and dishes with sauces

• Give the child plenty to drink

• Choose foods rich in vitamin C and copper

• Supplement the diet with wheatgerm and brewer's yeast, rich in group B vitamins and trace elements

• Give the patient plenty of garlic and onion, known for their anti-infective action

Some foods rich in vitamin C

Citrus fruits (lemon, orange, grapefruit), green vegetables (celery, green cabbage++, cress, spinach, sorrel, parsley, horseradish), fruit, especially red fruit (strawberries, raspberries, redcurrants), and others (pineapple, blackcurrants++, guava, kiwi++), potatoes, green peppers, tomatoes…

Some remedies based on vitamin C

Synergisti-C (Thorne) which contains

650mg ascorbic acid, 400mg Echinacea angustifolia, 100mg Baptisia tinctoria and 100mg hesperidin:
– Available in containers of 60 capsules
– Take one to two capsules twice daily
Biocare vitamin C (citrus free) 500mg containing magnesium ascorbate and bilberry:
– Available in containers of 180 veg capsules
– Take one to two capsules daily
Lamberts® Rutin+C+bioflavonoids (containing vitamin C 500mg, citrus bioflavonoids 100mg, rutin 50mg and hesperidin complex 30mg):
– Available in containers of 90 capsules
– Take one to two capsules daily

• You can take natural Vitamin C in chewable form – Lamberts® Vitamin C 100mg:
– Sold in containers of 90 tablets
– One to three tablets daily

• You can use natural vitamin C found, for example, in Weleda® sea buckthorn juice:
– Available in 200ml bottles
– One tablespoon in the morning provides about 30mg of the vitamin

Homeopathy

Sulfur to encourage eruption.

Six tablets at 7c, to be sucked once a day between meals.

Rhus toxicodendron, while vesicles are present.
– Four tablets at 5c to be sucked like sweets, two or three times a day between meals
– Vegetable origin: the poisonous sumac
– Homeopathic remedy for vesicles filled with clear fluid
– Characteristic sign: relieved by very hot water

• You can use Arnica-Heel® (Heel), Arnica D3, Rhus toxicodendron D6, Bryonia D4...
– Available in drop bottles of 30 and 100ml
– In general, ten drops three times daily.

Oligotherapy

Essentially **copper** or a **copper/gold/silver** combination.

• The combination can be found in many brands and presentations: colloidal minerals such as Organic Minerals (Colloidals) which contains 70+ trace minerals:
– Available in 946ml bottles
– Take 1–3 caps just before breakfast and/or evening meal
– Children 1 teaspoon daily for each 20lbs of body weight
Or Maximol (Ionized colloidals):
– Available in 500ml bottles
– Take ½ capful once or twice daily on an empty stomach

Herbal treatment

Echinacea, an excellent anti-infective agent.

Eleutherococcus and **ginseng** both very good general tonics for adults.

Prescription: For an adult, you can ask for a mixture of the dried extracts of these three plants to be made up, 100mg of each for a No. 2 capsule (the size of the capsule that the herbalist will prepare) Take three capsules a day (adults) for six days..

• You can use Echinacea complex (Bioforce) tincture which contains Echinacea purpurea...
– Available in 50ml bottles of oral drops
– Adults – 15 drops in a little water, three times daily . Children 6–12 years old – eight drops to be taken in a little water, three times a day. Children 2–5 years old – 4 drops in a little water, three times daily

Plant essential oils

Eucalyptus, niaouli, thyme linalol may be used in children. Their main activity is antibacterial.
– One drop of one of them to be taken in a spoonful of honey, twice a day

• You can use Lehning® Gouttes aux essences:
– Composed of cinnamon, cloves, lavender, mint, thyme...
– Available in 45ml and 90ml bottles
– Twenty drops to be taken four times a day (adult dose), or five to ten drops three times a day (children's dose), diluted in a small drink

Convalescence

Time to recover from an infection is obligatory and, depending on the illness, this period can be protracted and tiresome. Many types of treatment are effective in lessening the intensity of symptoms and shortening its course.

Dietary advice

• Do away with alcohol

• Choose foods containing vitamin C, mainly found in citrus fruits (lemons, oranges, grapefruit...), green vegetables (celery, sorrel, parsley, horseradish, green cabbage++), fruit (blackcurrants++, kiwis++, strawberries, raspberries, redcurrants...)

• Eat foods (garlic, onion) and condiments (thyme, cinnamon, mint, oregano...) known for their anti-infective action

• Add stimulating foods such as ginger, or foods rich in amino acids, vitamins and minerals... such as pollen

Two natural foods for convalescence

Royal jelly
– The virtues of this luxurious honey, secreted by young worker bees during their second week of life, have been known since the 17th century. This jelly is called 'royal' because it is intended

for the queen bees, which live much longer as a result. It is one of the foods richest in trace elements (calcium, copper, iron, phosphorus, and potassium), vitamins (A, B, C, D, and E), and essential amino acids;

– It stimulates immunity and thus helps fight infection. It is recommended in extreme fatigue and for convalescence

– If you are lucky enough to live near a beekeeper you may obtain it fresh. Take only a little at a time because it is very concentrated. Otherwise, you can buy sealed vials – airtight because it deteriorates easily. Take one vial at breakfast for a few days, at intervals.

Pollen
– A fine yellow-orange granular powder, composed of thousands of microscopic grains, the male seed of flowers collected by some bees when gathering nectar. Mixed with honey, it is used to feed the larvae, which is why the property of vitality has always been attributed to it in folk medicine. In fact it contains a number of minerals (copper, iron, magnesium, potassium, silicon...), amino acids (glutamic acid, methionine...), vitamins A,B,C, and E, and a substance (superoxide dismutase) which acts against the liberation of free radicals

– You will find pollen in a pharmacy or in health food shops, as capsules or in larger containers. On retiring to bed, pour a teaspoonful of pollen into half a glass of water, cover it, let it stand overnight, and take the mixture in the morning at breakfast

Homeopathy

Silicea, Sulfur iodatum
– Four tablets of each of these remedies at 7c to be sucked like sweets between meals, once a day, for two or three weeks

Silicea

– Mineral origin: silica, once extracted from quartz or flint
– A homeopathic remedy for protracted infections
– For a thin patient, tired, shivering, and deficient in essential minerals

Sulfur iodatum

– Chemical origin: sulphur iodide
– Homeopathic remedy for the effects of eruptive infections
– Characteristic sign: small swellings persist for some time after the infection

• You can use Cruroheel® (Heel), which contains Acidum silicum D6, Mercurius praecipitatus D8....
– Available in containers of 50 and 250 tablets
– In general, one tablet to be dissolved under the tongue three times daily. In acute disorders, initially one tablet every 15 minutes over a period lasting up to two hours

Oligotherapy

Essentially **copper**.

Trace elements are normally provided by the diet, which should be varied and of good quality. When there is a deficiency, copper can be given as a preparation.

Dietary sources of copper

Copper is present in small quantities nearly everywhere, except in milk, which contains very little.
It is found especially in liver++ (calf, sheep), seafood (lobsters, oysters, scallops, fish roe) and seaweed, almonds and nuts, certain vegetables (avocados, mushrooms), cereals (whole wheat, whole rice, soya), dried fruits, green vegetables, plums, cocoa, tea…

• Copper remedies: found in various forms and brands, e.g. colloidal minerals such as Organic Minerals (Colloidals) which contains 70+ trace minerals:
– Available in 946ml bottles
– Take 1–3 caps just before breakfast and/or evening meal
– Children 1 teaspoon daily for each 20lbs of body weight
Or Maximol (Ionized colloidals):
– Available in 500ml bottles
– Take ½ capful once or twice daily on an empty stomach

Herbal treatment

Eleutherococcus and **ginseng** for their stimulant properties.

Oak for its revitalizing action.

Possible prescriptions: Ask for a 30ml bottle of mother tincture of one of the first two remedies to be prepared. Take 25 drops in a little water three times a day. You can also ask for a 30ml bottle of oak buds macerated in glycerine at 1x. Take 25 drops in a little water three times a day.

Eleutherococcus

Eleutherococcus or Siberian ginseng is a plant of the ginseng and ivy family, but is native to the plains of Siberia where it grows in abundance. It is widely used by athletes from the countries of the former Soviet Union and Asia because it increases resistance to physical and mental fatigue.

Ginseng

A mythical plant known and venerated for four thousand years and for a long time the exclusive preserve of the Chinese emperor and nobility, ginseng has numerous properties. It is rich in ginsenosides, whose total concentration and relative proportions give it its activity and specificity. It also contains group B vitamins, vitamin C, minerals, and amino acids. It is primarily known as a tonic, a physical stimulant, an activator of the body's natural defence reactions, an aphrodisiac, anti-stress, antidepressant, and revitalizing remedy… Panax, the name of the main variety (from the word panacea) truly indicates its range of activity. The use of ginseng has two main contraindications: young children and arterial hypertension. It is normally perfectly well tolerated, but in high doses (more than 2 grams of powder) may cause agitation, nervousness or insomnia. It may also cause arterial hypertension with vertigo and headaches, or even trigger allergic reactions.

Oak

The oak, a common very tall forest tree, sturdy and much exploited for shipbuilding, relieves tiredness and possesses tonic, revitalizing, and immunostimulant properties. It is very useful during convalescence.

You can also use Red Kooga, a mixture of ginseng and multivitamins and minerals.
– Sold in boxes of 32 tablets
– Adults (over 12 years old) – one tablet to be taken each day

Plant essential oils

Mint, nutmeg, rosemary for their stimulant properties.
– Two drops of one of them to be taken in a little honey twice a day

Mint

Mint's activity is due to menthol, an alcohol extract of its essence, which gives it digestive and analgesic (pain-relieving) properties. It also stimulates the psyche… and sexuality.

Nutmeg

The nutmeg, brought to Europe in the 16th century, is a general stimulant, even of sexuality, but it can rapidly prove toxic. Use with caution.

Rosemary

This shrub is recognizable from afar by the beauty of its slender leaves, the colour of its flowers, and its penetrating smell. It fights fatigue, strengthens the memory, stimulates the circulation, and calms the nerves.

Complementary remedies are not only useful, but also indispensable in the treatment of most infectious illnesses.

They should be tried at the start to prevent the establishment of symptoms and to minimize their effect.

When the disease has become established they are useful in speeding recovery by augmenting defensive reactions.

In convalescence they are irreplaceable for speeding patient recovery.

They sometimes offer an alternative, or an invaluable, effective complement to antibiotic treatment, which is useless if the infection is viral.

Digestive disorders

Digestive disorders are often linked with stress, the main effect of which is nervous block, which slows the disposal of ingested food, causing a range of symptoms: bloating, heaviness, slow digestion, sleepiness after meals, burning stomach pains, belching, flatus, pain of varying severity, spasm. Echography and endoscopy allow the causes to be seen clearly, aiding an accurate diagnosis, but the classic treatments offered, though increasingly effective, have not in the least detracted from the usefulness of complementary remedies.

The Mouth: Bad breath, bad taste – Mouth ulcers

The Digestive tract: Stomach pain and heartburn – Difficult digestion – Food poisoning – Nausea, vomiting – Gut pains – Problems with wind (belching and flatulence) – Diarrhoea – Constipation – Colitis

Liver and bladder: Hepatitis – Bilious attack – Gall bladder pain, biliary colic

The mouth

Bad breath, bad taste

Bad breath is common, extremely unpleasant, and sometimes a real social handicap. It has various causes that can be dealt with immediately:

• Lack of hygiene in the mouth, especially the teeth, with multiple caries and tartar deposits

• Gums in poor condition, trapped food particles

• Chronic nose or sinus infection

• Airway problems mainly associated with smoking tobacco

• Digestion: the breath is tainted by food – garlic, onion, alcohol; dyspepsia (poor digestion); constipation; some slimming diets

• Occasionally, organic disease such as chronic gastritis, intestinal disorders, diabetes, pulmonary or renal infection

A bad taste in the mouth may have the same causes, but there may also be some psychological reason, or simply an occasional or habitual hangover.

Some plain advice

The following are necessary, but not always enough:

• Be meticulous about oral hygiene: use mouthwash regularly, but be careful because excessive use can lead to fungal infection

• Use toothpicks after meals to dislodge food particles stuck between the teeth

• Be careful about what you eat, drink, and smoke

• Ask your dentist or your doctor to look for any infection

Homeopathy

Mercurius solubilis, Nux vomica

– Four granules of each of these remedies at 5c to be sucked like sweets, three to four times a day between meals

Mercurius solubilis

– Mineral origin: mercury, quicksilver
– Homeopathic remedy for bad breath

Nux vomica

– Vegetable origin: the fruit of the Strychnos nux-vomica tree
– Homeopathic remedy for a coated tongue due to excess

• You can use Nux vomica-Homaccord® (Heel), which contains Nux vomica, Lycopodium, Bryonia and Colocynthis in various potencies...
– Available in drop bottles of 30 and 100ml
– In general, ten drops three times daily

Oligotherapy

Zinc

Trace elements are normally supplied by the diet, which should be varied and of good quality. When there is a deficiency, zinc can be given as a supplement.

Dietary sources of zinc

Zinc is widespread in seafood, oysters++, other shellfish, and fish. However it is also found in meat, egg yolk, cereals, wholemeal bread, brewer's yeast, nuts, some vegetables (broccoli, mushrooms, spinach, and haricot beans).

• Zinc preparations: there are various forms and brands, such as Organic Minerals (Colloidals) which contains 70+ trace minerals:
– Available in 946ml bottles
– Take 1–3 caps just before breakfast and/or evening meal
– Children 1 teaspoon daily for each 20lbs of body weight
Or Maximol (Ionized colloidals):
– Available in 500ml bottles
– Take ½ capful once or twice daily on an empty stomach
Or Lamberts® Zinc Plus Lozenges containing zinc (as citrate) 2 mg, vitamin C 100mg and bee propolis 5mg:
– Available in packs of 100 lozenges
– Adults can take up to 7 lozenges per day, children 3 lozenges per day

Herbal treatment

Echinacea, myrrh, marigold

– Possible prescription: Ask your herbalist to prepare a 30ml bottle of a mother tincture of one of these plants. Use a few drops diluted in water as a mouthwash three or four times a day.

Echinacea

The coneflower is a plant native to North America. It has antiviral and stimulant properties well known to the Native Indian tribes. It can be used at the start of an infection to make it less serious and shorten its course, but is equally effective in preventing recurrent winter ailments.

Myrrh

Myrrh is a thick yellow resin obtained from the balsam tree, a spiny plant that grows in hot countries. It is used throughout the Orient to treat infections of the mouth, throat and digestive tract.

Marigold

Thought of as 'a great plant for little skin problems', marigold is actually antiseptic, and heals and cleans.

• Chewing fresh mint leaves, or using infusions based on thyme, mint, or fennel seed can be helpful

Fennel

Fennel is an aromatic plant native to the Mediterranean basin. Its seeds help with digestion, alleviate some pains, reduce gas... and clear the breath. These properties explain its inclusion in various commercial infusions.

• Chew a coffee bean to sweeten the breath, or chew liquorice sticks (not the sweets) which cleans the teeth at the same time

Mouth ulcers

Ulcers appear as small, superficial, red-edged craters, white or yellow inside, almost always less than half a centimetre in diameter. Situated inside the cheeks, on or under the tongue, inside the lips or on the gums, they are very painful and troublesome. Mouth ulcers affect one in ten people at all ages in life. They can sometimes appear singly, are usually benign and, as a rule, last for six to ten days before disappearing without trace. So far, no conventional medical treatment has proved effective in preventing recurrence.

Care with food

The cause of the ulceration is not fully understood, but almonds, chewing gum, spices, strawberries, Gruyère cheese, honey, nuts, grapefruit, raisins, tobacco, and tomato skin are often responsible for its appearance.

Oligotherapy

Copper, gold, and silver the magic trio for the treatment of infection.

• You can take a copper/gold/silver combination as Organic Minerals (Colloidals) which contains 70+ trace minerals:
– Available in 946ml bottles
– Take 1–3 caps just before breakfast and/or evening meal
– Children 1 teaspoon daily for each 20lbs of body weight

Or Maximol (Ionized colloidals):
– Available in 500ml bottles
– Take ½ capful once or twice daily on an empty stomach

Magnesium, selenium
Trace elements are normally supplied in the diet, which should be varied and of good quality. When there is a deficiency, as is often the case with magnesium, the element can be given as a supplement.

Dietary sources of magnesium

Present in almost all foods, but unfortunately particularly in those rich in calories. Magnesium is found mainly in citrus fruits, bananas, whole cereals (oat flakes, bran…), cocoa and chocolate, shellfish (winkles, shrimps, oysters, clams…) and oily fish, snails, figs, hard cheeses, dried fruit and nuts (almonds, peanuts, hazelnuts, walnuts…), vegetables (spinach, dried haricot and green beans, split peas, soya…), wholemeal bread.

Dietary sources of selenium

Found mainly in foods of animal origin: meat (liver, kidneys), sea fish (herring, tuna etc.), shellfish (oysters), eggs. It is also found in whole cereals, wheatgerm, brewer's yeast, brazil nuts, some vegetables (garlic, broccoli, carrots, mushrooms), but its concentration can vary considerably according to the type of soil.

In countries where a lot of fish is eaten (Japan, Venezuela, Sweden…) the supply of selenium is generally sufficient or more than enough.

• Magnesium and Selenium medications: there are many different forms and brands such as Organic Minerals

(Colloidals) which contains 70+ trace minerals:
- Available in 946ml bottles
- Take 1–3 caps just before breakfast and/or evening meal
- Children 1 teaspoon daily for each 20lbs of body weight

Or Maximol (Ionized colloidals):
- Available in 500ml bottles
- Take ½ capful once or twice daily on an empty stomach

A preventive treatment could consist of one dose of selenium taken in the morning, one dose of magnesium in the afternoon, and one dose of copper/gold/silver morning and evening for a month. All these would be found in a colloidal supplement taken daily as recommended.

Homeopathy

Borax, Mercurius corrosivus

Borax

- Chemical origin: sodium borate
- Homeopathic remedy for mouth ulcers

Mercurius corrosivus

- Chemical origin: mercuric chloride or corrosive sublimate
- Homeopathic remedy for ulceration in the mouth

You can take Lehning® Agnus cactus Complex 2, which contains Apis 4x, Mercurius corrosivus 4x, Belladonna 4x...

- Available in 30ml bottles of oral drops
- Fifteen drops to be taken in a little water three or four times a day

Herbal treatment

Echinacea, marigold

POSSIBLE PRESCRIPTION: Ask your herbalist for a 30ml bottle of a mother tincture of echinacea, for its antiseptic role. Take 25 drops (for an adult) in a little water, three times a day for some days.

- You could also ask your herbalist to prepare a 30ml bottle of a mother tincture of marigold. Pour 15 drops into half a glass of warm boiled water and use it as a mouthwash three or four times a day.

Echinacea

Echinacea, or coneflower, is native to North America, and known by the Native American tribes for its great antiseptic properties. It stimulates the immune defences and has antibacterial and antiviral activity.

Marigold

Marigold (*Calendula officinalis*), originally native to Egypt, is used for its antiseptic, wound healing, and depurative properties. It is the remedy par excellence for all cuts – 'a great plant for little skin problems'.

- You can take Echinaforce (Bioforce), a tincture of Echinacea purpurea:

- Available in 50ml and 100ml bottles of oral drops
- Fifteen drops to be taken in a little water, three times a day by adults, seven drops three times a day by children (6–12 years old)

The digestive tract

Stomach pain and heartburn

These are very common symptoms, usually trivial and mild, and are most often linked with stress, and sometimes with taking medicines (aspirin, anti-inflammatory drugs), as well as with alcohol.

The symptoms suggest a diagnosis of hiatus hernia, gastritis, or ulcer; fibroscopy will reveal any possible lesions and may alsoconfirm the diagnosis.

Care must be taken to avoid prolonged self-medication without medical advice before a diagnosis has been made.

Some essential dietary advice

• Some foods are forbidden: chips and fried food, food cooked in oil or butter, offal and game, oily fish (anchovies, eel, mackerel, sardines, salmon, tuna), pickles, cauliflower, overripe cheese, jams, creams, confectionery, pastries (particularly commercially made ones), and strong alcoholic drinks

• Other foods to avoid are: crustaceans, eggs (fried, omelettes, scrambled), mushrooms, pulses, canned foods (meat), fresh soft bread

• Some other foods are allowed or recommended: cooked or dried vegetables, cereals and starchy foods, boiled eggs, lean meat and fish (bass, hake, sea bream, pollack, dab, sole), butter and

Helicobacter Pylori

Named after its helical shape, Helicobacter was discovered by Australian researchers in 1983. They found the organism living in the human stomach at a time when this environment, which contains concentrated hydrochloric acid, was believed unfavourable to bacterial growth. Most often the stomach becomes infected during the first five years of life, though the method of transmission (possibly saliva, stools, or gastric fluid) is unknown. Once established in the stomach, Helicobacter resists the hostile environment and the infection becomes chronic. The infection is universally distributed, without distinction between sex and race, but shows a preference for developing countries. A large proportion of people in the West carry the bacteria but, mysteriously, few people end up suffering from an ulcer. Long seen as the archetypal psychosomatic illness, gastric ulcer is in fact an ordinary infection that can generally be cured by antibiotics and antisecretory treatment. Vaccination is planned for the future.

unrefined oil, milk and all fresh, non-fermented cheeses, fresh fruit, fruit tarts

Oligotherapy

Magnesium

Trace elements are normally supplied by the diet, which should be varied and of good quality. When there is a deficiency, which is frequent in the case of magnesium, it can be taken as a supplement.

Dietary sources of magnesium

Present in almost all foods, but unfortunately particularly in those that are rich in calories. Magnesium is found mainly in citrus fruits, bananas, whole cereals (oat flakes, bran…), cocoa and chocolate, shellfish (winkles, shrimps, oysters, clams…) and oily fish, snails, figs, hard cheeses, dried fruit and nuts (almonds, peanuts, hazelnuts, walnuts…), vegetables (spinach, dried haricot and green beans, split peas, soya…), wholemeal bread.

• Magnesium preparations: there are many different brands and presentations, such as Organic Minerals (Colloidals) which contains 70+ trace minerals:
– Available in 946ml bottles
– Take 1–3 caps just before breakfast and/or evening meal
– Children 1 teaspoon daily for each 20lbs of body weight
Or Maximol (Ionized colloidals):
– Available in 500ml bottles
– Take ½ capful once or twice daily on an empty stomach

Chocolate

Foods that contain plenty of magnesium are also rich in calories, but it should be borne in mind that a 100g bar of chocolate, which is a fair amount, provides fewer calories than a medium-sized portion of chips.

• If necessary, you can take higher doses of magnesium by using Magasorb® (Lamberts) containing 150mg of magnesium (as citrate):
– Available in containers of 60 and 180 tablets
– one to three tablets daily

Homeopathy

Arsenicum album, Nux vomica

Four tablets of each of these products at 5c, to be sucked like sweets, alternately, three to four times a day between meals. The intervals should be increased when there is improvement.

Arsenicum album

– Chemical origin: arsenic oxide
– Homeopathic remedy for burning pains
– Specific sign: eased by warmth
Arsenic, once used to treat syphilis, is a deadly poison. When ingested it is most often fatal, causing agonizing pain throughout the digestive tract, with vomiting and convulsions.

Nux vomica

– Vegetable origin: the fruit of the Strychnos nux-vomica tree

Natural healing

– Homeopathic remedy for digestive disorders due to overindulgence
– Special psychological profile: irritable, bad tempered, cannot bear contradiction
Strychnine, which is highly toxic to the nervous system, is extracted from nux vomica seeds.

• You can use Gastricumeel® (Heel) which contains Carbo vegetabilis D6, Nux vomica D4, Argentum nitricum D6, Acid arsenicosum D6, Pulsatilla D4 and Antimonium crudum D6:
– Available in packs containing 50 and 250 tablets
– In general, 1 tablet to be dissolved under the tongue 3 times daily. In acute disorders initially 1 tablet every 15 mins

You can also add a constitutional remedy decided upon after consultation with your homeopath, in this case it will often be Argentum nitricum, Lycopodium, Sulfur.

Herbal treatment

Angelica, green anise, fennel for use in treating digestive pain.

Hawthorn, lime, valerian antispasmodic.

POSSIBLE PRESCRIPTION: Ask your herbalist to prepare a 30ml bottle of a mother tincture of a mixture of angelica and fennel. Twenty-five drops to be taken in a little water to relieve pain.

Anise

Anise, native to the Mediterranean basin, has considerable digestive properties. It reduces colic, relieves nausea, assists digestion and is effective against flatulence. For these reasons it is used both in the kitchen and in medicine.

Fennel

Fennel seed is used to treat abdominal pains and stomachache, and to relieve flatulence.
It is also mildly diuretic and is therefore sometimes used in slimming regimes.

Lime

To ancient civilizations, the lime tree was sacred because of its extraordinary longevity. Its leaves are mainly used in the evening because of their sedative properties, but they are also useful in dealing with digestive disorders and spasm.

You can use Weleda® digestive tea:
– Composition: Yarrow, anise, caraway, fennel, and camomile
– One infusion to be taken after meals

Acupuncture

Acupuncture finds a place here because of its sedative action and its undisputed effectiveness against pain. Though it may be difficult to organize acupuncture when the slightest pain appears, it can and should be a part of the fundamental treatment.

TREATMENT SCHEDULE: the programme of sessions is variable according to the frequency and intensity of the episodes of pain. The sessions can be weekly, monthly or three-monthly.

Difficult digestion

These very ordinary ailments are often connected with the hectic lives we lead, or with current difficulties, as witnessed by everyday expressions such as "I can't stomach it", or "I have a gut feeling".

Difficulty with digestion usually involves a feeling of heaviness in the stomach, but can also be accompanied by pain or nausea. The discomfort is often linked with an accumulation of air or gas in the stomach following too heavy a meal, or having eaten too quickly, In an anxious person, it can also be due to difficulty in emptying the gall bladder following a fatty meal. The pain can often be relieved by releasing the gas.

Dietary advice

It is essential to change some bad eating habits:

- Cut out badly tolerated foods: dairy products, cereals, or even fibre-rich foods can cause the symptoms to worsen
- If you suffer from gas, avoid the foods that cause it: aubergines, carrots, celery, cabbage, haricot beans, onions, and potatoes. Leave out apricots, citrus fruits, bananas, raisins, and apple, prune and grape juice; do not eat fresh bread, especially the soft part, or drink carbonated drinks, or use chewing gum
- Avoid stimulants such as tobacco and coffee

Your habits could change for the better:

– You eat too much, too quickly, in a noisy place, and you swallow too much air

– You eat sitting badly, as at the bar in a bistro or pub

– You chew incorrectly, swallowing your food before it is sufficiently soaked in saliva, the first essential stage in digestion

– You drink too much at meals, often carbonated drinks. This swells the stomach and dilutes the gastric juice so necessary to the second stage of digestion

– You start work too soon after your meal. This blocks digestion or slows it down. The best thing for proper digestion is to walk a little

Oligotherapy

Magnesium

Trace elements are normally supplied in the diet, which should be varied and of good quality. When there is a deficiency, as is often the case with magnesium, the element can be given as a supplement.

Dietary sources of magnesium

Present in almost all foods, but unfortunately particularly in those rich in calories. Magnesium is found mainly in citrus fruits, bananas, whole cereals (oat flakes, bran...), cocoa and chocolate, shellfish (winkles, shrimps, oysters, clams...) and oily fish, snails, figs, hard cheeses, dried fruit and nuts (almonds, peanuts, hazelnuts, walnuts...), vegetables (spinach, dried haricot and green beans, split peas, soya...), and wholemeal bread.

• Magnesium preparations: there are many different forms and brands, such as Organic Minerals (Colloidals) which contains 70+ trace minerals:
– Available in 946ml bottles
– Take 1–3 caps just before breakfast and/or evening meal
– Children 1 teaspoon daily for each 20lbs of body weight
Or Maximol (Ionized colloidals):
– Available in 500ml bottles
– Take ½ capful once or twice daily on an empty stomach

Homeopathy

Antimonium crudum, Nux vomica
Four granules of each of these products at 5c, to be sucked like sweets, alternately, two or three times in succession, between meals.

Antimonium crudum

– Chemical origin: antimony sulphide
– Homeopathic remedy for digestive disorders in heavy eaters
– Specific sign: condition worsened by acidic dishes, vinegar

Nux vomica

– Vegetable origin: the fruit of the Strychnos nux-vomica tree
– Homeopathic remedy for digestive disorders due to overindulgence
– Special psychological profile: irritable, bad-tempered, cannot bear contradiction

• You can use use Gastricumeel® (Heel) which contains Carbo vegetabilis D6, Nux vomica D4, Argentum nitricum D6, Acid arsenicosum D6, Pulsatilla D4 and Antimonium crudum D6:
– Available in packs containing 50 and 250 tablets
– In general, 1 tablet to be dissolved under the tongue 3 times daily. In acute disorders initially 1 tablet every 15 minutes

Herbal treatment

Artichoke, boldo, and **fumitory**, which activate the gall bladder.

POSSIBLE PRESCRIPTION: Ask your herbalist to prepare a 30ml bottle of a mother tincture of artichoke. Twenty-five drops to be taken in a little water in cases of difficult digestion, repeated if improvement is slow.

Artichoke

The numerous medicinal properties of the artichoke have been exploited since antiquity.

It is particularly active in ridding the liver of its toxins. It encourages digestion by activating the secretion of bile. Its purifying and diuretic properties also make it useful in patients who are slimming.

General advice on dealing with a hangover

– Do not go without eating. Try to eat something, even a little: a cup of coffee and some bread and honey will help to get you off to a good start

– Water is a must: drink it to eliminate alcohol

– Take a fruit juice cure: this will help you to burn off the alcohol still left circulating in the blood

– Take some bouillon: the salt and potassium are useful

– Avoid greasy fried food and alcohol

– Next time: avoid white wine, champagne, cognac, and mixtures. Vodka is relatively well tolerated

– There is a single homeopathic remedy, to be taken time and again – Nux vomica. Four granules to be taken at 5c, to be sucked three or four times during the day

Boldo

The boldo is a small tree native to Chile. Its leaves have an aroma close to that of mint, and it is used in many digestive or laxative preparations.

Fumitory

Fumitory is also called widows' weed because its sharp aroma readily brings tears to the eyes, even in a dry-eyed widow. A more useful property is its ability to stimulate the secretion of bile. It is also depurative, diuretic, and laxative.

• You can finish off your meal with mint tea, provided it is not too sweet

Plant essential oils

Anise, cumin, peppermint

POSSIBLE PRESCRIPTION: Obtain from your herbalist a bottle containing one of these three essential oils and add 1ml of it to your digestive infusion.

Cumin

Cumin, from Egypt, has a fairly strong, sharp smell. It is mainly used in North African and Indian cookery and to give an aroma to some breads. Just like caraway and anise, it reduces flatulence, stimulates digestion and eliminates intestinal spasm.

Peppermint

The essential oil of peppermint has antibacterial activity because it contains a great deal of menthol.

Acupuncture

This form of therapy has a place here because of its sedative effect. If organizing sessions to deal with each hangover or minor digestive problem may seem difficult, acupuncture should nonetheless be part of the constitutional treatment.

TREATMENT REGIME: The programme of sessions will vary with the frequency and intensity of the condition. Sessions could be weekly, monthly, or three-monthly.

Food poisoning

As much due to eating food of doubtful freshness as to indulgence in fruit or frozen dishes, food poisoning is frequently described as "a little gut infection" or "bad indigestion".

It may involve a temperature, combined with digestive disorders such as nausea, vomiting, diarrhoea, and abdominal pains. It is normally resolved quickly and without aftereffects, but close attention should be paid to young children, the aged, and those with weak immune systems.

General advice

• Drink, drink, drink – water, bouillon, Coca-Cola. Drink plenty, but only a little at a time

• You should 'refuel' gradually, choosing easily digested foods

Oligotherapy

Zinc

Trace elements are normally supplied in the diet, which should be varied and of good quality. When there is a deficiency, zinc can be given as a supplement.

Dietary sources of zinc

Zinc is widespread in seafood, oysters++, other shellfish, and fish. However it is also found in cereals, some vegetables (broccoli, mushrooms, spinach, haricot beans)... brewer's yeast, walnuts, wholemeal bread, egg yolk, and meat.

• Zinc preparations: there are various forms and brands such as Organic Minerals (Colloidals) which contains 70+ trace minerals:
– Available in 946ml bottles
– Take 1–3 caps just before breakfast and/or evening meal
– Children 1 teaspoon daily for each 20lbs of body weight

Caution

In all the following cases, seek medical advice without delay. Dehydration must be prevented or treated.

• If the symptoms arise after eating wild fungi, canned food, or seafood

• If you notice difficulty in swallowing, speaking, or breathing

• If there is a high temperature

• If there is intense thirst

• If there is continual vomiting

• If diarrhoea is abundant or persistent

• If micturition is weak

Or Maximol (Ionized colloidals):
– Available in 500ml bottles
– Take ½ capful once or twice daily on an empty stomach

Or you can take Zinc picolinate (Thorne) which contains 30mg of zinc:
– Available in containers of 60 or 180 capsules
– Take 1 capsule daily, preferably on an empty stomach

Homeopathy

• Aconite: start with Aconitum-Homaccord® (Heel) which contains Aconitum D2, D19, D30, D200, Eucalyptus D2, D10, D30 and Ipecacuanha D2, D10, D30, D200:
– Available in drop bottles containing 30 and 100ml
– Generally ten drops to be taken three times daily. Initially ten drops every 15 minutes

• Paratyphoïdinum B – six granules at 7c just once a day for two or three days

• Arsenicum album – four granules at 5c, two or three times a day for several hours or days, increasing the intervals between doses as improvement occurs

Or you can take Diarrheel® (Heel) which contains Acidum arsenicosum D8, Argentum nitricum D8, Colocynthis D6, Veratrum D4…
– Available in packs of 30 and 200 tablets
– In general, one tablet to be dissolved under the tongue three times daily. In acute disorders, initially one tablet every 15 minutes

Aconitum napellus

– Vegetable origin: the plant aconite, also known as wolf's bane because the poison it contains was once used in hunting
– Homeopathic remedy for infections that are sudden in onset
– Two characteristic signs: mental and physical agitation

Paratyphoïdinum B

– Animal origin: prepared from bacterial cultures of *Salmonella paratyphi* B.
– Homeopathic remedy for food poisoning with abundant diarrhoea

Arsenicum album

– Chemical origin: arsenic oxide
– Homeopathic remedy for food poisoning with acid indigestion
– Characteristic sign: condition improved by warmth

• You can use Lehning® China Complex 107, which contains Arsenicum album 6x, Belladonna 3x, and Nux vomica 4x
– Available in 30ml bottles of oral drops
– Twenty drops to be taken in a little water three times a day between meals; ten drops a day for children

• You can also add a constitutional remedy decided upon after consultation with your homeopath, in this case it will often be Lycopodium, Nux vomica, Sulfur

Changing the intestinal flora

Probiotics

– When ingested, these micro-organisms can restore the bacterial balance of the intestine. They control the proliferation of harmful bacteria, restore the intestinal flora, reinforce defence reactions, stimulate the immune system, and produce vitamin C;

– They can be found in natural yoghurts containing live bacteria (*acidophilus*, *casei*, *bifidus*), but also in the form of vials, capsules, tablets, and preparations in the pharmacy and in health food shops

– Take one or two doses a day during an infection, when travelling abroad, or following antibiotic treatment

POSSIBLE SIDE EFFECTS: Mild, but sometimes troublesome wind.

• You can use Acidophilis Extra (Lamberts) – each capsule contains 4 billion live bacteria:

– Available in containers of 30 and 60 capsules

– Take two capsules daily, one in the morning and one in the evening with glass of water or with a meal

• You can also take Replete (Biocare) – a seven-day intensive probiotic combination of L. acidophilus, B. bifidum and L. bulgaricus:

– Available in packs of 7 sachets

– 1 sachet per day

Herbal treatment

Lady's mantle, carob, and **purple** loosestrife for their intestinal antiseptic action.

POSSIBLE PRESCRIPTION: Obtain from your herbalist a 30ml bottle of mother tincture of purple loosestrife. Twenty-five drops to be taken in a little water, two or three times a day.

Lady's mantle

In former times, the alchemists referred to the dew that collected on the large leaves of this plant as 'heavenly water'. Lady's mantle is astringent, and can stop bleeding, slow menstrual flow, and halt diarrhoea.

Carob

This plant, from hot, temperate climes, affects the digestive tract in a number of ways. It encourages emptying of the stomach, relieves abdominal pain, and soothes the irritated colon.

When taken fresh it is a laxative, yet when used dry it soaks up bacteria and acts as an antidiarrhoeal.

Purple loosestrife

This plant is astringent and antiseptic, and very effective in treating diarrhoea and menorrhagia.

Plant essential oils

Ceylon **cinnamon** bark, and **caraway**, both antiseptic.

POSSIBLE PRESCRIPTION: Ask your herbalist to prepare 12 capsules of a mixture of 0.01g Ceylon cinnamon, 0.01g essential oil of caraway, and enough colloidal silica excipient for a No.2 capsule (the size of the capsule that the herbalist uses for the ingredients). One capsule to be taken twice a day for six days.

Cinnamon

Used as a spice and as a medicinal plant. Long considered to be one of the most precious aromatic plants, cinnamon is largely used to provide an aroma in confectionery, in punch, desserts etc. It is a very effective antiseptic.

Caraway

Caraway has an antispasmodic action that is very useful in relieving flatulence and colic. Very commonly used in food in northern European countries, it is a particular ingredient of Munster cheese.

Nausea, vomiting

Nausea is a common symptom experienced by everyone sometime or other, often referred to as 'feeling sick'. It may persist as nausea alone, or end in its logical conclusion, vomiting. Both are most often linked with the ingestion of foods that are poorly tolerated by the body, or to stress, but can sometimes indicate an underlying illness. Neither should ever be taken lightly and if they persist, a doctor should be consulted.

CAUTION: You should not treat nausea and vomiting yourself unless you are sure of the cause and are quite certain the condition is not serious.

General advice

- Drink moderately in small amounts: weak tea, fruit juice, bouillon, infusions. These can be hot, warm, or at room temperature

- Start eating again very gradually, taking easily digested foods and avoiding anything greasy or fried

- If the vomiting persists, and is severe enough to prevent drinking, you should consult a doctor. There may be a risk of dehydration, for which treatment is imperative.

Homeopathy

Nux vomica, ipecacuanha – in that order.

– Four granules of each of these products at 5c, to be sucked like sweets, alternately, three to four times a day between meals, increasing the intervals as improvement occurs

Nux vomica

– Vegetable origin: the fruits of the Strychnos nux-vomica tree
– Homeopathic remedy for digestive disorders due to overindulgence
– Specific sign: improvement after a short sleep

Ipecacuanha

– Vegetable origin: the dried root of a shrub from the tropical forests of Brazil, the ipecacuanha
– Homeopathic remedy for nausea, with or without vomiting

– Specific sign: the tongue is clean, not coated

• You can use Lehning®Nux Vomica Complex 49, which contains Arsenicum album 6x, Ipeca 4x, and Nux vomica 3x:
– Available in 30ml bottles of oral drops
– Fifteen drops to be taken in a little water three times a day, between meals; ten drops three times a day for children

• You should also add a constitutional remedy decided upon after consultation with your homeopath; in this case it will often be Lycopodium, Nux vomica, Sulfur

Herbal treatment

Ginger, mint, rosemary useful in treating nausea.

Dill, lemon balm, lime useful in treating vomiting.

POSSIBLE PRESCRIPTION: Ask your herbalist to prepare a 60ml bottle of a fresh whole-plant suspension of lemon balm. A half-teaspoonful to be taken in a little water, twice a day.

Thanks to a method of cold stabilization, fresh whole-plant suspension provides the full therapeutic effect naturally present in the whole plant.

Lemon balm

Lemon balm sometimes known as 'bee balm' has been used since antiquity as a 'passport to longevity', thanks to its physical and mental stimulant properties. But above all, it is famous as the principal component of a digestive preparation made since the 17th century in the Carmelite monastery in Rue Vaugirard in Paris, and distributed under the name 'Eau de Melisse des Carmes'. Lemon balm is antispasmodic, encourages the secretion of bile, and helps digestion. These qualities led to its inclusion in the two famous liqueurs, Chartreuse and Benedictine.
Eau de Melisse des Carmes is a mixture of the leaves and flowers of lemon balm, angelica root, lemon zest, and some aromatics (coriander, ground nutmeg and cinnamon, and cloves), macerated in wine. It is basically used like an alcoholic liqueur as an aid to digestion, but can also be used externally on small cuts and abrasions, because it is antiseptic.

Travel Sickness

Standard homeopathic remedy: **Cocculus**.

Four granules at 5c to be taken a few minutes before departure, and again at the start of and during the journey.

• You can take Cocculus-Homaccord® (Heel), which contains Cocculus and Petroleum in various potencies:
– Available in drop bottles containing 30 and 100ml
– In general, ten drops three times daily. In acute disorders, initially ten drops every 15 minutes

Dill

The seeds of dill, a plant related to anise and fennel, are mainly used as a spice in sauerkraut and marinades. They help with digestion, relieve flatulence and freshen the breath.

Ginger

A spice, condiment and remedy all in one, ginger is widely used throughout Asia. It is a useful digestive aid, but above all has a reputation as an aphrodisiac. It is used in Chinese cooking because it provides an aroma, is spicy, stimulates the senses, and helps the digestion. You can easily obtain ginger from the more exotic groceries. Grate it finely and add it to some cooked dishes (e.g. chicken).

Plant essential oils

Basil, camomile, cumin

POSSIBLE PRESCRIPTION: You can obtain a 1ml bottle of one of these essential oils in solution from your herbalist. When symptoms appear, take one drop in an infusion of mint.

Basil

Basil, an ingredient of 'pesto', should be used fresh, because when dried it loses its medicinal properties.
It has a light neurosedative action but is primarily a good digestive remedy, assisting digestion, relieving nausea and vomiting, easing pain, and reducing flatulence.

Camomile

Camomile has many medicinal properties. It is a mild antispasmodic and can be used to treat infant colic as well as gastric or intestinal pain in adults. It encourages digestion and therefore is found in a number of digestive infusions. It can be used to treat nausea and vomiting, and its sedative properties make it useful in nervous conditions, irritability, and minor problems with sleep.

Gut pains

About three or four per cent of medical consultations concern gut or stomach pains. The priority is to arrive at as accurate a diagnosis as possible and to decide whether it is serious, and the degree of urgency. In most cases it is not serious.

• If you have had these symptoms before and recognize them, you may know that they can be dealt with simply using a previously tried remedy or something quick and effective. Nevertheless, it will pay to follow the advice below:

• Be suspicious if:
– you are relatively old
– you are male
– the pain is intense, median, and impairs sleep
– the gut is very hard, and painful when breathing

– you have not had a bowel motion and are not normally constipated
– you have a temperature
– you are vomiting repeatedly
– you have serious diarrhoea
– there is blood in the stools
– you are losing weight
CAUTION: In the above cases, do not treat yourself. Go to your doctor without delay.

Homeopathy

There are three types of pain in the gut: due to cramps, burning, and flatulence.

Stomach cramps

Colocynthis, Magnesia phosphorica

Colocynthis

– Vegetable origin: bitter apple
– Homeopathic remedy for violent, intermittent, cramp-like pains
– Characteristic sign: relieved by pressure on the affected region

Magnesia phosphorica

– Chemical origin: magnesium phosphate
– Homeopathic remedy for unbearable, intermittent neuralgia
– Characteristic sign: improved by warmth

Burning pains

Arsenicum album, Iris versicolor

Arsenicum album

– Chemical origin: arsenic anhydride
– Homeopathic remedy for burning pains
– Characteristic sign: improved by warmth

Iris versicolor

– Vegetable origin: iris
– Homeopathic remedy for burning in the mouth, on the tongue, and in the stomach or the intestine
– Characteristic sign: hyperacidity

Pain due to flatulence

Carbo vegetabilis, China

Carbo vegetabilis

– Vegetable origin: wood charcoal
– Homeopathic remedy for flatulence in the pit of the stomach
– Specific sign: worsened by warmth

China

– Vegetable origin: cinchona bark
– Homeopathic remedy for distension throughout the intestine
– Two specific signs: improvement with warmth and firm pressure

Four granules of one of these remedies at 5c, to be sucked like sweets, alternately, between meals. The intervals should be increased as improvement occurs.

• You can use Gastricumeel® (Heel) which contains Carbo vegetabilis D6, Nux vomica D4, Argentum nitricum D6, Acid arsenicosum D6, Pulsatilla D4 and Antimonium crudum D6:

– Available in packs containing 50 and 250 tablets
– In general, one tablet to be dissolved under the tongue three times daily. In acute disorders initially one tablet every 15 minutes

Herbal treatment

Angelica, anise, and **fennel** – for pain.

Anise, fennel and **mint** – for wind.

Hawthorn, lime and **valerian** – for spasm.

Anise

A plant native to the Mediterranean basin. It has numerous digestive properties: it reduces colic, relieves nausea, aids digestion, and is effective against wind. For these reasons it is used both in the kitchen and in herbal remedies.

Fennel

Fennel seed is used in treating abdominal pain, relieving stomachache and flatulence. It is also mildly diuretic, and is sometimes used in slimming diets.

Lime

This familiar tree is both antispasmodic and mildly sedative. It encourages sleep and combats the symptoms of stress, which makes it useful in treating abdominal pain of nervous origin.

Valerian

The remarkable sedative properties of valerian have been known since antiquity. It encourages sleep and is mainly used to treat the symptoms of anxiety. At the same time it is very effective against spasm and cramps. Its only defect is its smell.

• You can use Valerian/Hops Complex (Bioforce), a mixture of valerian and hops:
– Available in drop bottles of 50ml
– Take 20 to 30 drops in a little water, half an hour before bed

• You can also drink one or two infusions per day of anise, boldo, fennel, dandelion, or mint
– One teaspoonful of the plant (bought loose from a herbalist) to one cup of water

Problems with wind (belching and flatulence)

Belching

Aerophagy (meaning 'eating air') results in the accumulation of too much air in the stomach. Air is normally swallowed during eating and usually escapes of its own accord, but sometimes accumulates as a pocket of compressed gas. Belching then occurs in isolation, or may occur along with bloating and a feeling of fullness in the stomach. Belching is most often the result of eating too much food containing a lot of air (ice cream, croissants, meringues, scrambled egg, soft bread, soufflés), or carbonated or mineral waters. People who chew gum or are under stress may also take in abnormal amounts of air. Those who suffer from aerophagy should avoid foods that tend to be swallowed without chewing: mashed potato, stew, soup, compote, whipped cream desserts.

Belching is good news for baby after breast-feeding, reassuring to the mother who awaits or even provokes it. In the Middle East it is considered polite, a sign of contentment showing that the meal has been appreciated. However, we find it unacceptable, especially in public.

Homeopathy

Carbo vegetabilis, China

Carbo vegetabilis

– Vegetable origin: wood charcoal
– Homeopathic remedy for flatulence in the pit of the stomach
– Characteristic sign: relieved by belching

China

– Vegetable origin: cinchona bark
– Homeopathic remedy for distension throughout the intestine
– Characteristic sign: not relieved by belching

• You can take Lehning® Basilicum Complex 96, which contains China 3x, and Lycopodium 4x:
– Available in 30ml bottles of oral solution
– Take 20 drops in a little water 15 minutes after meals and when the condition is troublesome

• You should also add a constitutional remedy decided upon after consultation with your homeopath; in this case it will often be Argentum nitricum, Kalium carbonicum, Lycopodium

Herbal treatment

Artichoke, boldo, fumitory activate the gall bladder, assist digestion and so help avoid the formation of gas.

Possible prescription: Ask your herbalist to prepare a 30ml bottle of a mother tincture of artichoke. Twenty-five drops to be taken in a little water when digestion seems sluggish.

Artichoke

Used since antiquity for its many medicinal properties, artichoke is particularly active in eliminating liver toxins. It encourages digestion by stimulating the secretion of bile. Its depurative and diuretic properties permit its use in slimming diets.

Fumitory

Fumitory is also called widows' weed because its sharp aroma readily brings tears to the eyes. It also stimulates the secretion of bile and is depurative, diuretic and laxative.

• You could finish your meal with a mint tea, provided it is not too sweet and not accompanied by highly calorific pine nuts

The Origin of Gas

The gas in the digestive tract has three sources: swallowed air, air in the food (much nitrogen and oxygen), and a great deal of hydrogen and carbon dioxide produced by bacterial fermentation in the colon.

When food containing carbohydrates that are indigestible or only partly digestible in the intestine are eaten, there is an increase in the fermentation processes taking place in the colon. This produces symptoms of pain and distension, and an increase in the amount of fermentation gas released though the anus (flatulence). Inadequate evacuation is in itself a source of discomfort and embarrassment. Patients who complain of distension may well be suffering from an excess of intra-abdominal gas, but they often show reduced tolerance to it, which explains the pain.

The daily output of gas in a normal subject varies from 200 to 2000ml in 24 hours, with an average of 600ml, involving ten to twelve emissions, or farts – some more discreet than others.

The role of stress

Stressed subjects swallow air by eating too quickly, by talking, chewing gum, or smoking. The intestine contracts spasmodically to move it; the passage of these pockets of air through the liquid contents of the large intestine causes rumbling noises.

Gas down below, or flatulence

This symptom, the most frequent in gastroenterology, mainly affects women. It is due to the presence of too much gas in the intestine and colon, or to difficulty in getting rid of it. The established medical term is tympanites. The condition reveals itself as local or generalized distension, sometimes painful, with excessive rectal emission of gas. The rumblings in the gut actually come from the colon, though patients often imagine they are in the stomach. The development of this condition is unpredictable, and closely linked with the environment and to personal equilibrium.

Homeopathy

China, Raphanus niger

– Four granules of one of these two remedies at 5c, to be sucked like sweets, two or three times a day between meals. The intervals between doses should be increased as improvement occurs

Raphanus niger

– Vegetable origin: horseradish
– Homeopathic remedy for distension of the gut, with no release of gas

• You can use Lehning® China compound 107, which contains China 3x, Arsenicum album 6x, and Nux vomica 4x:
– Available in 30ml bottles of oral solution
– Twenty drops to be taken in a little water after meals and when the condition is troublesome

• You should also add a constitutional remedy decided upon after consultation with your homeopath; in this case it will often be Argentum nitricum, Lycopodium, Nux vomica

Minerals

Clay, carbon

Clay is a sedimentary rock taken orally as a 'sponge' to adsorb intestinal germs. You can obtain clay of excellent quality, ground, as granules and as a powder, from health food shops and pharmacies;
– Take one dessertspoonful of finely ground clay in a half-glass of water, once or twice a day

• You can use Argiletz® Fine Green Clay:
– Available in 300g boxes
– Add one teaspoon to a glass of water and stir well. Allow to stand overnight and next morning drink the clay milk or just the clear water before breakfast

Charcoal

Charcoal is one of the most powerful absorbent substances, capable of retaining bacteria, viruses, gas, and toxins. It is therefore almost indispensable as a natural 'intestinal bandage' for the treatment of diarrhoea, aerophagy, and gas distension. It is perfectly well tolerated, but can sometimes cause constipation.

• You can use Bragg's medicinal charcoal:
– Available in boxes of 250 tablets
– Take three or four tablets after meals, three times a day. Not recommended for children under twelve

Herbal treatment

Anise, fennel, mint

Mint

Peppermint is the most valued of all the varieties of mint because it is very rich in the essential oil that makes it so fine and so effective.

• If you are in a restaurant, you may be able to get a mint infusion at the end of your meal
• If you are at home, you can have an infusion of thyme, star anise, or fennel, or add some fennel or coriander seeds to the main dishes

Diarrhoea

This is the natural method the body uses to get rid of irritant or harmful substances in the intestine, but it may become pathological and troublesome if the stool is too abundant, too frequent or too loose. It is caused by an infection, viral in 80 per cent of cases, which explains why antibiotics are usually ineffective.

Diarrhoea normally takes a favourable course, needs no further examination, and presents no special problems apart from transient discomfort.

In Third World countries diarrhoea is a veritable scourge and, because of the considerable loss of water and minerals it entails, the most common cause of death in children under five.

General advice

Of vital importance:

• An absolute necessity for rapid rehydration with water and bouillon

'Holiday Tummy'

Caused by a change in eating habits during a trip, leading to the secretion of toxins by the intestinal bacteria, resulting in diarrhoea. It can be contracted in any country, not necessarily in the Far East.

Here are the foods responsible for the formation of gas:

– Much gas from these vegetables: artichokes, aubergines, carrots, celery, mushrooms, cauliflower, cucumber, broad beans, haricot beans, onions, potatoes, salsify, and soya

– Little gas from asparagus, avocado, leeks, lettuce, tomatoes, and cooked legumes

– Much gas from the cereals in pastries, bread

– Little gas from rice

– Much gas from apricots, citrus fruits, bananas, apples, prunes, raisins, rhubarb, fruit skins, apple, plum, and grape juice

– Little gas from peanuts, hazelnuts, walnuts, and grapes

– Much gas from milk

– Little gas from these dairy products: fermented cheese, yoghurt

– Much gas from paprika

The consumption of broad beans was once more or less forbidden in convents because the noises that resulted disturbed the services.

• Go on a starvation diet because the intestine needs to rest, then a diet that

Natural healing

produces little residue, to reduce the volume of the stools:

– For a few days you must rule out vegetables (especially haricot beans and cabbage), fruits, fat, fatty meats, dairy products, bread, potatoes, and pastries

– You may eat rice, cooked carrots, fruit jellies, Coca-Cola (surprisingly, an antidiarrhoeal), infusions, tea, coffee, and plenty of liquids (tap water, natural bouillon, vegetable broth, and sweet broth with no pulp)

• Seek medical advice quickly:
– if the diarrhoea does not stop in 48 hours
– if it is accompanied by abdominal pain
– if it is accompanied by signs of extreme weakness
– if the patient cannot drink
– if you see blood, mucus, or pus in the stools

Oligotherapy

Zinc
Trace elements are normally supplied by the diet, which should be varied and of good quality. When there is a deficiency, zinc can be given as a supplement.

Dietary sources of zinc

Zinc is widespread in seafood, oysters++, other shellfish, and fish. However it is also found in cereals, some vegetables (broccoli, mushrooms, spinach, haricot beans)... brewer's yeast, walnuts, wholemeal bread, egg yolk, and meat.

• Zinc preparations: there are various forms and brands: Organic Minerals (Colloidals) which contains 70+ trace minerals:
– Available in 946ml bottles
– Take 1–3 caps just before breakfast and/or evening meal
– Children 1 teaspoon daily for each 20lbs of body weight
Or Maximol (Ionized colloidals):
– Available in 500ml bottles
– Take ½ capful once or twice daily on an empty stomach
Or you can take Zinc picolinate (Thorne) which contains 30mg of zinc:
– Available in containers of 60 or 180 capsules
– Take 1 capsule daily, preferably on an empty stomach

Homeopathy

Arsenicum album, Podophyllum

Arsenicum album

– Chemical origin: arsenic oxide
– Homeopathic remedy for severe diarrhoea
– Characteristic sign: improved by warmth

Podophyllum peltatum

– Vegetable origin: the root of a North American plant, the May apple
– Homeopathic remedy for summer diarrhoea

– Two characteristic signs: improved by warmth and by lying on the stomach

– Four granules of each of these products at 5c, to be sucked like sweets, alternately, throughout the day, increasing the interval when improvement occurs

• You can almost automatically add Paratyphoïdinum B:
– Six granules at 6c, when the diarrhoea starts, then once a day for three or four days

Paratyphoïdinum B

– Animal origin: prepared from bacterial cultures of Salmonella paratyphi B
– The specific homeopathic remedy for food poisoning with abundant diarrhoea

• If the bout of diarrhoea seems serious, call your doctor and take four granules of Veratrum album 5c every ten minutes while you wait.

Veratrum album

– Vegetable origin: white hellebore
– Homeopathic remedy for abundant diarrhoea with extreme weakness
– Characteristic sign: cold sweats

You can take Diarrheel® (Heel) which contains Acidum arsenicosum D8, Argentum nitricum D8, Colocynthis D6, Veratrum D4...
– Available in packs of 30 and 200 tablets
– In general, 1 tablet to be dissolved under the tongue 3 times daily. In acute disorders, initially 1 tablet every 15 minutes

Hellebore

This herbaceous plant was once used to cure madness; now it is simply used as a purgative and vermifuge.

Modifiers of the intestinal flora

Probiotics

Ingested live, these micro-organisms are taken to repopulate the intestinal ecosystem. Living with us in our bodies, in perfect harmony, are a great number of bacteria (about one kilogram of body weight), some of which are even indispensable. Friendly bacteria, which invade the colon from birth, control harmful bacteria by secreting lactic acid. This makes the intestine hostile to the development of other colonies of harmful guests. Benign bacteria also produce substances with antibiotic properties, hence the name 'probiotics'. When present in appropriate numbers and balance, they carry out their policing action efficiently. As soon as their numbers change (due to age, change of diet, stress, or antibiotic treatment) the defences are lowered and clinical symptoms of illness may appear. When this happens, restoration of the intestinal flora becomes necessary.

PROPERTIES: Probiotics control the reproduction of harmful bacteria and restore the intestinal flora. They strengthen defence reactions and increase the ability to combat infection by stimulating the immune system and producing vitamin C. They also pre-digest proteins and in particular, lactose, improving digestion and assimilation. They produce vitamins in group B, and may prevent cancer of the colon.

The digestive tract is host to numerous bacterial species. More than 400 germs have been identified in the faeces. The largest, dominant group is represented by the genera Bifidobacteria and Bacteroides. Least represented are the genera Lactobacilli, Enterococci, and Enterobacteria (colibacilli). Other potentially pathogenic germs are Corynebacteria, Klebsiellas, Proteus, and Staphylococci. Probiotics help to maintain the balance of this internal flora.

METHOD OF USE: You can find probiotics in natural yoghurt containing live bacteria (acidophilus, casei, bifidus), and also in vials, capsules and tablets, in pharmacies and health food shops. Take one or two doses a day during an infection, while travelling abroad, or after antibiotic treatment.

POSSIBLE SIDE EFFECTS: Mild but troublesome gas

• You can use Acidophilis Extra (Lamberts) – each capsule contains 4 billion live bacteria:
– Available in containers of 30 and 60 capsules
– Take two capsules daily, one in the morning and one in the evening with a glass of water or with a meal

• You can also take Replete (Biocare) – a seven-day intensive probiotic combination of L. acidophilus, B. bifidum and L.bulgaricus:
– Available in packs of seven sachets
– one sachet per day

Minerals

Clay and **charcoal** have a long history of effectiveness against flatulence and diarrhoea.

Clay

Clay is a sedimentary rock taken orally as a 'sponge' to adsorb intestinal germs. You can obtain clay of excellent quality, ground, as granules and as a powder, from health food shops and pharmacies
– One dessertspoonful of finely ground clay should be taken in a half-glass of water, once or twice a day

• You can use Argiletz® Fine Green Clay:
– Available in 300g boxes
– Add one teaspoon to a glass of water and stir well. Allow to stand overnight and next morning drink the clay milk or just the clear water before breakfast

Charcoal

Charcoal is one of the most powerful adsorbent substances, capable of retaining bacteria, viruses, gas, and toxins. It is therefore almost indispensable as a natural 'intestinal bandage' for the treatment of diarrhoea, aerophagy, and gas distension. It is perfectly well tolerated, but can sometimes cause constipation.

• You can use Bragg's medicinal charcoal:
– Available in boxes of 250 tablets
– Take three to four tablets after meals, three times a day
– Not recommended for children under twelve

Herbal treatment

Carob, blueberry, purple loosestrife

POSSIBLE PRESCRIPTIONS:
– You can take an infusion of purple loosestrife three times a day, for rehydration and as a treatment
– Ask your herbalist to prepare 15 capsules of a mixture of dried extracts of carob, blueberry, and purple loosestrife, 100mg of each for a No.2 capsule (the size of the capsule that the herbalist will use for the ingredients). One capsule to be taken three times a day for five days
– A decoction of dried blueberries is effective against diarrhoea

The decoction is prepared by cutting the plant into pieces and boiling it in water for 15 minutes. After filtering, it may be drunk hot or cold.

Blueberry

The tannins present in these bluish-black berries are antidiarrhoeal, antiseptic, and have a beneficial effect on intestinal pains and spasm. By contrast, the ripe berries are mildly laxative.

Purple loosestrife

Nicknamed 'the colic herb', purple loosestrife is a hardy plant that lives in humid locations; it grows readily by the sea under willow trees. It is an antiseptic and of course, effective against diarrhoea.

Constipation

One of the most frequent conditions in gastroenterology, affecting ten per cent of the population of the Western world, inexplicably mostly women.

Constipation can be defined as a slowing of intestinal transit leading to the delayed, irregular, and difficult evacuation of too few stools. Normally food takes four or five hours to travel from the mouth to the beginning of the colon, and the residues can remain there for 24 to 36 hours before evacuation through the anus. Every day, about a litre and a half of liquid produced by digestion reaches the entrance to the colon.

The main function of this two-metre long tube is to concentrate the liquids, then expel 100ml to 150ml of stools composed of 80 per cent liquid and 20 per cent 'dry weight'. If the colon concentrates the contents too much, the stools will be low in volume, dry and hard: the term constipation is used when there are less than three stools per week, with a daily weight of less than 35 grams.

General advice

There are three essential elements:

• Educating the patient to adopt a new, healthy way of life, by acquiring new eating habits and new treatments

• The education of the patient is fundamental: the evacuation of stools is easier when the need for it is felt

There is a moment in the day, often in the morning, when this desire is at a maximum. This moment should not be allowed to pass, because evacuation will become more difficult later, so much so that a vicious circle may be established in which the rectum gradually becomes distended, its tolerance to stools increases, and the constipation gets worse.

• The diet should be rich in fibre, because the volume of the stools partly depends on the amount of fibre ingested. Choose from the following foods and drink plenty of water

Foods rich in fibre (per 100g)

– All Bran®: 27g
– Dried coconut: 23g
– Dried figs: 18g
– Wheatgerm: 17g
– Dried prunes: 16g
– Almonds: 15g
– Wholemeal bread: 8g
– Haricot beans: 8g
– Raspberries: 7g
– Oat flakes: 7g
– Hazelnuts: 6g
– Rye bread: 5g
– Walnuts: 5g

At the start, bran may cause flatulence, especially if not taken gradually. Raise the amount to twenty grams a day in increments of five grams every five days.

• You can use Solgar Apple Pectin Powder:
– Available in 113g bottles
– Take ½ teaspoon in an 8 ounce glass of water

Advice for children

• Give the child a little orange juice and vegetable broth

• Train the child to go to the toilet regularly, preferably after a meal

• Encourage physical exercise

• Explain that one should not hold oneself in

• Give the child paraffin oil, which slows the absorption of water and increases hydration of the stools

Oligotherapy

Magnesium almost as a matter of course, the more so because in large doses it is laxative. Trace elements are normally supplied in the diet, which should be varied and of good quality. When there is a deficiency, as is often the case with magnesium, the element can be given as a supplement.

Dietary sources of magnesium

Present in almost all foods, but unfortunately particularly in those rich in calories, magnesium is found mainly in citrus fruits, bananas, whole-grain cereals (oat flakes, bran...), cocoa and chocolate, shellfish (winkles, shrimps, oysters, clams...) and oily fish, snails, figs, hard cheeses, dried fruit and nuts (almonds, peanuts, hazelnuts, walnuts...), vegetables (spinach, dried haricot and green beans, split peas, soya...), wholemeal bread.

• Magnesium preparations: there are many different brands and forms: Organic Minerals (Colloidals) which contains 70+ trace minerals:
– Available in 946ml bottles
– Take 1–3 caps just before breakfast and/or evening meal
– Children one teaspoon daily for each 20lbs of body weight
Or Maximol (Ionized colloidals):
– Available in 500ml bottles
– Take ½ capful once or twice daily on an empty stomach

• You can take higher doses of magnesium by using remedies such as as Magasorb® (Lamberts) Containing 150mg of magnesium (as citrate):
– Available in containers of 60 and 180 tablets
– one to three tablets daily

Homeopathy

Alumina, Lycopodium

– Four granules of one of these products at 5c, to be sucked like sweets, two or three times a day, increasing the interval as improvement occurs

Alumina

– Mineral origin: aluminium oxide from the ore, bauxite
– Homeopathic remedy for constipation or when even small, soft stools are difficult to expel

Lycopodium clavatum

– Vegetable origin: the spores and powder of lycopodium, or stag's horn club moss
– Homeopathic remedy for constipation with spasm
– Characteristic sign: swelling of the lower part of the gut after meals

• You can take Proctheel® (Heel), which contains Lycopodium D4, Alumina D8, Sulfur D6 and Phosphorus D6
– Available in drop bottles of 30ml
– ten drops three times daily

• You should also add a constitutional remedy decided upon after consultation with your homeopath, in this case it will often be Lycopodium, Nux vomica, Sulfur...

Herbal treatment

Watch out for irritant plants such as aloes, black alder, cascara, bladderwrack, rhubarb, and senna, because they carry a risk of laxative colitis. However, they are found in many commercial preparations and should not be taken for long periods of time.

Natural healing

Psyllium seeds are fine, as are **isphagul** and **mallow**.

Artichoke, dandelion and **rosemary** increase the amount of bile secreted, aiding digestion.

Artichoke

Artichoke is highly effective in ridding the liver of its toxins. It activates the secretion of bile, thus providing a mild laxative effect.

• You can use Cynara Artichoke, a dried artichoke extract (320mg):
– Available in packs of 30 capsules
– One capsule daily, preferably before meals

• You can also use Lamberts® Artichoke 8000mg:
– Available in containers of 60 tablets
– One tablet daily, preferably before meals

Dandelion

The dandelion leaf we can eat is diuretic, and the root is a potent depurative that helps the liver and kidneys to eliminate toxins more easily.

• You can ask your herbalist to prepare a 60ml bottle of a fresh whole-plant suspension of dandelion and/or artichoke. A half-teaspoonful to be taken in a little water, twice a day

Thanks to a method of cold stabilization, fresh whole-plant suspension provides the full therapeutic effect naturally present in the whole plant.

Rosemary

This shrub is recognizable from afar by the beauty of its slender leaves, the colour of its flowers and its penetrating smell. Rosemary is an outstanding general and cerebral stimulant, improving both concentration and memory. In addition, its effect on biliary secretion gives it a very useful laxative action.

• You can use Dr. Gillian McKeith's Liver Tone powder, containing dandelion, artichoke, milk thistle, psyllium, slippery elm bark and the amino acid taurine:
– Available in 200g bottles of powder
– Adults take ½ teaspoon mixed in water or fruit juice daily and build up to 1 teaspoon twice daily. Take before meals.
– You can take Herba Naturelle tincture of rosemary leaf:
– Available in bottles of 50ml
– Take as directed

• You can take a dessertspoonful of psyllium seed in a glass of water in the evening before going to bed. For a constipated child, give an infusion prepared with one teaspoonful of mallow flowers.

Psyllium

This plant originated in southern Europe and North Africa. Its mucilaginous seeds contain the main laxative ingredient.

Mallow

Mallow, which can be recognized by its pretty mauve-coloured flowers, is found everywhere in Europe. It is extremely effective in calming a cough, and eases the respiratory tract during an infection. It is also used in poultices to soothe inflamed skin through its emollient action.

• You can use Solgar Psyllium Husk Fibre:
– Available in 280g bottles
– One tablespoon daily in an 8 ounce glass of water. Take between meals and drink plenty of water throughout the day

Colitis

The term colitis means inflammation of the colon, the lowest part of the digestive tract, between the small intestine and the rectum. The condition may present five types of symptom. They can appear singly or together: pain or colic, gas, discomfort at gut level, diarrhoea, and the need to empty the colon several times a day. Colitis may be accompanied by nervous disorders such as lack of energy and listlessness, irritability, and aggressiveness.

Some doctors look on colitis as the intestinal equivalent of an outburst of tears, leading one to think it could be due to adverse situations: professional or emotional frustration, nervous strain, various problems in coping with life generally – all of which could easily cause attacks, or make them worse.

Colitis is very common, affecting close to a quarter of the population in the West and representing half of all gastroenterological consultations. It is found mainly in the 20–40 age group, among people living in an urban environment, two-thirds of them women, but it also appears in children as abdominal pain and intermittent diarrhoea.

It is a mysterious ailment, generally harmless, but very difficult to cure whatever type of treatment is chosen. The majority of patients suffer one attack a week; one-third have a bout every day. Eighty per cent of patients describe it as a nuisance, but five per cent see it as a real handicap with repercussions on quality of life, either in the family or at work.

General advice

Nowadays people eat too quickly without chewing their food enough, in an atmosphere that is too tense. They do not eat enough fruit, fresh vegetables, and pulses; instead they eat too many refined foods such as sugar, and animal protein, which bring about harmful changes in the intestinal flora.

You should:
– take the time to eat peacefully, chewing your food thoroughly in a calm atmosphere
– avoid drinking during meals

– hold back from foods that are too sweet, too refined
– favour cereals

Specific advice

There is no such thing as an ideal diet for colitis: everyone has to learn to identify, limit, or even do without the foods that give them trouble or tend to irritate the colon wall. The problem is that they are not the same for everybody.

Nonetheless, it is possible to make some recommendations that bring some improvement during an attack. You should:
– give your intestine a rest for two or three days with a low residue diet. Steamed or braised foods are permissible, but fried food, dishes with sauce, and spices are not. Gassy drinks, chewing gum, and the middle of fresh bread are not advisable because they cause flatulence;
– over a few days follow an interim diet comprising cooked and refined products;
– then resume a normal diet.

Eating with an irritable bowel

• Meat and cooked pork products:
– eat grilled lean meat, grilled or roast poultry, cooked ham
– do not eat cold meats in general, offal, fatty meat (pork, mutton), meats in sauce, fatty poultry (goose, turkey, duck), game

• Fish:
– eat grilled or baked fish, shellfish
– do not eat oily fish (herrings, mackerel, salmon, tuna)

• do not eat chips

• Dairy foods:
– you may use fresh butter on food, and powdered skimmed milk
– do not have fresh milk, whipped cream, ice cream, or milky coffee

• Eggs:
– no soft- or hard-boiled eggs

• Bread, pastries, confectionery:
– you may eat toasted stale bread, biscuits, rice, pasta, semolina, dry pastries
– no fresh or warm bread, pastry, ravioli, or greasy noodles

• Vegetables:
– you may eat steamed or boiled vegetables, steamed or boiled potatoes
– no garlic, artichokes, mushrooms, cabbage, cauliflower, cucumbers, shallots, pulses, peas, mashed potatoes, radishes, onions, or salsify

• Fruit:
– you may eat fruit, cooked or uncooked, jellied, very ripe, crystallized, as juice...
– no almonds (or almond paste), bananas, peanuts, green fruit, melon, walnuts, hazelnuts, oranges, pistachio nuts

• Drinks:
– you may drink still mineral water, tea, infusions, a little red wine
– no carbonated drinks (water, cider, fruit juice, soda) or iced drinks, rosé wines, champagne

• You can eat honey

• No cocoa or chocolate

Some definitions

The term 'colic' means abdominal pains.

Functional colitis:
– painful episodes occur three or four times a year
– the illness is of at least two years' duration

Irritable bowel:
– pains relieved by passing stool
– frequent or loose stools at the start of the attack
– visible distension of the abdomen
– mucus oozing from the rectum
– a feeling of incomplete evacuation

Oligotherapy

Trace elements are normally supplied by the diet, which should be varied and of good quality. When there is a deficiency, which is frequent in the case of magnesium, it can be taken as a supplement.

• Magnesium medications: there are many different brands and forms: Organic Minerals (Colloidals) which contains 70+ trace minerals:
– Available in 946ml bottles
– Take 1–3 caps just before breakfast and/or evening meal
– Children 1 teaspoon daily for each 20lbs of body weight
Or Maximol (Ionized colloidals):
– Available in 500ml bottles
– Take ½ capful once or twice daily on an empty stomach

CAUTION: Colitis is very sensitive; magnesium can sometimes make it worse and should be taken progressively, with care.

The role of the colon

The colon can be thought of as a reservoir with three important functions:

– It absorbs some substances, e.g. water

– It transforms food into faeces by means of its bacterial flora

– It fills by contraction, transferring the faeces (everything that has not been assimilated by the small intestine) to the rectum

Homeopathy

Carbo vegetabilis, and **China** when gas is the main problem.

Colocynthis and **Magnesia phosphorica** when diarrhoea predominates.

Nux vomica when the problem is constipation.

Ignatia when diarrhoea and constipation alternate.

– Four granules of one or more of these remedies at 5c, to be sucked like sweets, two or three times a day between meals

You can use Gastricumeel® which contains Argentum nitricum D6, Carbo vegetabilis D6, Arsenicum album D6,

Natural healing

Antimonium crudum D6, Pulsatilla D4 and Nux vomica D4:
– Available in tablet form (50 and 250 tablet packs)
– One tablet dissolved under the tongue three times daily

You can also add a constitutional remedy decided upon after consultation with your homeopath; in this case it will often be Lycopodium, Nux vomica, Sulfur.

Herbal treatment

Camomile and **purple loosestrife** to treat spasm.

Camomile
Camomile has many digestive properties. It is a mild antispasmodic and can be used to treat infant colic as well as gastric or intestinal pain in adults. It encourages digestion and therefore is found in a number of commercially available digestive infusions. It can be used to treat nausea and vomiting, and its sedative properties make it useful in nervous conditions and irritability. The popular apple-flavoured German variety is pleasant to take.

POSSIBLE PRESCRIPTION: Take one dessertspoonful of camomile flowers for one cup of boiling water. Leave it to infuse for ten minutes before drinking it, covering it carefully to prevent the escape of the highly volatile active ingredients (essential oils).

– Ask your herbalist to prepare 30ml of a mother tincture of purple loosestrife. Twenty-five drops to be taken in a little water two or three times a day during an attack

Anise, fennel, and **mint** for the treatment of gas.

• If the meal is eaten in a restaurant, you may be able to get a mint infusion after the dessert

• If you are at home, you can take an infusion of thyme, star anise or fennel, or add some fennel or coriander seeds to the main dishes

Plant essential oils

Camomile
POSSIBLE PRESCRIPTION: Obtain from your herbalist a bottle of 2ml of essential oil of camomile in solution. One or two drops to be taken in an infusion after a very hearty meal.

The liver and the gall bladder

Hepatitis

Hepatitis is a condition in which the liver becomes inflamed, mostly because of a virus, but sometimes because of medicines or toxic substances, generally alcohol. At least five viruses, A, B, C, D, and E are responsible for five types of hepatitis, all of which are differentiated by their respective modes of infection, development, and prevention.

Some simple facts about the function of the liver and the gall bladder

The liver

Cone-shaped, with an average weight of a kilo and a half, the liver is a veritable chemical factory of great sophistication. It produces a number of substances of great importance, among them the albumen in the blood, the immune proteins that defend the body, and the coagulation factors so vital in stopping bleeding.

To the despair of some patients, the liver also makes cholesterol, which is indispensable to cell formation and structure. It performs as a substantial central sugar supply, releasing it as and when it is needed.

Refuse collection is another of the liver's duties: it neutralizes and discharges toxic substances and drugs whose accumulation might prove harmful to the body.

The liver can also regenerate itself – within certain limits. There are close to 150 medicines that are supposed to soothe, purge, or detoxify the liver.

The gall bladder

The gall bladder is oval in shape, and located below the liver. Its function is to concentrate the bile and release it through the bile duct, which leads from the liver to the intestine.

The litre of bile produced every day carries away the bile acids and waste produced by the liver, as well as aiding digestion of fats in the food when they reach the intestine. If the bile is too concentrated, cholesterol gallstones may form.

These small stones form quite often, are usually trivial and produce no symptoms as long as they remain peacefully in the gall bladder, which they can do for long periods of time. If their presence is revealed by echography, this does not mean their removal is an absolute necessity. Treatment is indicated only if they decide to migrate into the bile duct, causing the intense pain of biliary colic.

Natural healing

The five types of hepatitis

• Hepatitis A spreads through direct contact or in dirty water. It is easily contracted in countries where hygiene is dubious, but also in close communities, and in summer holiday resorts. Those affected are only contagious during the incubation period, which is 15–60 days. In the West, with improvements in hygiene, there are fewer and fewer viruses in circulation, but people are becoming more and more susceptible to the Hepatitis A virus. Vaccination has been available for some years

• Hepatitis B is transmitted through blood (blood transfusion, improperly sterilized syringes), or through sexual contact, as are Hepatitis C and D. In 60 per cent of cases this disease affects young people between 15 and 30. The virus persists in the blood for a long time. Of the many hundreds of thousands, possibly millions, of chronic virus carriers in the world, around ten per cent will develop complications

• Hepatitis C is mainly transmitted through blood or soiled material. It mainly occurs after transfusions or is contracted by drug addicts

• Hepatitis D can only occur in persons already infected with hepatitis B. It can therefore be prevented by vaccinating against hepatitis B

• Hepatitis E is not common in the West. It is very severe in pregnant women, and is seen especially in India, Nepal, and North Africa.

The symptoms of the disease

At the start the symptoms are often not very suggestive of hepatitis in particular: fever, aches, and headaches, which might be attributed to a bout of 'flu. Nor are the digestive upsets involved (nausea and vomiting) any more specific. A diagnosis of hepatitis is strongly suspected when jaundice appears, accompanied by darkened urine and light-coloured stools. However, these signs are absent in 90 per cent of cases, which means that most of the time the disease is not noticed.

A diagnosis is possible when blood is taken: transaminase levels are found to be raised.

The disease normally progresses towards recovery with a disappearance of symptoms and when examination indicates the restoration of normal biological values. Most fortunately, complications are rare.

Recovery from hepatitis A is almost always without after-effects. Hepatitis B and C sometimes become chronic and may even produce cirrhosis. The classic treatment based on interferon is sometimes necessary to arrest development, but the virus does not disappear. Currently, there are vaccines against hepatitis A and B, but not against hepatitis C.

Dietary advice

The diet is self-imposed because the symptoms of the disorder spontaneously suppress the desire for certain foods.

Homeopathy

Phosphorus

Four granules at 15c, to be sucked like sweets, once a day between meals, for some weeks.

Research with humans and laboratory animals has shown that phosphorus may be useful in encouraging the normalization of transaminase levels.

Phosphorus

– Mineral origin: white phosphorus
– Specific homeopathic remedy for hepatitis

Herbal treatment

Artichoke and **milk thistle** provide powerful protection and regeneration for the liver.

• You can use Cynara Artichoke, a dried artichoke extract (320mg):
– Available in packs of 30 capsules
– One capsule daily, preferably before meals

• You can also use Lamberts® Artichoke 8000mg:
– Available in containers of 60 tablets
– One tablet daily, preferably before meals

• You can ask your herbalist to prepare 45 capsules made from a heat vaporization of milk thistle, 200mg for a No.2 capsule (the size of the capsule that the herbalist will use for the ingredients). One capsule to be taken three times a day for some weeks. (It is a little expensive, but useful.)

Artichoke and milk thistle

The artichoke came originally from North Africa. Its leaves contain chemical substances that protect the liver and stimulate the formation and secretion of bile. Milk thistle seeds contain silymarin, a substance that protects the liver from toxins and thus speeds recovery from hepatitis.

• You can take Lamberts® Milk Thistle 3000mg, which contains 70mg of silymarin:
– Available in containers of 90 capsules
– One capsule to be taken daily

• You can also take S.A.T.® (Thorne) which contains milk thistle 150mg, artichoke extract 150mg and turmeric extract 150mg:
– Available in containers of 60 capsules
– Take 1–3 capsules 3 times daily

Bilious attack

There is a tendency among some people to deny overeating and blame something else for a bilious attack. In truth, there are many explanations for such a condition: the stomach doesn't empty properly, the gall bladder is lazy, the colon is too full, there is a hormonal problem (premenstrual syndrome), migraine, etc. Whatever it is, it affects young women between 30 and 40 in particular. They tend to be anxious, over-careful, suffer migraines, work very hard, and are by temperament pessimistic.

The attack starts on awakening with a feeling of illness accompanied by nausea, pains in the area of the liver and solar plexus, pallor, and sweating or a cold feeling. It usually ends with bilious vomiting. Even if the cause is not entirely clear, it would be difficult to deny the pains in the region of the liver or gall bladder that are a source of complaint. Many remedies that reduce spasm are useful or even indispensable in relieving the symptoms.

Dietary advice

This is simple, effective and easy to put into practice: a watery diet composed of vegetable broths and fruit juice followed by 24 hours of a light diet, with boiled potatoes, lean meat, preferably grilled, or poached fish.

Homeopathy

Nux vomica, almost as a matter of course.

Carduus marianus, Chelidonium

– Four granules of one of these remedies at 5c, to be sucked like sweets, two or three times a day between meals

Nux vomica

– Vegetable origin: the fruit of the Strychnos nux-vomica tree
– Homeopathic remedy for digestive disorders due to overindulgence
– Specific sign: improved by a short sleep

Carduus marianus

– Vegetable origin: the milk thistle
– Specific homeopathic remedy to encourage liver drainage

Chelidonium majus

– Vegetable origin: celandine
– Homeopathic remedy for hepatic pain
– Specific sign: pain spreading towards the right shoulder blade

• You can use Chelidonium-Homaccord® (Heel), which contains Chelidonium and Belladonna in various potencies:
– Available in drop bottles of 30ml and 100ml
– In general ten drops three times daily. In acute disorders, initially ten drops every fifteen minutes

Herbal treatment

Artichoke, boldo, fumitory

POSSIBLE PRESCRIPTION: Ask your herbalist to prepare a 30ml bottle of a mother tincture of one of these plants. Twenty-five drops to be taken in a little water, two or three times a day.

Artichoke

Eating artichoke stimulates liver function: several of its constituents increase the secretion of bile, accelerating the process of detoxification. It is thus a depurative.

• You can use Cynara Artichoke, a dried artichoke extract (320mg):
– Available in packs of 30 capsules
– One capsule daily, preferably before meals

• You can also use Lamberts® Artichoke 8000mg:
– Available in containers of 60 tablets
– One tablet daily, preferably before meals

Gall bladder pain, biliary colic

This is a very sharp stabbing pain, felt under the ribs in the region of the gall bladder. It is worsened by breathing movements and by the pressure exerted during clinical examination. It is often due to the presence of gallstones which, when they migrate, trigger episodes of biliary colic. The diagnosis is confirmed by echography, and the treatment is medical, and occasionally surgical. The pain is sometimes so intense that it is completely justifiable, and sometimes essential, to use orthodox painkillers.

Homeopathy

Belladonna, almost automatically.

Chelidonium, Magnesia phosphorica

Belladonna

– Vegetable origin: the deadly nightshade or belladonna
– The homeopathic remedy for severe pain that comes on suddenly and finishes abruptly
– Two specific signs: it is eased by resting, and aggravated by the slightest jolt

Chelidonium

– Vegetable origin: celandine
– The homeopathic remedy for hepatic pain
– Specific sign: pain spreading towards the right shoulder blade

Magnesia phosphorica

– Chemical origin: magnesium phosphate
– Homeopathic remedy for intermittent, unbearable neuralgia
– Specific sign: symptomatic improvement when the patient doubles up

Carduus majus the remedy for congestion.
– Four granules at 4c to be sucked like sweets, twice a day.

Carduus majus

– Vegetable origin: the milk thistle
– Homeopathic remedy for liver drainage

• You can use Hepeel® (Heel), which contains Chelidonium D4, Carduus marianus D2, Lycopodium D3, Nux moschata D4, China D3...
– Available in containers of 50 and 250 tablets
– One tablet dissolved under the tongue three times daily

• You should also add a constitutional remedy decided upon after consultation with your homeopath; in this case it would often be Lycopodium, Nux vomica, Sepia

Herbal treatment

Artichoke, boldo, fumitory, dandelion

POSSIBLE PRESCRIPTION: Ask your herbalist to prepare a 30ml bottle of a mother tincture of one of these plants. Twenty-five drops to be taken in a little water, two or three times a day.

Boldo

The Boldo is a tree native to the Andes cordillera. Its leaves stimulate digestion and the secretion of bile in particular. This bitter tonic is an ingredient of a tisane that is good for the liver, but which unfortunately also contains senna and black alder, both irritating to the colon.

Fumitory

Fumitory is an effective stimulant of biliary secretion. It is also an aperitif, a depurative, a mild laxative, and a sedative.

Dandelion

Dandelion has a powerful depurative action and stimulates the production of bile. This hardy plant also has the property of preventing the formation of gallstones and dissolving small ones that have already formed.

You can ask your herbalist to prepare a 60ml bottle of a fresh whole-plant suspension of dandelion and/or artichoke. A half-teaspoonful to be taken in a little water, twice a day. Thanks to a method of cold stabilization, fresh whole-plant suspension provides the full therapeutic effect naturally present in the whole plant.

• You can take Herba Naturelle, tincture of fumitory:
– Available in bottles of 50 and 100ml
– Take as directed

• You can also use Metabolics, tincture of boldo:
– Available in bottles of 30, 100, 250 and 500ml
– Take as directed

Head pain and dysfunction

Humankind may have been trying to find ways to overcome pain for centuries, but it has only been in recent years that a new awareness of the need to manage pain better has emerged. Complementary medicines have an important contribution to make here – acupuncture, mesotherapy, and osteopathy are especially helpful in pain relief.

Recent discoveries

Pain has been with us since humans first evolved, but it is only in the last 30 years or so that researchers have taken a scientific, rather than a purely philosophical, interest in it. In particular, two almost simultaneous discoveries have transformed our understanding of the mechanisms of pain:

– The 'gate control' theory is based on the discovery of receptors at skin level, sensitive to pain, touch, temperature, and pressure. These receptors send a message to the brain when they are stimulated, transmitting through different nerve fibres that deliver their message at different speeds. Since the nerve fibres that transmit the sensation of touch work faster than those that transmit pain, a tactile sensation will be perceived first. In addition, once at its destination, the tactile message 'closes the gate' on the pain message behind it, preventing it from reaching the brain's processing centres. Thus, when we hit ourselves against something, we instinctively rub the painful part so as to activate the gate which, temporarily at least, prevents our brain from receiving the pain message. Similarly, the nurse who gives a little tap to the buttock before giving an injection is also making use of this physiological mechanism, in order to make the needle slightly less painful

– The discovery within our nervous system of morphine-like substances known as endorphins (a contraction of 'endogenic morphines'). Natural methods of pain control, including, of course, acupuncture, are effective precisely because they are able to stimulate generous amounts of endorphin production

It has been found that children, and even newborn babies, are capable of experiencing pain, even if they do not express it as an adult would. Not long ago, for example, circumcisions were performed without anaesthetic because it was believed that infants were too young to feel pain. The change in mentality and practice is slowly but surely taking place in the medical profession, and pain is finally being taken seriously and treated effectively, no matter what the age of the patient.

Pain

Pain, along with tiredness, accounts for the majority of patient visits to doctors in general practice. Two simple, but related definitions can be offered here:

– pain is an unpleasant sensation felt in some part of the body

– pain is a subjective experience that cannot be shared or imparted, may be difficult to pinpoint, and cannot be measured. But at the same time, it should be seen as an important alarm signal, the body's way of protecting the organism by alerting it to a particular danger and localizing it. Once it has performed this function, it can be eliminated. Only one medical situation brings on inexplicable and unproductive pain, and that is childbirth.

It was only in 1846 that a Scottish gynaecologist, Dr. Simpson, broke with the biblical injunction that "in sorrow thou shalt bring forth children", with his pioneering use of anaesthetics in midwifery. His medical colleagues protested, maintaining that the pain of childbirth is the moral guarantee of a mother's love for her child. The clergy were also up in arms at the idea of a painless delivery, refusing to baptize children born in such conditions. It was almost a century before any real change in thinking took place, brought about firstly by the development of preparatory classes in pain-free childbirth, then by the widespread use of epidural injections.

Acupuncture

Pain is the main indication for the use of acupuncture.

TREATMENT SCHEDULE: one session once or twice a week, depending on the nature of the symptoms and/or their intensity. Some pain reduction will usually be felt within the first few sessions.

Mesotherapy

This treatment is effective for most types of pain.

TREATMENT SCHEDULE: one session once or twice a week, depending on the nature of the symptoms and/or their intensity. Again, some pain reduction will usually be felt within the first few sessions.

I would place this technique in the category of reflex therapies, as it uses tiny injectable doses of traditional medicines or homeopathic blends, and it strikes me as being similar to acupuncture, both in its areas of application and in its results. This therapy is not common in Britain and if it is used, it is only by GPs who have studied homeopathic medicine.

Transcutaneous Electrical Nerve Stimulation (TENS)

TREATMENT SCHEDULE: a brief training session should be sufficient to learn how to use the equipment, after which it can be applied daily as needed.

Osteopathy and chiropractic

This treatment is appropriate for pain in the spine or joints.

– TREATMENT SCHEDULE: Two or three sessions, one week apart.

Heat

Heat acts as an antispasmodic and a relaxant. Hot compresses on stomach cramps, a warm bath for lumbago, poultices for a backache, moxas for rheumatic pain, warm air from a hairdryer for a stiff neck, an infrared lamp for a frozen back, are just some of the ways heat can be applied.

Cold

Cold has an anaesthetic effect on pain. Some of the best-known remedies are an ice cube held against a bruise, running cold water on a burn, an ice pack for tendinitis, cold drinks given after a tonsillectomy, and the magic sponge or cold spray offered by the sports medicine specialist.

Homeopathy

There is no one specific homeopathic remedy for pain. But there are several treatments that are useful for different types of pain:

• **Aconite**: for violent, unbearable pain that has come as a shock

• **Belladonna**: for violent, inflammatory, throbbing pain such as migraine or headaches that accompany a high temperature

• **Berberis**: for the tearing, burning pain of renal colic

• **Bryonia**: for pain made worse by the slightest movement

• **Cactus**: for constrictive pain in the head and heart area

• **Chamomilla**: for teething pains

• **Cantharis**: for the pain of cystitis, for painful, burning sensations when urinating

• **Capsicum**: for the pain of earache and the feeling that the ear will burst

• **Chelidonium**: for pain at the tip of the right shoulder blade, made worse by movement and touch, improved by heat

• **Colocynthis**: for very violent, cramping pain

• **Ignatia**: for variable pain, with some spasms, and contradictory symptoms

• **Magnesia phosphorica**: for acute, cramping, biting pain that causes the patient to double over

• **Rhus toxicodendron**: for pain made worse by rest or immobility, improving on first movement

– Dosage: four 5c tablets of one, or several, of these remedies, which are to be sucked slowly like sweets, three or four times a day

Herbal remedies

Once again, there is no one specific herbal treatment for pain, except for toothache, for which cloves are the recommended remedy. But numerous plants have a localized effect on certain kinds of pain, such as marigold (Calendula) and phytolacca for sore throats, arnica and wild rosemary for bruises, and St. John's wort (Hypericum) for nervous disorders. Certain plants, such as angelica and camomile, are effective against spasms. And others are beneficial for rheumatic pain, namely devil's claw, horsetail, meadowsweet, and white willow.

Cloves

Cloves, much used here in the West to flavour certain dishes, are also a very useful medicine thanks to their anaesthetic and antiseptic properties. If you suffer from a toothache while travelling, you can soothe it by placing a dried clove next to the affected area. Even more effective is a drop of essential oil of cloves on a piece of cotton wool.

Plant essential oils

Basil, camomile and **tarragon** are digestive antispasmodics.

Cloves for dental pain.

Cajuput for certain rheumatic pains.

The Cajuput Tree

The properties of this aromatic tree from Southeast Asia are comparable to those of its relative, the niaouli tree of New Caledonia. Its essential oil is sometimes used as an ingredient in ointment for treating the pain of osteoarthritis.

Oligotherapy

Magnesium is recommended for its muscle-relaxing properties.

Headaches and migraine

Headaches are a cripplingly painful condition that has plagued mankind since ancient times. Originally thought to represent a punishment from the gods, in the Middle Ages they were believed to be caused by an accumulation of 'bad humours', while by the beginning of the 20th century they were thought to have psychological causes. We now think that headaches may have their origins in our evolutionary past, in our transition to bipedal status. Although we are gradually discovering more about headaches and how to treat them, unfortunately a complete cure still eludes us.

Headaches and their less common form, migraines, are one of the most frequent reasons why people consult their doctor. Migraine sufferers – two-thirds of whom are women – tend to live with the condition over a long period of time, consult numerous doctors, swallow many different medicines that often cause unpleasant side effects, and anxiously await any new developments in treatment.

Natural healing

Is it a migraine? If so:

– the pain is only on one side of the head (hemicranial)

– it is a throbbing headache, due to its vascular nature

– the pain comes in bouts, after which you are free of symptoms

– the pain must be accompanied by stomach upset, neurological (and/or mood) disorder, or visual disturbances, which account for the three main varieties of migraine

– you have a family history of migraine

What triggers a migraine?

We are a little more knowledgeable about the factors that set off an attack, and some can thus be prevented or avoided:

– a strong emotional reaction

– a sudden change of pace in your daily routine

– some foods and alcoholic drinks

– skipping a meal

– sensory overstimulation (such as loud music or bright, flashing lights at a concert)

– sudden physical activity

– a rapid change of temperature from heat to cold (moving, for example, from a sauna to a cold shower)

Quite clearly migraine is a very particular and multifaceted condition, which is painful, occasionally incapacitating, and difficult to treat. Doctors now have a better grasp of the illness and its seriousness, but standard tests rarely show any abnormality and we still do not understand its true cause.

Acupuncture and mesotherapy

It makes sense that these two treatments should have a role to play here because of their soothing action and because of their undeniable effectiveness against pain. They are just as helpful for headaches originating in the neck as for tension headaches or migraines, whether at the onset of the pain or as part of an ongoing course of treatment.

TREATMENT SCHEDULE: the number and timing of the sessions is a personal choice, depending on the frequency and severity of the attacks. You may opt for weekly, monthly, or even quarterly appointments;

These two methods may be used individually or in combination. They are also recommended in cases for which manipulation is unsuitable or if the patient does not want it.

Osteopathy and chiropractic

If you are dealing with headaches that have recently developed, and that do not respond to simple treatments, it can be helpful to consult an osteopath

The Menstrual Cycle, Hormones, and Migraine

– Migraines often start with the onset of puberty, returning each month at the start of the period or mid-cycle at ovulation. They may be accompanied by weight gain, water retention, breast tenderness, and anxiety – they are thus part of the general premenstrual syndrome

– These migraines mostly disappear during pregnancy, only to reappear sometime after the baby is born

– They are somewhat less predictable after menopause: most gradually disappear, but some persist, or may even worsen

– Contrary to what one might expect, surgical removal of the ovaries does not always eliminate migraine headaches

– The influence of the contraceptive pill remains unclear – it should theoretically relieve this kind of migraine, but does not always do so. There is clearly a link between migraine and hormones, but copious research on the subject has so far come to some very contradictory conclusions

or chiropractor. There might be an osteopathic lesion or something 'out of place' in the spine that could be resolved by the appropriate manoeuvre. You should, however, consult a doctor before undergoing any manipulation, just to rule out any contraindications to this treatment.
TREATMENT SCHEDULE: three sessions, ten days apart, are generally enough to solve the problem.

Manipulation of the spine is the preferred treatment for cervicodorsal (neck and upper back) pain that can bring on headaches. It is obviously not the right treatment for migraines, but tension headaches that are brought on, aggravated or prolonged by one's state of nerves can be improved by osteopathy or chiropractic treatment. So once again, an accurate diagnosis is essential, as is the choice of the most appropriate technique.

Homeopathy

Cyclamen is helpful for migraines with visual disturbances, **Iris versicolor** is best for those that bring on a stomach upset, and **Belladonna** is good for the common forms of migraine with throbbing pain.
TREATMENT REGIME: four 5c tablets of any of these treatments, to be sucked slowly three or four times a day, between meals.

Cyclamen europaeum

– Vegetable origin: the plant's knob-shaped tuber is used for this remedy

– This is the homeopathic treatment for visual-disturbance migraines
– A specific indication: the headache comes on at menstruation

Iris versicolor

– Vegetable origin: the whole flag iris plant is used, with its blue, purple, or white flowers
– The homeopathic treatment to use for migraines accompanied by acid, burning vomiting
– The specific indication: everything feels as though it is on fire – the tongue, mouth, stomach, anus...

Belladonna

– Vegetable origin: the fresh leaves and flowers of the deadly nightshade plant
– The homeopathic treatment to use for throbbing pain
– A specific indication: the violent, sudden onset of the symptoms

• You can also use Spigelon® (Heel), containing Belladonna D3, Spigelia D3, Bryonia D3, Gelsemium D3...

• Available in boxes of 50 and 250 tablets. Also available in drop bottles of 30 and 100ml

• Tablets: In general, one tablet to be dissolved under the tongue three times daily, In acute disorders, one tablet every 15 minutes

• Drops: In general, ten drops three times daily, in acute disorders, ten drops every 15 minutes

Homeopathy is an approach that pays a lot of attention to the symptoms of the individual, to the causes that trigger an attack, to the small details and particular indications normally overlooked by conventional medicine. It is a worthwhile treatment to use if you wish to tailor your management of headaches, and especially migraines, to your own needs, but it does require an in-depth consultation with a professional homeopath to determine the constitutional remedy that will get to the root of the problem.

If you are keen to try self-treatment, however, the following remedies may be helpful:

• **Ignatia**: for headaches that come on after a setback; the pain feels like a nail embedded in the skull; most common in patients who are anxious by nature and prone to changeable moods

• **Gelsemium**: for headaches that come on following a fright; the pain feels like a vice tightened round the head; it occurs mainly in patients who are emotional and given to attacks of nerves

• **Nux vomica**: the headache is brought on by eating the wrong foods, or by consuming too much coffee or alcohol; the predominant symptoms are of stomach upset. This sort of headache affects mainly angry and authoritarian personalities

– Four 7c tablets of one of these treatments, to be sucked slowly, once or twice per day

Oligotherapy

Magnesium is an almost automatic recommendation in the treatment of headaches. This trace element usually comes from the diet, which should be varied and of high quality. In cases of deficiency, which often occurs with magnesium, it can be given as a medicinal supplement.

Dietary sources of magnesium

Present in almost all foods, but mostly in the calorie-rich ones, unfortunately. The best sources of magnesium are: citrus fruits, bananas, whole-grain cereals (oat or bran flakes), cocoa and chocolate, shellfish (winkles, shrimps, oysters, and clams) and oily fish, figs, hard cheeses, nuts (almonds, peanuts, hazelnuts and walnuts), vegetables (spinach, dried and green beans, maize, split peas, and soya beans), and whole-grain bread.

• Magnesium treatment: this is available in various brands and formats, such as Organic Minerals (Colloidals) which contains 70+ trace minerals:
– Available in 946ml bottles
– Take 1–3 caps just before breakfast and/or evening meal
– Children 1 teaspoon daily for each 20lbs of body weight
Or Maximol (Ionized colloidals):
– Available in 500ml bottles
– Take ½ capful once or twice daily on an empty stomach

• You can also take higher doses of magnesium by using remedies such as Magasorb® (Lamberts) containing 150mg of magnesium (as citrate):
– Available in containers of 60 and 180 tablets
– one to three tablets daily
POSSIBLE PRESCRIPTION: one dose of magnesium twice a day, for several days or weeks.

Herbal remedies

Feverfew, St. John's wort

– Ask your herbalist to make up 20 capsules containing 200mg of dried St. John's wort extract; take one capsule twice a day with a little water

Feverfew

This herb's beneficial properties are comparable to those of aspirin: its leaves bring down fever, help headaches and migraines, reduce rheumatic symptoms, and stimulate menstrual flow.

St. John's wort

Used during the Middle Ages in cases of dementia to ward off 'evil spirits', it is currently one of the few plants known to have antidepressant properties. But it has also long been known for its effectiveness in dealing with pain

• You can treat yourself with 'Nature's Plus' Feverfew; each capsule contains 250mg of feverfew:
– Sold in containers of 60 capsules
– One capsule to be taken daily

• Another alternative is Petadolex ® (Thorne), which contains butterbur

(another important herb in the treatment of migraine):
– Available in containers of 50 gelcaps
– 1 gelcap twice daily with meals

Several other groups of plants can be suggested for alleviating different types of headache.

• Plants that soothe the nervous system, such as **angelica**, **hawthorn**, and **birdsfoot**
• Plants that act on circulatory problems, such as **garlic**, **ginkgo**, and **melilot**
• Plants that act on the gallbladder, such as **artichoke**, **milk thistle** and **fumitory**
• Plants that act on the digestion, for example, **mint** and **fennel**

– You can ask your herbalist to make up a 30ml vial of mother tincture of one of these plants. Take 25 drops in a little water, 2–3 times per day;

SAMPLE HERBAL PRESCRIPTION: ask your herbalist make up a 60ml vial of one of the following plants in a whole fresh-plant suspension. Take half a teaspoonful in a little water, twice a day.

Ginkgo

This plant increases blood flow to the brain, which brings better concentration and memory, and increased vitality. It also helps in treatment of headaches and migraines.

Mint

This is one of the main ingredients of Tiger Balm, a Chinese product which has very good local effects on headaches.

The whole fresh-plant formulation restores the full natural therapeutic effect of the plant. Artichoke, hawthorn, and melilot are available in this form.

Plant essential oils

True **Lavender**

HERBAL PRESCRIPTION: one or two drops applied locally

Lavender

This herb is grown all over the world, mostly for its delicate perfume. But it is also known for its therapeutic benefits in soothing, aiding digestion, and combating infection. Its essential oil provides very effective pain relief.

Memory problems

Being unable to find your glasses or car keys, or forgetting the phone number of the relative you rang only last night might be amusing at the age of 20, when you can put it down to having too many things on your mind. When it happens at the age of 60, it is hard not to worry about the possibility of Alzheimer's disease. But most memory problems are not nearly that serious.

Oligotherapy

The main trace elements useful against memory loss are **phosphorus** in particular, but also **magnesium**, **selenium**, and **zinc**. Trace elements are usually found in the diet, which should be varied and of high quality. In cases of deficiency, they can be given as medicinal supplements.

Dietary sources of phosphorus

The highest concentrations of phosphorus can be found in dairy products ++, but also in bananas, whole-grain cereals (such as corn-flakes), brewer's yeast, cocoa and chocolate, sparkling drinks, green, leafy vegetables (such as artichokes, asparagus, carrots, celery, mushrooms, cabbage, parsley, and soya beans), pulses such as haricot beans, lentils and peas, nuts and dried fruits (almonds, peanuts, dates, figs, hazelnuts, and walnuts), eggs, fish ++, potatoes, and meat (especially poultry ++).

Dietary sources of magnesium

Magnesium is found mainly in citrus fruits, almonds, cereals (oat flakes), chocolate, fish and shellfish, figs, nuts (hazelnuts and walnuts), vegetables (especially maize), whole-grain bread, and soya beans.

Dietary sources of selenium

Selenium is mostly found in animal products, such as meat (especially liver and kidney), saltwater fish (herring and tuna), shellfish (oysters), and eggs. Other sources include whole-grain cereals, wheatgerm, brewer's yeast, brazil nuts, and some vegetables (garlic, broccoli, carrots, and mushrooms).

Dietary sources of zinc

Zinc is plentiful in seafood, fish, oysters ++, and other shellfish, but also in meat, egg yolk, cereals, whole-grain bread, brewer's yeast, nuts, and some vegetables (broccoli, mushrooms, spinach, and beans).

• Phosphorus and magnesium treatment is available in various brands and forms – such as Organic Minerals (Colloidals), which contains 70+ trace minerals:
– Available in 946ml bottles
– Take 1–3 caps just before breakfast and/or evening meal
– Children 1 teaspoon daily for each 20lbs of body weight
Or Maximol (Ionized colloidals):
– Available in 500ml bottles
– Take ½ capful once or twice daily on an empty stomach

• You can also take Citramins® (Thorne), a citrate-bound multi-mineral formula containing selenium, zinc, magnesium, potassium and others:
– Available in containers of 90 capsules.
– One capsule three times daily

• You could also try Soya Lecithin 1100mg (Lamberts), which contains soy lecithin and vitamin E:
– It comes in containers of 120 capsules
– One to four capsules daily

A natural food

Lecithin

ORIGIN: Lecithin is one of the phospholipids, substances that are both water-soluble and fat-soluble. Lecithin is manufactured by the liver in order to disperse and dissolve fats. It is present in high concentrations in the vital organs (the brain, the heart, the liver, and the kidneys) and delivers beneficial unsaturated fatty acids to nerve cells. Because it is rich in phosphorus and amino acids, it assists in the development of the nervous system and fulfils a regulatory role in various disorders. It calms the nerves, enhances memory, helps concentration, and promotes good sleep

– It can be found principally in liquid egg yolk, nuts, and soya beans, or in sunflower, safflower, and flaxseed oils

– You can buy it from a herbalist or at a health food shop, most commonly as a soy extract. Take one teaspoonful twice a day

Vitamins

Mainly from the **B vitamin complex**

Dietary sources of B vitamins

These are plentiful in the outer layer of cereal grains (wheatgerm ++, oat flakes), green, leafy vegetables, legumes (such as beans, lentils, peas), brewer's and baker's yeast, whole-grain bread, fish, meat (especially heart, liver, or kidney), and dairy products.

• You could also try Vitamin B-100 Complex (Lamberts) a mixture of vitamins B1, B2, B3, B5, B6, B12, folic acid, PABA, choline and inositol:

– Sold in containers of 60 and 200 tablets

– One tablet to be taken in the morning

If you don't use it, you lose it...

The faculty of memory is located at various, unevenly distributed points in the brain at birth, but from that point on, its function is much more a question of daily intellectual activity, motivation, and general health, than of how old you are.

Regular, constant mental activity (whether you are at work or doing crossword puzzles) will keep the brain young. Conversely, lack of attention, anxiety, or depression may bring on mental decline, because when the mind is elsewhere, the brain is unable to 'imprint' experiences.

Herbal Remedies

Garlic, ginkgo, and **melilot** are beneficial for the circulation.

Ginseng and **oak** are excellent tonics for the body and mind.

HERBAL PRESCRIPTION: ask your herbalist to make up a 30ml bottle of mother tincture of ginkgo or ginseng. Take 25 drops in a little water three times a day for several days.

Melilot (sweet yellow or bee's clover)

Bees love melilot's clusters of yellow flowers – as the name might suggest, for *meli* is the Greek word for honey.

Oak

This mythical tree is a symbol of strength and long life, for it has been vital in the history of ship-building and it can live for several hundred years. Its bark is known for its astringent properties (i.e., it helps reduce secretions and lessen bleeding), and this has made it a popular remedy for mucous and skin problems.

Ginkgo biloba

Also known as the maidenhair tree, the ginkgo was considered sacred in the temples of Asia. Its leaves have unquestionable benefits for the circulation of the blood, thus also improving memory, helping mood swings and slowing down the ageing of the brain.

• You could also try Pure-Gar (Lamberts) containing garlic powder in 500mg capsules:
– Available in containers of 90 capsules
– 1–3 capsules daily for several weeks

• You can take Ginkgo Biloba 6000mg (Lamberts), a high strength extract of ginkgo biloba:
– Available in containers of 90 tablets
– One tablet to be taken daily

Garlic

Garlic came originally from the steppes of Central Asia, and was used in Upper Egypt to sustain the builders of the pyramids and protect them from infection. Its one drawback is its smell.

Homeopathy

Acidum phosphoricum and **Kalium phosphoricum**
– Four 5c tablets of one or both of these remedies, to be sucked like sweets between meals, twice a day for several weeks.

Acidum phosphoricum

– Chemical origin: phosphoric acid
– This is the homeopathic remedy for nervous exhaustion
– A specific indication: lack of mental alertness

Kalium phosphoricum

– Chemical origin: potassium phosphate
– This is the homeopathic remedy for emotional exhaustion
– A specific indication: physical fatigue

• You could also try Nervoheel® (Heel), containing Acidum phosphoricum D4, Ignatia D4, Sepia D4, Kalium bromatum D4
– Available in containers of 50 and 250 tablets
– 1 tablet to be dissolved under the tongue 3 times daily

• Several constitutional remedies (Calcarea phosphorica, Lycopodium, or Phosphorus, for example) are helpful against memory loss, but before taking them you need to have an in-depth consultation with your professional homeopath.

Natural healing

Calcarea phosphorica

– Chemical origin: tricalcic phosphate
– A characteristic indication: tendency to tire very quickly

Lycopodium clavatum

– Vegetable origin: the dust spores of the lycopodium or club moss plant
– A characteristic indication: tendency to be irritable in the late afternoon

Phosphorus

– Mineral origin: white phosphorus
– A characteristic indication: extreme sensitivity

Back, spine, and joint problems

The human body is a marvellous mechanism, an assemblage of 206 bones bound together by joints, held in place by tendons, and set in motion by muscles. But these delicate components wear out, seize up, become swollen, and eventually make their presence felt through pain or malfunction. Stiff neck, lumbago, sciatica, and degenerative osteoarthritis are terms we all know and fear. Patients often find the medical treatments currently offered (such as anti-inflammatory medicines or injections) to be too harsh, or simply unhelpful, and come to fear and avoid them. Natural therapies – especially osteopathy, chiropractic, acupuncture, mesotherapy, but also oligotherapy and herbal medicine – are an excellent alternative, or the ideal complement, to orthodox medical treatments.

Back pain – Osteoarthritis – Osteoporosis – Tendinitis – Sprains – Muscle cramps

Back pain

A few years ago, back pain was called (perhaps a little dramatically), 'the disease of the century'. Actually, it is not strictly speaking a disease, but a symptom – a precise diagnosis is needed, for the pain has many causes. It is very often due to poor functioning of the spinal column and of the muscles and/or ligaments that support it. Back pain is extremely common, accounting for almost as many visits to the doctor as ear, nose, and throat problems. Men whose backs are strained by their work, or by the long journey needed to get to work (driving ++), tend to complain of lumbar (or lower back) pain. Women, on the other hand, are more prone to pain in the cervical (neck) and dorsal (upper back) areas. Factors such as an uncomfortable sitting position at work, housework, and stress (++) can trigger or aggravate this pain.

Problems with rheumatic ailments cause millions of people per year to see their doctor, with pain as their only symptom in common. Back pain can generally be divided into the following categories:
– lumbago, accounting for two thirds of the cases
– sciatica, in 20 per cent of the cases
– cervical pain, in 20 per cent
– dorsal pain, in 10 per cent

Preventive measures

These are of vital importance and can be divided into five groups:

• **Movement**
– You should try to spare your back whenever possible, always seeking out a comfortable position for it
– Avoid any movement that causes pain, and treat pain signals as a warning
– Be wary of leaning forward, the familiar 'touch your toes' position from gym lessons, as it opens up the spaces between the vertebrae and may cause the disc to come into contact with the annulus fibrosus
– Be careful with twisting movements, for example, when you turn round to pick up a file or answer the telephone
– Be careful when stretching up to reach something, such as when putting a book back on a high shelf
– Crouch down on your knees when reaching down to the floor, and take the weight on your hands when you get up again, ungraceful though it might look. Strengthen and maintain the muscles of the abdominal wall; when you use your abdominal muscles, you reduce the pressure exerted on the discs by one-third

• Choice of exercise: any form of exercise is more or less injurious to the back, but be especially careful about weightlifting, judo, and tennis. Swimming, on the other hand, is highly recommended

• Equipment: you should avoid long walks or sports activities when you do not have suitable shoes, and wear warm clothing if it is cold

- Mattress and furniture: these should be 'firm', neither too soft nor too hard
- Dietary measures: your diet should be balanced and varied, and should include sufficient portions of magnesium and calcium. Keep your weight under control, as excess weight only increases the strain on the back

Three principles derived from the sport of weightlifting should always be used when lifting heavy objects: (1) keep as close to the load as possible; (2) keep your back straight; (3) lock the muscles of the back when making the lift.

Manipulation of the spine

This is at the heart of many treatments, whether they are called osteopathy, chiropractic, or occasionally vertebrotherapy. Osteopathy and chiropractic are both very popular in Britain and the US. Osteopathy is possibly better known, but chiropractic often seems more attractive because it is perceived as more gentle. Both are generally pleasant experiences and practically risk-free, contrary to what might be said or imagined.

TREATMENT SCHEDULE: three sessions one week apart should be quite sufficient in most cases.

All these manipulation methods require both 'brains' and 'brawn': a competent practitioner, the right diagnosis, complete technical mastery, and trained hands.

Acupuncture

This is one of acupuncture's most appropriate applications, and it should be systematically suggested for back pain.

TREATMENT SCHEDULE: it can be used for acute episodes at a relatively intensive rate of one session every two or three days, reducing the frequency once improvement has begun.

Mesotherapy

This therapy can be used alone or in combination with others. The micro-injections of diluted treatments directly into the affected area act relatively quickly in having an effect on spasms and muscle pains.

TREATMENT SCHEDULE: two sessions several days apart should be enough in most cases.

Acupuncture and/or mesotherapy are an excellent alternative when the patient's condition rules out manipulation of the spine, whether temporarily or permanently.

Pool exercise

This mild form of exercise can be recommended to patients of all ages, because, as Archimedes demonstrated, water supports and relieves the burden on the back, while still allowing it to exercise full mobility. As well as health spas, more and more fitness centres are also offering this type of therapy.

Pain sufferers can be divided into two basic groups

– The 10- to 20-year-old age group: the rapid growth that takes place during puberty is behind the growing pains and the deformities that may develop at this stage. Scoliosis (in which the spine takes on a lateral 'S' shape) and kyphosis (rounded shoulders) may well distort the body, but do not cause as much pain as might be imagined

– The 20- to 50-year-old age group: here the pain is the result of sedentary work, sitting in front of a computer screen, for example, or of a movement that places stress on an intervertebral disc no longer able to absorb shock as it used to. A disc at the base of the lumbar column supports more than 50 pounds of pressure in a lying position, over 300 pounds of pressure in a sitting position, and more than 1,000 pounds of pressure when we lean forward. If the disc moves out of place or 'slips' as a result of this pressure, we say that it has herniated

Stiff neck

Its medical name is torticollis, a term derived from the Latin *tortum collum*. Its literal meaning, 'twisted neck', is actually a perfect description of the symptoms. It is a reflex freezing of the muscles at the base of the neck, a painful spasm that is the equivalent of 'neck lumbago'. The pain affects otherwise healthy people, coming on with no prior warning, after a simple movement or effort, an awkward position held a little too long, after catching a chill or being in a draught. The head is twisted and tilted to one side, locked into position, since any attempt to change it causes intense pain. It does not last beyond a few days, as there are effective treatments for it. If the pain persists or recurs, you should consult a doctor.

Lower back pain

The frequency of this condition and the resulting socioeconomic effects make this a significant health problem. In the West, it accounts for millions of visits to a doctor in a year, and it temporarily disables more people under the age of 50 than any other disease or injury. In this age group, it is most often caused by some pathology of the disc, and may or may not be accompanied by hernia. Among those over the age of 50, it is usually related to osteoarthritis or a narrowed lumbar canal. Its symptoms are well known: an awkward movement or strain triggers intense pain in one side of the lower back, which is made worse by coughing, and perhaps the sensation of having 'seized up'.

Homeopathy

Bryonia

– Four 5c tablets, to be sucked slowly, four times a day between meals

Bryonia alba

– Vegetable origin: the fresh root of white bryony
– The homeopathic remedy for pain made worse by the slightest movement
– Two specific indications: the pain eases when pressure is applied or when the patient lies on the painful side

• You can also try Bryaconeel® (Heel), containing Bryonia D4, Aconitum D4 and Phosphorus D5:
– Available in packs of 50 and 250 tablets
– In general one tablet to be dissolved under the tongue three times daily. In acute disorders, initially one tablet every 15 minutes
Or you can take Rheuma-Heel® (Heel), containing Bryonia D4, Rhus toxicodendron D6, Arnica D4...
– Available in packs containing 50 and 250 tablets
– One tablet to be dissolved under the tongue three times daily

Herbal Remedies

Devil's claw and **white willow**

These two plants can be prepared and packaged by your herbalist, either individually or combined in a mother tincture, powdered in capsules, or as dried extracts.

SAMPLE PRESCRIPTION: obtain a 30ml bottle of mother tincture of white willow (known as the 'aspirin plant'), and take 30 drops in a little water twice a day. You can also massage your back with a devil's claw gel made up by your herbalist.

Devil's claw (harpagophytum)

This creeping perennial from southwest Africa has long been used by the 'witch doctors' of Namibia to relieve rheumatic pain. It comes by the name 'devil's claw' because its fruits catch the hooves of unwary antelope.

White willow

This plant has been used empirically since antiquity to treat rheumatic pain and fever. Its effectiveness comes from its high salicylic acid content – this is the main ingredient of aspirin, first synthesized from the plant in the 19th century.

• You could also try 'Bioforce' Devil's Claw in tincture form:
– Available in drop bottles of 50ml
– Take 15 drops in a little water, three times daily before meals

• Alternatively you could take AR-ENCAP® (Thorne), which includes extracts of devil's claw, turmeric and Boswellia as well as glucosamine sulphate and MSM:
– Available in containers of 240 capsules
– Take four capsules twice daily

Oligotherapy

Magnesium is highly recommended for its muscle-relaxing properties.
This trace element usually comes from the diet, which should be varied and of high quality. In cases of deficiency, which often occurs with magnesium, it can be given as a medicinal supplement.

• Magnesium treatment: this is available in various brands and formats, such as Organic Minerals (Colloidals) which contains 70+ trace minerals:
– Available in 946ml bottles
– Take 1–3 caps just before breakfast and/or evening meal
– Children 1 teaspoon daily for each 20lbs of body weight
Or Maximol (Ionized colloidals):
– Available in 500ml bottles
– Take ½ capful once or twice daily on an empty stomach

• In the case of serious muscle spasm, you could try a higher-dose magnesium supplement, such as Magasorb® (Lamberts) containing 150mg of magnesium (as citrate):
– Available in containers of 60 and 180 tablets
– One to three tablets daily

Here is an outline of the different treatments suitable for different pain symptoms, given in the order in which they should be applied:

Treatments for stiff neck

1) rest, 2) heat, 3) acupuncture and/or mesotherapy to relax the muscles and soothe the pain, 4) very gentle massage, 5) herbal and other supplements to ease the symptoms, 6) manipulation as a subsidiary treatment.

Treatments for lower back pain

1) manipulation of the spine, 2) acupuncture and/or mesotherapy, 3) complementary remedies.

Treatments for lumbago

1) rest, 2) heat, 3) acupuncture and/or mesotherapy, 4) complementary remedies, 5) manipulation as a subsidiary treatment.

Treatments for sciatica

1) rest, 2) heat, 3) medical treatment, 4) acupuncture and/or mesotherapy, 5) manipulation, but for sciatic pains rather than for the sciatica itself.

Lumbago

The word 'lumbago' is used to describe a muscle spasm in the lumbar region, often associated with an intervertebral disc starting to slip out of place. It often comes on with no warning, after unusual stress on the back, or if the person simply bends down. The sudden, stabbing pain pins the patient in an 'analgesic' position from which he or she is unable to move, for fear of an instant return of the pain. Lumbago gets better within five to ten days, but readily recurs and may develop into sciatica.

Sciatica

Sciatica accounts for about three per cent of patient visits to general practitioners, and fifty per cent of a rheumatologist's caseload. It affects men more than women, and especially those aged between 30 and 50. It generally comes on as a result of a lifting motion (perhaps performed without due care), that displaces the intervertebral disc. This in turn irritates the nerve root and triggers the symptoms.

Sciatica begins as an unbearable, knife-like pain in any part of the sciatic nerve, which runs the length of the leg from the buttock down to the foot. The pain is made worse by the slightest strain, by coughing, sneezing, or having a bowel movement. It may be accompanied by neurological symptoms, such as loss of muscle strength or sensation, which make walking difficult, if not impossible. Medical treatment is the only solution in 95 per cent of cases.

The disc

The disc is a gelatinous component that sits between two vertebrae in order to cushion the pressure from the movements of the spine. Any sort of shock is liable to push the disc's nucleus out of its membranous envelope and up against the ligament behind. The pain comes from the contact between these two structures, not unlike that produced when the dentist's drill hits a nerve.

Osteoarthritis

This extraordinarily common affliction affects, to a greater or lesser degree, about one in three of those in middle age, and four out of five people over the age of sixty-five.

Osteoarthritis is linked with the ageing process, and is thus not a preventable condition at this time (although the process can be slowed considerably with proper diet and supplementation). It is the combination of deterioration, repair and the subsequent inflammation of the joint cartilage, bones, and surrounding tissues which leads to the familiar painful, creaking, misshapen joints.

Arthritis may be felt as nothing worse than the odd twinge, or sometimes become a debilitating pain when the person gets up to walk or changes position. Rest usually helps, and it does not usually disrupt night-time sleep. It develops at a variable rate, but may well degenerate into a severe, chronic condition that is marked by flare-ups (especially in spring and autumn) and swollen, painful joints.

Being overweight aggravates arthritis because of the extra mechanical stress put on the hips and knees (a fact that applies equally well to physical activity and to injuries). Heredity plays a role too, since some of us inherit poor cartilage to begin with, and thus develop the disease earlier than others.

X-rays will confirm the diagnosis and can show up the bone spurs on the vertebrae, which are the result of the bone's rebuilding process. So-called chondro (i.e., cartilage)-protector treatments have only a palliative effect at the moment (this means that they cannot actually rebuild lost cartilage). Arthritis was long neglected by researchers because it was considered simply inevitable, but more scientists are taking an interest in it now, which leads one to hope for a breakthrough in the near future.

Outline of the different treatment options for arthritis, in order of preference:

1) physical measures,
2) complementary remedies for both on-going treatment and flare-ups,
3) acupuncture and/or mesotherapy to ease acute pain,
4) physiotherapy to help maintain mobility.

Physical measures

• Rest diminishes the pain and allows the cartilage to regenerate

• Heat is equally beneficial, in all its forms (whether warm water, heat packs, or a warm climate)

• Moderate physical activity nourishes the cartilage

• It is vital to keep one's weight down in order to reduce the stress placed on the joints

The pains of growing old

All our body tissues show signs of wear over time. Bones, and the cartilage that covers them, lose their flexibility and elasticity, become more brittle, shrink, crack, calcify, and become less able to regenerate and heal after an injury.

The more demands one places on a joint, through, for example, repetitive manual labour or strenuous athletic activity, the greater the risk that arthritis will develop. This applies particularly to the hips, knees, back, and fingers. The wrists and shoulders seem to come off more lightly.

Dietary advice

- Eliminate dairy products temporarily from your diet when your arthritis flares up
- Limit red meat to no more than two meals per week, and eat more poultry instead
- Avoid smoked or cured meats
- Eat oily fish three times per week
- Avoid butter, margarine, vegetable fats, and fried foods

Acupuncture

This treatment is more effective for acute arthritic pain than for long-term prevention.

TREATMENT REGIME: three sessions 72 hours apart should bring noticeable relief.

Mesotherapy

Mesotherapy can be used instead of acupuncture treatment, or as a complement to it.

TREATMENT REGIME: two sessions per week are in order during an acute episode.

I would place this technique in the category of reflex therapies, as it uses tiny injectable doses of traditional medicines or homeopathic blends, and it strikes me as being similar to acupuncture, both in its areas of application and in its results.

Homeopathy

Bryonia, Rhus toxicodendron

– Four 5c tablets of one of these remedies, to be sucked slowly between meals

Bryonia alba

– Vegetable origin: the fresh root of white bryony
– The homeopathic remedy for pain made worse by the slightest movement
– Two specific indications: the pain eases when pressure is applied or when the patient lies on the painful side

Rhus toxicodendron

– Vegetable origin: sumach, or poison ivy
– The homeopathic remedy for pain improved by a change in position
– A specific indication: the pain is made worse by rest

• You could also try Zeel® (Heel), containing Rhus toxicodendron D2, Arnica Montana D2, Solanum dulcamara D2, Sulphur D6 and Sanguinaria Canadensis D2:
– Available in packs of 50 and 250 tablets
– 1 tablet to be dissolved under the tongue 3–5 times daily

• It is also important that you combine these treatments with a constitutional remedy, to be chosen after consultation with a professional homeopath. Some likely choices are Natrum sulfuricum, Kalium carbonicum, or Tuberculinum residuum.

Herbal remedies

Meadowsweet, white willow

These two plants can be prepared and packaged by your herbalist, either individually or combined in a mother tincture, powdered in capsules, or as dried extracts.

Possible prescription: obtain a 60ml bottle of mother tincture of either of these plants, and take 30 drops in a little water three times a day for several weeks.

Meadowsweet (queen of the meadows)

Its regal name reflects its importance in medicinal treatment in the past, for it was used to treat practically every illness. Some of its effectiveness is due to its salicylic acid content (the main ingredient of aspirin).

White willow

White willow bark is rich in natural aspirin, which makes it useful against rheumatic pain, as well as for bringing down a fever.

You could also try meadowsweet in a whole fresh-plant suspension (this formulation's cold stabilization process restores the full natural therapeutic effect of the plant). Have your herbalist make up a 60ml bottle, and take half a teaspoonful in a little water twice a day. This treatment is for adults only.

• Another alternative is 'Herba Naturelle' tincture of Meadowsweet:
– Available in bottles of 50ml and 100ml
– Twenty drops in a little water three times daily

Plant essential oils

Yellow birch, Roman camomile, and **wintergreen** all contain anti-inflammatory ingredients.

• Obtain a 1ml bottle of one these essential oils from your herbalist, and take two drops twice a day in a little honey. (I should warn you that the Roman camomile oil is effective, but expensive.) You could also add two drops of essential oil to a teaspoonful of macerated blackcurrant flower buds in glycerine at a dilution of 1x, for full effect.

Oligotherapy

Cobalt and **manganese** are almost automatic recommendations for arthritic pain, as are **fluorine** and **sulphur**.

Trace elements are usually found in the diet, which should be varied and of high quality. In cases of deficiency, they can be given as supplements.

Dietary sources of cobalt

The best food sources of cobalt are shellfish, meats, and vegetables (mushrooms, white cabbage, onions, and radishes).

Dietary sources of fluorine

Fluorine is found principally in plants and table water, tea ++, beer, seaweed, cereals, vegetables (such as asparagus, carrots, celery, cabbage, spinach, radishes, salsify or oyster-plant, and tomatoes), leafy greens (endive, lettuce, and watercress), saltwater fish, and cherries.

Dietary sources of manganese

Manganese is plentiful in cereals, vegetables and dried fruits, almonds, soya beans, fish and shellfish, and snails.

Dietary sources of sulphur

The main food source of sulphur is eggs, but it can also be found in meat and fish, garlic, onions, and dried beans.

• Trace element remedies: these are available in various brands and formats, such as Organic Minerals (Colloidals) which contains 70+ trace minerals:
– Available in 946ml bottles
– Take 1–3 caps just before breakfast and/or evening meal

– Children one teaspoon daily for each 20lbs of body weight
Or Maximol (Ionized colloidals):
– Available in 500ml bottles
– Take ½ capful once or twice daily on an empty stomach

• You could also try Arkopharma® cod liver oil + multivitamins, which contains fish oil plus vitamins A, C and the B vitamins:
– Available in containers of 90 capsules
– One capsule to be taken per day with a glass of water

• Alternatively you could take Seven Seas® cod liver oil plus vitamins; each 525mg capsule contains fish oil plus vitamins A, D and E:
– Available in containers of 120 capsules
– One capsule to be taken daily with a glass of water

Vitamins

Primarily from the **B group**

Dietary sources of B vitamins

These are found largely in whole-grain cereals, brewer's yeast, wheatgerm, meat (especially liver), fish and seafood, vegetables (such as asparagus, mushrooms, Brussels sprouts, spinach, and lentils), whole-grain rice, and pasta.

• You could also try Vitamin B-100 Complex (Lamberts) a mixture of vitamins B1, B2, B3, B5, B6, B12, folic acid, PABA, choline and inositol:
– Sold in containers of 60 and 200 tablets
– One tablet to be taken in the morning

Note: A dessertspoonful of brewer's yeast taken at midday and in the evening will also provide these vitamins.

Osteoporosis

This is the term used to describe the loss of bone mass and of calcium, which results in brittle bones that are liable to fracture. Osteoporosis constitutes a 'silent menace' to one quarter of post-menopausal women, involving thousands of cases per year of compressed spinal column, wrist fractures, and femur fractures.

Fractures caused by osteoporosis primarily affect the vertebrae and wrists among people aged between 65 and 74. For those aged over 80, the upper femur is the most likely site for such injuries. A bone densitometry test can provide you with an accurate, reliable, and sensitive measurement of bone mass.

Risk factors

– Any family history of osteoporosis
– The early onset of menopause
– A calcium-deficient diet during childhood and throughout adulthood
– Heavy smoking or drinking
– A medical history of cortisone-based treatments
– Being underweight (for once, fat serves a useful purpose by helping protect the body from calcium loss)
– Lack of physical exercise

Preventive measures

- A daily supply of calcium in the diet from childhood onwards
- Regular, moderate physical exercise
- Giving up cigarettes and alcohol
- A daily supply of calcium and vitamin D for elderly people
- Hormone replacement therapy (HRT)

Bone calcium is enriched by a moderate exercise regimen of one hour three times a week. If you over-train, you will actually cause calcium to leach from the bones.

Dietary advice

- Limit the amount of meat and animal products you eat
- Eliminate margarine and vegetable fats, and use a little butter instead
- Take one tablespoonful per day of a mixture of olive and rapeseed oils
- Include oily fish regularly in your diet

The trace element for bones

Calcium

You can get most of what you need from cheese and dairy products, as well as from mineral water (Volvic, Vittel). Adults require about 800mg of calcium per day, but older people need 1,500mg.

Calcium found in dairy products

One glass of semi-skimmed milk (250ml) contains 370mg
One portion (50g) of Cheddar cheese: 360mg
One portion of Gruyère cheese: 250mg
One portion of Gouda: 225mg
One pot of yoghurt: 160–190mg
One portion of goat's cheese: 30–50mg

Calcium found in still mineral water brands

Talians: 596mg per litre
Hépar: 555mg per litre
Contrex: 486mg per litre
Vittel: 202mg per litre
Ashe Park 122mg per litre
Evian 78mg per litre
Volvic 115mg per litre
Panna 32mg per litre
Highland Spring 35mg per litre

Calcium found in sparkling mineral water brands

Salvétat: 253mg per litre
Quézac: 241mg per litre
Badoit: 190mg per litre
Perrier: 14 mg per litre
Pellegrino 208mg per litre
Highland Spring 35mg per litre
Ashbrook 14mg per litre

• You could also try Chewable Calcium with Vitamin D and FOS tablets(Lamberts), each of which contains 400mg of calcium:
– Sold in containers of 60 tablets, to be sucked
– One to two tablets to be taken per day. For adults. Children (4 years and over) chew one tablet daily

The vitamin for osteoporosis

Vitamin D

Dietary sources of vitamin D

The best sources of this vitamin are to be found in oily fish liver (such as that of halibut and cod), eggs, cheese (such as Brie and Emmental), and meat.

• You can take Oscap Plus (Thorne), which contains vitamin D, calcium, magnesium, boron, horsetail, vanadium, ipriflavone, folate, vitamin K, vitamin B6 and vitamin B12:
– Available in containers of 180 capsules
– Take two capsules three times daily

We can get up to 800mg of calcium per day from our diet, but this is insufficient for our increased needs in old age. And while sunlight and diet together can provide 5mcg of vitamin D, sunlight is not always available and our diet alone will provide only up to 2.5mcg of the vitamin, which is also insufficient. Thus, it is quite easy (and common) to suffer from a double deficiency, which only weakens the bones further.

Homeopathy

Silicea

– Two 7c pills to be sucked slowly like sweets, once a day for several weeks

Silicea

– Mineral origin: pure silica, which used to be extracted from quartz
– The homeopathic remedy for mineral loss
– Two typical indications: a tendency to tire easily (both physically and mentally), and a sensitivity to cold

• You could also try New Era Silica tissue salt, which contains Silicea 6x:

– Available in containers of 450 tablets

– Adults dissolve four tablets under tongue; children take two tablets. three doses to be taken daily

• It is also important that you combine these treatments with a constitutional remedy, to be chosen after consultation with a professional homeopath. Some likely choices are Calcaria phosphorica and Sulfur iodatum

Herbal remedies

Horsetail is known for its ability to restore minerals.

POSSIBLE PRESCRIPTION: ask your herbalist to make up a 60ml bottle of this herb in a whole fresh-plant suspension (this formulation's cold stabilization process restores the full natural therapeutic effect of the plant). Take half a teaspoonful in a little water twice a day.

Horsetail

This plant does not flower, but reproduces by means of spores. Its long, fluted stem is the source of its active principles, the most important of which is silica. In fact, horsetail is one of the best sources of plant minerals we know of. In the past, the plant was attached to horses' tails to help the animals drive off flies, hence its name.

Tendinitis

This is a common condition relating to pain in the tendon where it connects with the bone. The most frequent victim is the athlete over 30, as it often comes on after unaccustomed activity, or exercise performed without sufficient training or adequate equipment. However, even D.I.Y. or gardening can bring it on.

It causes pain that is triggered or made worse by tensing, or even touching, the affected tendon. The areas most vulnerable to tendinitis are the shoulder, where it causes what we call 'frozen shoulder', the elbow ('tennis elbow'), the tendons of the kneecap, and the ankle, where it may cause an inflamed Achilles tendon.

If tendinitis comes on for no apparent reason, if it does not respond to treatment, or if it keeps recurring, you should control your levels of uric acid, and see if there might be some unsuspected source of dental irritation that is causing it. A full X-ray of the teeth should reveal any problem areas.

Important advice

• Be sure to warm up properly before starting any athletic activity

• Be careful to do some 'cooling-down' stretches when you have finished. No dancer or athlete finishes a performance or competition without stretching afterwards

• Always use the appropriate equipment

• Do not play tennis in jogging trainers

(which do not provide the stability you need for lateral movements), or go for a run in tennis shoes (which are too heavy, and unsuitable for running)

• Avoid borrowing your friends' equipment – someone else's tennis racquet may be too tightly strung for you, for example, or the handle may be too big or too small

Dietary advice

Some doctors and sports trainers hold that it is an excess of acid that either causes, or at least supports, tendinitis and other pains and inflammations. It makes sense, then, to counterbalance your diet with alkaline foods (which will neutralize the acids), following the rules set out by naturopaths:

• You should avoid fatty meats (such as pork, mutton, and lamb), smoked or tinned fish, cheeses (the stronger their flavour, the more acid they contain), fried foods, crisps, seasoned and roasted nuts, cakes, spicy foods, vinegar, refined sugar, syrup, jam, chocolate, honey, coffee, tea, cocoa, and alcohol

• You should limit your consumption to no more than two servings per week of the following foods: eggs, lean meats, yoghurt, acidic vegetables (watercress, sorrel, rhubarb, tomatoes), citrus fruits (oranges, lemons, grapefruit), acidic fruits (gooseberries, blackcurrants), fruit juice, and sweetened, prepared drinks

• You should eat plenty of fresh fish, raw and cooked vegetables, leafy greens, soya milk, cereals (for example, oats, muesli, whole-grain rice, rye bread, and tapioca), fresh, unroasted nuts (such as almonds and walnuts), low-fat fromage frais, bananas, pears, and alkaline mineral waters such as Badoit

This type of regimen should be followed for one month. If at the end of that time you notice an improvement, you can reintroduce the excluded foods from one of the groups twice a week. If the symptoms recur, resume the diet for a month.

The different treatment options for tendinitis, in order of preference:

1) rest, 2) cold treatments, 3) acupuncture and/or mesotherapy, 4) manual therapies, 5) kinesitherapy combined with physiotherapy, 6) herbal and homeopathic remedies – with a view to avoiding injections and perhaps surgery if at all possible.

Non-medicinal measures

• **Rest** is the rule, but you can still continue to exercise, as long as you avoid the movements that cause pain, prolong the inflammation and delay healing. As an example, tennis players can continue to practise, provided they avoid serves and backhands if those are the moves that cause pain

• Cold should be applied either by means of ice cubes (wrapped in a cloth

Natural healing

to protect the skin), or ice-water packs. A 10- to 15-minute treatment is invaluable when used right after exercise, but remember that ice cubes from the freezer chill the skin more quickly than cold packs from the fridge

Acupuncture

This treatment is highly recommended for tendinitis.

TREATMENT SCHEDULE: Three or four sessions, four to five days apart, may well be enough to bring about a noticeable improvement.

Mesotherapy

This is the complement to acupuncture, involving tiny injections of very diluted remedies into the painful area. The solution is not injected directly into the tendon, and no cortisone is used, unlike most orthodox medical injections. There is no set number of sessions.

TREATMENT SCHEDULE: Three sessions, one week apart, may be enough to end a bout of tendinitis that is still in its early stages.

Magnets (Magnet therapy)

The disadvantage of magnets is that their effectiveness is somewhat unpredictable. However, they are so simple and harmless to use that they are worth a try.

– Attach two or three small magnets to the affected area with adhesive tape or plasters and keep them on overnight

Manual therapies

These treatments (osteopathy, chiropractic, or vertebrotherapy) can sometimes identify an underlying structural problem, which they may be able to correct.

Kinesitherapy and physiotherapy

Using 'deep transverse friction massage' (DTFM) is effective, if not exactly enjoyable. Massage can be supplemented by other physiotherapy techniques and resources, such as medical lasers.

Herbal remedies

Horsetail and **white willow**

POSSIBLE PRESCRIPTION: Ask your herbalist to make up 30 capsules of 150mg of a blend of dried extract of horsetail and white willow for each No. 2 capsule (the size of the capsule that the herbalist will use for the ingredients). Take one capsule three times a day for ten days.

Horsetail

The non-flowering plant's active principles are contained in its long, fluted stem. It is especially rich in silica, which makes it the best-known plant remedy for mineral deficiencies.

White willow

Named for its silvery-white leaves, this tree's bark contains natural aspirin compounds. It is used both to bring down a fever and to treat rheumatic pains.

• Ask your herbalist to make up a 60ml

bottle of white willow in a whole fresh-plant suspension (this formulation's cold stabilization process restores the full natural therapeutic effect of the plant). Take half a teaspoonful in a little water twice a day

• Or 'Nature's Plus' Willow Bark; each capsule contains 500mg of White Willow.
– Available in containers of 30 capsules
– Take one capsule daily

Plant essential oils

Juniper, mint, and **wintergreen**

POSSIBLE PRESCRIPTION: Ask for a cream made up of the following ingredients: 1 gram of essential oil of juniper, 3 grams of essential oil of mint, 2 grams of essential oil of winter green, made up to 50 grams with carrier cream. This is to be applied two or three times per day for several days.

Homeopathy

Arnica and **Ruta graveolens**
– Four 5c tablets of one or both of these remedies to be sucked slowly like sweets two or three times a day for several weeks

Arnica montana

– Vegetable origin: the leopard's bane plant
– The specific homeopathic remedy for bruises and the after-effects of injuries

Ruta graveolens

– Vegetable origin: the sap of the rue plant, whose strong, unpleasant smell was believed to ward off the plague
– The specific homeopathic remedy for ligaments and tendons

• You could also try Arnica-Heell® (Heel), containing Rhus toxicodendron D6, Arnica D3, Bryonia D4, Dulcamara D4...
– Available in drop bottles containing 30 and 100ml
– Ten drops three times daily

• You could add a topical ointment such as Weleda Arnica ointment:
– Available in 25g tubes
– To be applied three or four times daily

Sprains

Sprains are usually the result of an injury to one or more of the ligaments that support a joint, most commonly the knee or ankle. They are marked by varying degrees of pain and swelling. Sprains should not be ignored, for that may prolong the pain, there may be

Treatments for sprains, in order of preference:

1) Arnica to be applied straight away,
2) ice packs,
3) immobilization,
4) acupuncture and/or mesotherapy,
5) homeopathy and herbal remedies.

functional impairments, and there is always the risk of a repeat injury.

Ice packs

An emergency measure to be applied as soon as possible in order to bring down the swelling, which is caused by blood released by the injured ligament.

– Half fill a plastic bag with ice. Add a little salt to the ice to make it melt faster, then wrap the bag in a towel and place it on the sprain for 15-minute periods. There is, of course, no need to use a thermometer, but ice treatments should bring the skin's temperature down to about 25° C

Immobilization

It is essential to immobilize a sprain both so as not to aggravate the injury, and also because immobility has an analgesic (pain-killing) effect.

– The best solution is a support bandage, such as those made by UniChem®, Boots or Elastoplast®. It is sometimes necessary to put a plaster cast on more serious sprains

Acupuncture

This treatment is beneficial both soon after the accident to relieve the pain, and later on to encourage healing.

TREATMENT SCHEDULE: two sessions per week for two or three weeks.

Mesotherapy

This can be used instead of acupuncture treatment, or as a complement to it.

– Minute quantities of various remedies can be delivered through intradermic micro-injections directly to the site of the injured ligament

TREATMENT SCHEDULE: two or three sessions at weekly or ten-day intervals.

Magnets (Magnet therapy)

The disadvantage of magnets is that their effectiveness is somewhat unpredictable. However, they are so simple and harmless to use that they are worth a try.

– Attach two or three small magnets to the affected area with adhesive tape or plasters and keep them on overnight

Homeopathy

Arnica can be used systematically in all its forms, whether as tablets, or a gel to be rubbed on, or as a topical mother tincture.
– Four 5c tablets every half-hour, four or five times immediately after the injury, then two or three doses per day over the next few days

Arnica montana

– Vegetable origin: the leopard's bane plant
– The specific homeopathic remedy for injuries of various kinds

• For pain relief, you could also try Rheuma-Heel® (Heel), containing Bryonia D4, Rhus toxicodendron D6, Arnica D4...

– Available in packs containing 50 and 250 tablets

– One tablet to be dissolved under the tongue three times daily

• A constitutional homeopathic remedy is also in order here, combined with physiotherapy to help strengthen the ligaments. Professional homeopaths often prescribe Calcarea fluorica and Natrum carbonicum

Herbal remedies

Horsetail and **meadowsweet**

• Both of these herbs should be obtained in a whole fresh-plant suspension (this formulation's cold stabilization process restores the full natural therapeutic effect of the plant). Ask your herbalist make up a 60ml bottle of either one of these herbal remedies, and take half a teaspoonful in a little water twice a day

Trace elements for tendons and ligaments

Known to most people as fluoride, the element added to water or toothpaste to help prevent tooth decay, fluorine is also the fundamental constituent of bones, tendons, and ligaments. It can thus be helpful in preventing repeated sprains.

Dietary sources of fluorine

Fluorine is found principally in plants and table water, tea ++, seaweed, salt-water fish, cereals, vegetables (such as asparagus, carrots, celery, cabbage, spinach, radishes, salsify or oyster-plant, and tomatoes), leafy greens (endive, lettuce, and watercress), cherries, and beer.

• Fluorine treatment: this is available in various brands and formats, such as Organic Minerals (Colloidals) which contains 70+ trace minerals:
– Available in 946ml bottles
– Take 1–3 caps just before breakfast and/or evening meal
– Children 1 teaspoon daily for each 20lbs of body weight
Or Maximol (Ionized colloidals):
– Available in 500ml bottles
– Take ½ capful once or twice daily on an empty stomach

Muscle cramps

This is the sensation of sudden, intense pain and involuntary tightening of a muscle, usually in the leg. It comes on with no warning, and usually lasts no more than a few seconds (a few minutes in more serious cases), but it leaves residual soreness in the affected muscle, and is liable to recur in the same place. It is improved by stretching the muscle or muscles involved. Although we do not know the exact cause of muscle cramps, hydration levels and certain minerals are known to be important factors.

Natural healing

Treatments for cramp, in order of preference:

1) One simple movement: stretching, 2) water,
3) homeopathy, 4) trace elements (copper and magnesium),
5) B vitamins, 6) brewer's yeast,
7) acupuncture.

One simple movement

When a cramp comes on, you must stretch the contracted muscle immediately. You often see this among soccer players, for example, when the match is extended into extra time.

Water

This is an essential treatment, and you must drink enough of it, especially after exertion. The best water to drink in the recovery phase after exercise is brands with high bicarbonate content, such as Badoit, or those with a high magnesium content, such as Vittel.

Homeopathy

Cuprum

– Four 5c tablets to be sucked slowly, two or three times in succession

Cuprum metallicum

– Mineral origin: metallic copper
– The specific homeopathic remedy for cramp

Oligotherapy

Copper in the first instance, but also **calcium, cobalt, magnesium, manganese**, and **potassium**

Trace elements usually come from the diet, which should be varied and of high quality. In cases of deficiency, they can be given as a medicinal supplement.

Dietary sources of calcium

The best sources of calcium are dairy products.

Dietary sources of cobalt

The best food sources of cobalt are mushrooms, white cabbage, shellfish (such as lobster), onions, radishes, and meat (especially liver).

Dietary sources of copper

Copper is to be found principally in seaweed, almonds, avocado pears, cocoa, cereals (especially in whole wheat and whole-grain rice), mushrooms, shellfish, veal and lamb liver ++, dried fruit and nuts, oysters, green vegetables, fish roe, and tea.

Dietary sources of magnesium

The best sources of magnesium are: citrus fruits, whole-grain cereals (oat or bran flakes), chocolate, fish and shellfish, oil-producing nuts (almonds, hazelnuts, and walnuts), vegetables (maize ++ and soya beans), and whole-grain bread.

Dietary sources of manganese

Manganese is plentiful in beetroot, cereals, chocolate, nuts (such as almonds, hazelnuts, and walnuts), wheatgerm, green vegetables, soya beans, egg yolk, and tea.

SAMPLE PRESCRIPTION: one dose of manganese-and-cobalt treatment in the morning, and one of manganese-and-copper treatment in the afternoon and evening, for two weeks. This should be combined with a magnesium supplement.

• You could also try Calcium-Magnesium Citramate (Thorne) which is a blend of calcium citrate-malate (80mg), magnesium citrate-malate (80mg) and malic acid (240mg):
– Available in containers of 240 capsules)
– Take one to three capsules three times daily.

Vitamins

Primarily the **B complex** vitamins

• You could try Berocca®, a blend of vitamins B and C, with calcium and magnesium:
– Available in a tube of ten effervescent tablets
– One tablet to be taken in the morning, dissolved in water, each day for ten days

The natural food for cramp

Brewer's yeast

– This is a living substance derived from a microscopic fungus, prepared up to now specifically as a supplement to the beer-brewing process. It is not the same as baker's yeast, and is better tolerated by the digestive system. It is an extraordinary food supplement, being low in fat, salt, sugar, and calories, but packed with essential proteins and amino acids, minerals (chromium, phosphorus, potassium, and selenium) and B vitamins. It is obtainable from health food shops and pharmacies in the form of tablets, capsules, and flakes (be warned, it tastes bitter). Take one dose three times a day

Acupuncture

This treatment is appropriate for cramp due to its muscle-relaxing effects.

There is an acupuncture point located on the calf, below the gastrocnemius muscle, especially favoured by rickshaw drivers in China. Stimulated at frequent intervals, it allowed them to ward off cramps – presumably one of the hazards of the job.

Gynaecological problems

Complementary therapies have much to offer the field of gynaecology, as they are appropriate for all ages and stages of a woman's life, namely puberty, pregnancy, and menopause. They can be used as a long-term treatment, as a complement to orthodox medical treatment, or as an actual alternative to what has become the systematic prescription of hormones. Soya and yam, in particular, have recently come to the forefront as elements in the more natural treatment of menopause.

Premenstrual syndrome – Painful, heavy periods – Pregnancy problems – Hot flushes and menopause

Premenstrual syndrome

Studies show that from 25 to 90 per cent of women suffer from this condition – and these figures represent only those women who seek treatment. This syndrome comprises varied and multiple symptoms that appear with each period, and subside when it has passed. The symptoms include painful swelling of the breasts or abdomen, temporary weight gain or simply water retention, pains in the stomach, abdomen or lower back, and mood disorders with increased irritability or temporary depression. Researchers have put forth numerous hypotheses to try to explain its onset, but none so far seems to provide all the answers.

Dietary advice

- Reduce your consumption of dairy products before and during your period, as they interfere negatively with oestrogens
- Avoid fats for the same reasons
- Cut down on your salt intake if you tend to retain water during this period
- Eat as much cereals and fibre as you can manage
- Eliminate alcohol and stimulants (tea and coffee) from your diet for this period

Acupuncture

Acupuncture helps regulate the menstrual cycle, calms the nerves, and helps circulatory problems – three good reasons to use it for this syndrome.
TREATMENT SCHEDULE: Initially, six sessions two weeks apart to bring the syndrome under control; the schedule can then be modified depending on the symptoms and the length of the cycle.

Homeopathy

Lac caninum for breast tenderness.
– Four 5c tablets to be sucked slowly like sweets, three to four times a day depending on the symptoms

Lac caninum

– Animal origin: the milk from a mother dog
– The specific homeopathic remedy for pre-menstrual breast pain and tenderness

Folliculinum for its regulating action.
– Four 7c tablets, to be taken once a day, beginning in the second half of the cycle
– If you show signs of hyperfolliculin (nausea, breast tenderness, heaviness in the legs, changes to the cervical mucus) or of marked psychological symptoms (irritability, mood swings), you could take six tablets at a strength of 15c or 30c in one dose
– If not, take this remedy as prescribed, at 7c, for its regulating properties

One homeopathic rule prevails, even

though it has not been scientifically confirmed:
– Low dilutions (5c) are said to have a stimulating effect
– Average dilutions (7c) are said to have a regulating effect
– High dilutions (15–30c) are said to have either regulating or curbing effects

Folliculinum

– Hormonal origin: diluted, dynamized oestrogen
– This remedy is considered the 'homeopathic hormone treatment'
– Folliculinum is often prescribed by professional homeopaths, but there is still some debate as to its effectiveness, the appropriate dilution to give, and the best time to prescribe it. Some propose it should be given mid-cycle at ovulation, while many give it at the end of the cycle

• You could also try Hormeel® S (Heel), containing Pulsatilla D4, Sepia D6, Viburnam opulus D3
– Available in drop bottles containing 30 and 100ml
– In general, 10 drops 3 times daily

• It is also important that you combine these treatments with a constitutional remedy, to be chosen after consultation with a professional homeopath. Some likely choices are Actaea racemosa, Nux moschata, or Pulsatilla

Actaea racemosa

– Vegetable origin: black cohosh or cimicifuga
– The homeopathic remedy for pain and nervous disorders aggravated by menstruation

Nux moschata

– Vegetable origin: nutmeg
– One of the homeopathic remedies for hysterical symptoms with mood and personality changes

Black cohosh or cimicifuga

This herbaceous plant grows in open woodlands and along fields in North America (Canada and the USA). The plant grows up to two metres tall, with large leaves bearing clusters of small white flowers. Herbal preparations use the plant's dried, fibrous roots and rhizomes, which have a narcotic smell and an acrid taste. Black cohosh was long considered a cure-all by the natives of North America, and used to treat menstrual problems and to hasten along slow deliveries (hence its other name of 'squaw root'), as well as for rheumatic pains, lung ailments, and agitation.

Herbal remedies

Chasteberry, evening primrose, and sage

PRESCRIPTION: Ask your herbalist to make up 30ml bottle of mother tincture of sage. Take 25 drops in a little water three times a day during the week before your period until it starts.

• You can also try Menosan (Bioforce) Sage drops:

Natural healing

– Available in tincture form in bottles of 50ml
– 15 to 20 drops in a little water, 3 times daily before meals

Sage

Sage, from the Latin *salvare*, to save, has been used as a cure-all since Greek and Roman times, as it helps treat stomach upsets as well as gynaecological problems. Sage has been discovered to contain plant hormones, whose properties help regulate the menstrual cycle and reduce hot flushes.

Evening primrose

This plant with large, yellow flowers grows in rocky soil in North America. The seeds have been pressed for their oil ever since scientific discoveries showed its medicinal use for a wide range of complaints. The key substance in the oil is gamma-linoleic acid, an unsaturated fatty acid responsible for various chemical reactions that are vital for good health. It has been found that borage also contains this acid, but whereas evening primrose primarily benefits gynaecological conditions, borage is more useful for skin complaints.

• Oil of evening primrose is available in Lamberts® 1000mg, which also contains vitamin E:
– Available in containers of 90 capsules
– One to three capsules daily

Vitex agnus castus or chasteberry

Its Latin name, 'agnus-castus', means chaste lamb, and it has been a symbol of chastity since the days of antiquity. The fruits of this pungent tree from Central Asia were used in medieval monasteries as a condiment to dampen sexual appetite (another name for it is 'monk's pepper'). Recent scientific findings show that it also affects the hormonal balance in women and can be used to regulate the menstrual cycle.

• You could try Bioforce Agnus castus in tincture form:
– Available in bottles of 50ml
– 15 to 20 drops in a little water twice daily

Wild yam

Wild yam was used for centuries in Central America for the relief of menstrual and ovarian pain. In 1936, Japanese researchers found that its effectiveness is due to a chemical substance found in the roots and tubers, diosgenin, a naturally occurring progesterone precursor. The plant has also been found to contain precursors of DHEA (dehydroepiandrosterone), a substance produced in the adrenal glands, which has been much in the news of late.

Painful, heavy periods

Menstruation is a natural occurrence and is not normally painful, except occasionally in young girls. Pain accompanies an ovulatory cycle, which is why women on the pill do not suffer from menstrual pain, and why gynaecologists offer this method of contraception as the treatment for it.

Under the influence of oestrogens, the tissue that lines the uterus thickens in preparation to receive an egg. If fertilization does not take place, the drop in hormone levels produces a contraction in the uterine vessels, and the mucous lining, no longer fed by blood vessels, begins to shed. Periods generally last from three to five days, and produce on average the equivalent of half a glass of blood (3–4 fluid ounces) – in some cases much more.

A simple measure: heat

Heat promotes blood circulation and relaxes the muscles.

One very simple, but truly beneficial, remedy is a hot-water bottle held against the stomach for a few minutes several times a day.

Acupuncture

Acupuncture's effectiveness against all kinds of pain makes it a suitable treatment here, even during menstruation.

TREATMENT: Two sessions ten days apart before your period is due, then again just before or as it starts.

Homeopathy

Colocynthis and **Magnesia phosphorica** for period pain.

Colocynthis

– Vegetable origin: the dried pulp of the colocynth or bitter apple
– The homeopathic remedy for violent but intermittent pain, such as cramps
– There are four characteristic modalities: the pain is improved by applying strong pressure, or heat, by a curled-up position, or by movement

Magnesia phosphorica

– Chemical origin: magnesium phosphate
– The homeopathic remedy for unbearable spasms that come and go abruptly
– A specific indication: the pain is improved by heat

Cyclamen and **China** for painful periods with heavy bleeding.

Cyclamen europaeum

– Vegetable origin: the corm of the plant
– The homeopathic remedy for the combination of pain and bleeding
– There are two characteristic modalities: the pain is made worse by fresh air, and improved by a warm room

China

– Vegetable origin: the bark of the cinchona tree, source of quinine

– The homeopathic remedy for haemorrhage
– A specific indication: there is dizziness accompanied by headache
– China is of historical interest because it was the first remedy tested by Samuel Hahnemann, the 'father' of homeopathy

– Four 5c tablets of one or several of these remedies to be sucked slowly three to four times a day, depending on the symptoms

• You could also try Lehning® Rosmarinus complex 24 whose ingredients include China 1x and Pulsatilla 3x:
– Sold in 30ml bottles of oral drops
– Fifteen drops to be taken in a little water three times a day while the period lasts

• It is also important that you combine these treatments with a constitutional remedy, to be chosen after consultation with a professional homeopath. Some likely choices are Actaea racemosa, Pulsatilla or Sepia

Pulsatilla

– Vegetable origin: the meadow anemone or windflower
– One of the homeopathic remedies for scanty, irregular periods with thick, dark blood
– Some specific character traits: a shy, emotional nature, very gentle but of changeable mood, inclined to sadness, cries easily, with a need for signs of sympathy

Oligotherapy

Iron ++

Dietary sources of iron

Iron is found mainly in black pudding, cocoa, spinach, soya flour, liver, beans, lentils, mussels, potatoes, red meat and offal, and wine.

• For those women who need iron for blood loss, but who dislike black pudding and red meat (the two foods that contain the most iron), supplements such as Floradix Liquid Iron Formula can help replace it:
– Available in bottles of 250ml and 500ml
– Take two teaspoons before morning and evening meals

• You could also try trace-element combinations such as Premtis® (Lamberts), which includes iron, magnesium, calcium, folic acid, copper, zinc, vitamin B12, B6 and others:
– Available in containers of 120 tablets
– Two tablets to be taken daily

Herbal remedies

Yarrow, evening primrose, sarsaparilla, sage, and **crampbark**

POSSIBLE PRESCRIPTION: Ask your herbalist to make up a 30ml bottle of mother tincture of yarrow. Take 25 drops in a little water three times a day from the night before your period is due to start until it ends.

Yarrow or milfoil

Yarrow is an aromatic, herbaceous plant with slender upright stalks and white or pinkish flowers in separate, narrow clusters. It is used first of all to heal wounds: its Latin name, 'Achillea millefolium', comes from the Greek hero Achilles whose tendon was apparently healed by this herb. Another of its common names, soldier's woundwort, is even clearer on the subject. But it is also a tonic and a sedative, a digestive stimulant and anti-spasmodic, a diuretic, and an anti-allergy remedy (useful for hay fever). It also relieves uterine cramps and painful periods.

• You could take Herba Naturelle Sarsaparilla:
– Available in bottles of 100ml
– 20 drops in a little water 3 times daily

• Evening primrose is available most often in the form of capsules obtainable from your pharmacy. Each capsule contains between 400 and 600mg of cold-pressed oil. Take one capsule two or three times a day during the second half of your cycle

• You could also try Lamberts® Evening Primrose Oil (1000mg), which also contains vitamin E:
– Available in containers of 90 capsules
– 1 to 3 capsules daily

Sarsaparilla

This climbing vine grows in the tropical forests of Latin America, Asia, and Australia. Used for many years to treat the skin eruptions of syphilis, it is still used in dermatology to treat cases of psoriasis and eczema. It is also a depurative (a purifying agent) and a diuretic, it stimulates the immune system, and also has a hormonal effect, which makes it useful for menstrual problems. Its root is still eaten in some countries for its stimulating and (some say) aphrodisiac effects.

Crampbark

Also known as viburnum, this North American shrub's bark and roots were used by the native people to treat dysentery. It is also considered the specific plant for painful periods, for its sedative effect on the uterus. It is also one of the ingredients in treatments for circulation.

There's iron and there's iron

There are two categories of iron:

– 'Heminic' iron represents only 10–15 per cent of dietary iron, but it is very well absorbed by the body. This kind is found in black pudding, meat, and fish

– 'Non-heminic' iron is found in greater quantities in the diet, but is less well absorbed (only 8 per cent of it). The main sources of non-heminic iron are cereals, vegetables, fruits, and dairy products. Priority should therefore be given to the first food group, since it provides more useable iron

Evening Primrose

A native of Virginia in the United States, evening primrose was first brought to Europe in the 17th century. Its almost magical curative properties meant that at first it was reserved for the king's personal use only. Only gradually did it eventually become available to all. These days, it is most commonly used by women, because its natural anti-inflammatory effects make it helpful against the more unpleasant aspects both of premenstrual syndrome (depression and irritability, breast tenderness, abdominal pain, water retention, headaches) and of menopause (hot flushes, skin changes, and mood disorders).

Oil of evening primrose and borage have attracted the attention of researchers, since both contain the 'good' kind of fatty acids, the unsaturated kind that are essential for optimum health. Evening primrose is particularly helpful for gynaecological conditions, while borage is more helpful for the skin.

Pregnancy problems

The special time of pregnancy is also often accompanied by some rather troublesome complaints – many of which can be helped or eliminated by complementary therapies, especially as they present no risks to the baby.

Diet

Being pregnant means an increased need for vitamins and minerals:

- You need more protein – from eggs, cheese, milk, and meat
- During the first six months, a pregnant woman requires 1,500mg of calcium per day, increasing to 2,000mg from seven months until delivery. You should eat plenty of skimmed milk, cheese, and yoghurt
- Take 30–50mg of iron each day, to avoid becoming iron-deficient
- Take a zinc supplement as well
- You need to supplement your folic acid (or vitamin B9): 15mg per day
- Make sure you get plenty of magnesium
- Vitamin D is another requirement; you need 400–1,000mg every day so as not to risk hypocalcaemia in the newborn baby

Oligotherapy and vitamins

If you do not wish to take trace-element remedies, you will need to get these elements and vitamins from your diet:

Calcium

Calcium is found not only in dairy products, but also in mineral waters, which can provide as much calcium as milk. Calcium also comes from green vegetables (broccoli, Brussels sprouts, spinach, green beans, and watercress), nuts (almonds and walnuts), and fish (such as shrimp, sardines, and salmon).

Iron

Iron is found mainly in black pudding, cocoa, spinach, soya flour, liver, beans, lentils, potatoes, red meat and offal, and wine.

Magnesium

The foods rich in magnesium are citrus fruits, almonds, cereals (such as oat flakes), chocolate, fish and shellfish, snails, figs, nuts (hazelnuts and walnuts), vegetables (especially maize), whole-grain bread, and soya beans.

Zinc

Zinc comes from broccoli, cereals, mushrooms, spinach, seafood, beans, oysters ++ and shellfish, brewer's yeast, nuts, egg yolk, fish, and meat.

Vitamin D

Vitamin D is found mainly in oily fish (especially halibut and cod ++), where it is concentrated in the liver, eggs, cheese (such as Brie or Emmental), and meat.

Vitamin B9

Folic acid is most plentiful in green or leafy vegetables, but also in offal, apricots, beer, carrots, cereals (whole wheat), beans, and eggs.

Relaxation methods

These are tremendously useful because, by learning to control your breathing, bodily sensations and mental processes, you can relax and thereby lessen your fear of the unknown and your anxiety over the delivery to come. This will make the actual delivery easier and less painful. 'Pain-free childbirth', however misnamed, draws on these relaxation methods to calm you in preparation for what is, after all, a natural process.

Morning sickness

Morning sickness is such a well-known symptom that for most people it is synonymous with pregnancy. It affects half of all pregnant women, and comes on most often in the morning soon after waking. Certain smells seem to induce nausea, even if they are not in themselves unpleasant (some examples are cheese, spices, cosmetics, and perfumes), and even if the woman quite likes them under normal circumstances. Fortunately, these stomach upsets usually disappear of their own accord about the fourth month.

Homeopathy

Nux vomica and Sepia

– Four 5c tablets of one or both of

these remedies to be sucked slowly two or three times a day, reducing the frequency once morning sickness begins to improve

Nux vomica

– Vegetable origin: nux vomica or poison nut
– The homeopathic remedy for nausea that comes on after eating
– A characteristic sign: the feeling that vomiting would bring relief

Sepia

– Animal origin: squid ink
– The homeopathic remedy for nausea brought on by the smell or even the sight of food
– A specific indication: a tendency to suffer from low moods or clinical depression

Skin problems

Pregnant women often look radiant, with glowing complexions. Pregnancy alters the skin's texture, drying it out somewhat as the production of sebum goes down. This is helpful for oily skins, which look less shiny.

– You may see some acne develop round about the fifth month, caused by higher hormone levels. Be careful not to abrade the skin with excessively harsh cleansing products

– The 'pregnancy mask' is formed of yellow or brown patches on the face that come on especially after exposure to the sun. This discoloration will fade gradually over time, but is liable to reappear with any further sun exposure. To avoid it, be sure to protect your skin by using a total sunblock

– The increased hormone levels occurring at the fifth month are also responsible for other instances of hyper-pigmentation, involving the whole body: the areolas of the breasts darken, and in 90 per cent of women a dark line develops from the navel down to the pubis

– Many women worry about stretch marks, although they are in fact fairly rare. They may appear on the thighs, abdomen, and breasts in the sixth month of pregnancy, in the form of purplish streaks that gradually fade to a pearly white after the baby is born. They were long thought to be caused by the stretching of the skin, but we now know they are related to an often-hereditary loss of the skin's elasticity. They do fade with time, but no treatment can get rid of them completely

These skin complaints are not really serious, but are still a cause of concern to expectant mothers. A few simple changes to your diet can help prevent them, or at least minimize them.

Back pain

This very common condition of pregnancy can be roughly divided into two phases:

– Back pain in the first trimester is easily treatable, as a common mechanical problem, by gentle manipulation of the spine or by acupuncture

– Back pain in later pregnancy is caused by the baby's growth as it presses on the epidural area, and is more difficult to treat. The best and simplest solution is to rest with the legs slightly elevated, on a systematic basis

Three outlines for treatment of back pain, in preferential order:

– Pain in early pregnancy:
1) manipulation, 2) acupuncture, 3) homeopathy

– Pain in mid-pregnancy: 1) rest, 2) acupuncture, 3) homeopathy

– Pain in the late stages of pregnancy: 1) rest with the legs slightly elevated, 2) homeopathy, 3) acupuncture

Homeopathy

Actaea racemosa and **Bryonia**

Actaea racemosa

– Vegetable origin: the black cohosh or cimicifuga plant
– The homeopathic remedy for pain in the upper back or trapezius area
– A characteristic sign: alternating states of depression and agitation

Bryonia alba

– Vegetable origin: the white bryony plant
– The homeopathic remedy for pain brought on by the slightest movement
– A characteristic indication: the pain is improved by rest

– Four 5c tablets of one or both of these remedies to be sucked slowly once or twice a day when the pain comes on

Constipation

This complaint affects almost every woman at some point during pregnancy, even those who do not normally suffer from it.

Homeopathy

Hydrastis and Nux vomica

– Four 5c tablets of one or both of these remedies to be sucked slowly once or twice a day during bouts of constipation

Hydrastis canadensis

– Vegetable origin: the root of the goldenseal plant
– The homeopathic remedy for constipation with no urge to have a bowel movement
– A specific indication: the stools are hard and fragmented

Haemorrhoids

The condition of pregnancy tends to dilate the veins and inhibit venous return, with the result that bouts of haemorrhoids are very common.

When they are troublesome, avoid too much wine at dinner and alcohol in general, as well as spicy foods and condiments.

Homeopathy

Aesculus hippocastanum and **Collinsonia**

– Four 5c tablets of one or both of these remedies to be sucked slowly once or twice a day when hemorrhoids are painful

Aesculus hippocastanum

– Vegetable origin: the horse chestnut
– The homeopathic remedy for congestion caused by haemorrhoids
– Two specific indications: the condition is made worse by heat and by prolonged standing

Collinsonia canadensis

– Vegetable origin: the horse balm plant
– The specific homeopathic remedy for haemorrhoids combined with constipation
– Stools are large and very difficult to evacuate

Heavy legs and varicose veins

A feeling of heaviness in the legs, puffiness after standing for any length of time, and the appearance or worsening of varicose veins are all common symptoms among pregnant women. To help these conditions, your diet should be rich in the following:

– **Vitamin E**, found principally in asparagus, spinach, whole-grain cereals, wheatgerm, cold-pressed oils such as olive oil, lettuce, and soya beans

– **Vitamin C**, which is plentiful in citrus fruits (lemons, oranges, and grapefruits), spinach, parsley, and tomatoes

– **Vitamin B3**, which comes mainly from black- and redcurrants, brewer's yeast, blackberries, and blueberries

Homeopathy

Hamamelis

You can take Aesculus composition (Heel) which contains Hamamelis D4 and Aesculus D1 among others:
– Available in drop bottles containing 30 and 100ml
– In general 10 drops 3 times daily. In acute disorders initially 10 drops every 15 minutes

Hamamelis virginiana

– Vegetable origin: a small shrub, the Virginian witch hazel
– The homeopathic remedy for congestion and inflammation of the veins
– A specific indication: the pain is made worse by heat

Herbal remedies

Witch hazel, horse chestnut, and **red vine leaf**

Possible prescription: Ask for a preparation of dried extracts of witch hazel and red vine leaf, 150mg of each in a No.2 capsule (the size of the capsule that the herbalist will use for the ingredients). Take one capsule in the morning and another at night for several days.

Minor infections

Homeopathy

Homeopathy is a particularly valuable treatment against infection, as it is not advisable to use antibiotics, especially tetracycline, during pregnancy.

Aconite, Belladonna, or **Ferrum phosphoricum**: any of these 'anti-fever' remedies can be used, to be chosen according the patient's symptoms.
– Four 5c tablets of one of these remedies to be sucked slowly, several times in succession, reducing the frequency once the infectious symptoms begin to improve

• You could also try an Aconite compound such as: Aconitum-Homaccord® (Heel) which contains Aconite D2, D19, D30, D200, Eucalyptus D2, D10, D30 and Ipecacuanha D2, D10, D30, D200:
– Available in drop bottles containing 30 and 100ml
– Generally 10 drops to be taken three times daily. Initially 10 drops every 15 minutes

• I recommend instituting preventive measures, as these will spare you most winter colds and infections

Oligotherapy

• **Copper** is the basic anti-infectious agent, and should be prescribed systematically at the first sign of infection. You can take this in colloidal form, such as Organic Minerals (Colloidals) which contains 70+ trace minerals:
– Available in 946ml bottles
– Take 1–3 caps just before breakfast and/or evening meal
– Children 1 teaspoon daily for each 20lbs of body weight

Or Maximol (Ionized colloidals):
– Available in 500ml bottles
– Take ½ capful once or twice daily on an empty stomach

You should get an accurate medical diagnosis for a fever, especially during pregnancy. But remember that being pregnant raises the body's temperature to about 37.4° in the morning and 37.8° at night.

Insomnia

This common problem typically gets worse in the later stages of pregnancy, but you should still not take sleeping pills, which are contraindicated anyway.

Homeopathy

Coffea
– Four 5c tablets to be sucked slowly at bedtime, to be repeated once or twice during the night if need be

Coffea cruda

– Vegetable origin: the coffee plant
– The basic homeopathic remedy for disturbed sleep
– Specific indications: identical to the

symptoms brought on by drinking too much coffee

Herbal remedies

Black horehound, California poppy, and **lime blossom**

Anaemia

This condition is to be expected among pregnant women and should be systematically treated with an iron prescription. You could either take iron supplements or increase your consumption of iron-rich foods (see above).

Fatigue in later pregnancy

It is hardly surprising that carrying several pounds of extra weight will make you more tired and breathless after any exertion. The answer is to listen to your body and reduce your activities.

Delivery

Homeopathy

Homeopathy can be used before, during, and after the delivery of the baby.

• **Actaea racemosa** and **Gelsemium**: these remedies should be started a few days before the baby is due to keep natural anxiety under control:
– Four 7c tablets of one or both of these remedies to be sucked slowly like sweets twice a day between meals

• **Arnica** and **China**: these should be started when the contractions begin, and continued for 48 hours to avoid or reduce bleeding:
– Four 7c tablets of one or both of these remedies, to be sucked slowly like sweets three or four times a day between meals
• **Caulophyllum**: during childbirth to make it easier:
– Four 5c tablets to be sucked slowly, three or four times during delivery

• **Sepia**: to prevent or treat post-partum depression:
– Four 7c tablets to be sucked slowly twice a day, for several days or weeks

Breast-feeding

• **Belladonna** and **Bryonia**: for engorged breasts.
– Four 5c tablets of one or both of these remedies to be sucked slowly between meals, three or four times a day for several days

• **Calcarea carbonica**: to stimulate falling milk production.
– Four 5c tablets to be sucked slowly between meals, two or three times a day for several days

Medicine and the menopause

In the last few years there has been an increasing tendency to treat the menopause as a medical issue, with the result that HRT is now much more widely prescribed, even though we cannot be sure that it is entirely harmless.

Each woman needs to draw up her own list of the pros and cons of this treatment, taking into account her needs, wishes, and expectations, and her individual risk factors, as well as the advantages, drawbacks, and risks of HRT, in order to make a fully informed decision.

Hormone replacement therapy is contraindicated in cases of breast and endometrial cancer, which would tend to confirm that it does carry some risk to those organs. Women seem in general to be aware of the potential dangers, and are showing some caution: millions of women are going through menopause or peri-menopause at this very moment, but only a small percentage are having HRT.

What are my real reasons for having HRT?

– Improving my quality of life, or, more specifically: the end of hot flushes, feeling happier and more optimistic, with fewer mood swings, a good or better quality of sleep, continuing to enjoy a good sex life, a more youthful-looking skin, being able to stay young longer

– Increasing my life expectancy, or, more specifically: preventing osteoporosis and reducing the risk of heart disease

– But the value of the treatment is in some doubt when we consider the possible risks to the breasts and endometrium

We, as doctors, have evidence to believe that this sort of treatment can help prevent some broken bones and heart disease. But there are also reasons to think that it is not risk-free, and that it might in some cases be dangerous. The decision as to whether or not to take hormone treatment is a difficult one, a very personal one, and it is finally the (informed) woman's choice.

Hot flushes and menopause

Menopause is defined as the cessation of the reproductive function, which means in concrete terms that menstruation stops, the ovaries cease functioning, and their hormones are no longer secreted. The consequences of this hormonal shortfall are well known, producing a group of symptoms that are typical at this stage in a woman's life. These include not only the familiar hot flushes, but also vaginal dryness that may result in pain during intercourse, drying skin inclined to look thin and dull, and a tendency towards low moods, if not outright depression. Two other conditions have long-term importance: the loss of calcium from the bones, which could lead to osteoporosis, and increased risk of heart disease.

Hot flushes generally start two years before menstruation comes to an end. They usually continue during the first three years of menopause in the form of a sudden sensation of uncontrollable heat. The flushing mostly affects the face and upper body, and is accompanied by sweating and sometimes trembling, lasting a few seconds or a few minutes. This may be repeated several times during the day or night, and can greatly hamper one's social, professional, or personal life. Hot flushes are connected with the drop in oestrogen secretion, which disturbs the body's heat control mechanism in the brain.

Here are some gentle, alternative solutions to help the body compensate for the missing hormones:

Diet and menopause

In women over the age of 50, there is a risk of deficiency in calcium, copper, fluorine, magnesium, phosphorus, selenium, zinc, and vitamins D and E. Such deficiencies can have effects on the whole metabolism, and must be compensated. Trace elements and vitamins usually come from the diet, which should be varied and of high quality.

A recent scientific study suggests that the reason Japanese women rarely suffer from hot flushes is that they eat much more soya and beans, foods that contain large quantities of oestrogen precursors or phyto (plant)-oestrogens.

Acupuncture

Acupuncture is helpful for several unwanted symptoms of menopause, such as hot flushes, mood disturbances, and weight gain.

TREATMENT SCHEDULE: one session every two weeks, to be adapted depending on the symptoms.

Homeopathy

Lachesis and **Sanguinaria** for hot flushes.

Lachesis mutus

– Animal origin: the venom from a South American snake
– One of the great homeopathic

menopause remedies, effective both for mood and for hot flushes
– A characteristic sign: talkativeness

Sanguinaria canadensis

– Vegetable origin: the roots of the Canadian bloodroot plant
– The homeopathic remedy for excess blood flow to the head
– A characteristic indication: the cheeks become red during hot flushes

– Four 7c tablets of one or both of these remedies to be sucked slowly two or three times a day

• You could also try Lehning® L25, which contains a blend of several remedies including Actaea racemosa 3x:
– Sold in 30ml bottles of oral solution

– Twenty drops to be taken in a little water two to three times a day

• It is important that you combine these treatments with a constitutional remedy, chosen after consultation with a professional homeopath. Some likely choices here are Lachesis, Sepia, or Sulfur

Herbal remedies

Evening primrose is the first choice.

• The seeds are cold-pressed to extract the oil, which provides the therapeutic benefit.
– It is obtainable from the pharmacy, herbalist, or health food shop, most often as capsules each containing between 400 and 600mg of evening primrose oil

– Two capsules to be taken per day for two weeks each month during perimenopause, three capsules per day during menopause

Other beneficial herbs include:

• **Black cohosh, sage**, or **soya** for their oestrogen-like action
• **Yarrow, sarsaparilla, chasteberry** and **yam** for their progesterone-like effects
• **Ginkgo, ginseng**, and **common periwinkle** for their anti-ageing benefits

POSSIBLE PRESCRIPTION: Ask your herbalist to make up a 60ml bottle of mother tincture of sage. Take 25 drops in a little water three times a day for several weeks.

Common periwinkle

This plant contains a substance that improves blood flow to the brain, promoting its oxygenation. It is also one of the ingredients in a renowned classical remedy for mental deterioration in the elderly.

• You could also try Nature's Plus Black Cohosh (extended release); each tablet contains 200mg of black cohosh:
– Available in containers of 30 tablets
– One tablet to be taken daily

• Another alternative is Isoflavone (Nutri):
– Available in containers of 60 capsules, each containing 60mg of isoflavones
– One to two capsules taken daily

• Or you could take MenoBalance®

(Bional), which contains soya extracts and extract of Angelica sinensis:
– Available in containers of 60 capsules
– One capsule twice daily with meals

Soya

Soya is a subtropical plant, probably first grown in Manchuria. After five thousand years of cultivation and use in Asia, it appeared in the West in the 18th century. Various states in the US now grow more soya than maize, and the country now leads the world in soya production. Although it is grown intensively almost everywhere, it does require a hot climate to flourish. Soya has provided the impetus to herbal therapies and natural medicines in the struggle to find an alternative to the monopoly of hormone replacement therapy (HRT).

Urinary problems

These might seem at first glance to be the domain of orthodox medicine, but herbs and homeopathy can play a very useful complementary role here. One very common problem is that of recurring bladder infections, which antibiotics treat very well in the short term, but which they seem unable to prevent. The observation, made in the 19th century, that 'the microbe is nothing, the terrain is all', remains equally valid today.

Cystitis – Kidney stones (renal colic) – Prostate problems

Cystitis

Cystitis describes a disorder of the bladder caused by (in most cases) E. *coli* bacteria from the area of the urethra (the bladder's evacuation tube). The term 'cystitis' is now more commonly heard today than 'bladder infection'.

Cystitis is a minor ailment, benign as a rule, but frustrating because it persistently returns. It is extremely common and young women are the most frequent victims (four per cent of women aged between 20 and 30 suffer from it at least once). Post-menopausal women can also be affected (since the loss of vaginal secretions tends to favour genital infections), as can pregnant women (one out of ten).

The symptoms are an urgent and repeated need to urinate, accompanied by burning, painful and stinging sensations during urination, a heavy feeling in the lower abdomen, and sometimes the passing of a little blood in the urine (known as haematuria). Two important negative signs distinguish cystitis from other bladder infections: there is no high temperature, and no pain in the lower back. A cytobacteriological urine test can confirm the presence of bacteria, and if the infection is sufficiently serious, antibiotics will be prescribed.

General advice

A better understanding of the processes that trigger or sustain the symptoms – that allow the contamination of the bladder or vagina by bacteria from the intestine – will go a long way towards improving or minimizing the infection:

- Both lack of attention to personal hygiene and (less obviously) too much of it can interfere with the balance of bacterial flora and promote infection
- Do not wear very tight clothing or synthetic underwear, which provide the closed, moist environment in which bacteria flourish
- Try to prevent or treat constipation, as it can cause a proliferation of intestinal bacteria
- Since sexual intercourse can help transmit bacteria from the vagina or anus to the bladder and thus trigger an infection, make it a practice to empty your bladder after sexual relations
- At the first sign of symptoms, make sure you drink a litre and a half of water each day in order to dilute your urine. Use drinking bottles so you know how much liquid you are getting
- Pass urine often – even if this is painful during periods of infection

Essential dietary advice

- Avoid alcoholic drinks for the period of the infection
- Avoid very strongly brewed coffee and tea
- Do not eat asparagus, watercress, or tomatoes
- Eat plenty of foods containing vitamin C, which is mainly concentrated in citrus

fruits (lemons, oranges, and grapefruit), green vegetables such as celery, sorrel, parsley, and green cabbage ++), and fruits such as blackcurrants ++ and kiwi fruit ++, as well as strawberries, raspberries, and redcurrants

• Supplement your diet with vegetables (such as garlic and onions) and herbs (thyme, cinnamon, mint, and oregano) known for their effectiveness against infections

Also take a tonic such as ginger or bee pollen. This second item can be obtained from your herbalist or health food shop, either in capsule form or in bulk from glass jars. To prepare it, put one teaspoon of pollen in half a glass of water before you go to bed, cover and leave overnight. Drink the mixture next morning with breakfast.

Bee pollen

This looks like a fine yellow-orange dust, made up of the thousands of microscopic specks which are the male flower seed normally picked up by certain bees as they search for nectar. In the hive it is mixed with honey and used to nourish the bee larvae, which is why popular wisdom has always attributed life-giving properties to the pollen. Indeed, it does contain numerous minerals (copper, iron, magnesium, potassium, and silica), amino acids (glutamine and methionine), vitamins A, B, C, and E, as well as superoxide dismutase, a substance that fights the formation of free radicals.

Oligotherapy

Copper or a combination of **copper, gold, and silver** for their anti-infective properties.

Magnesium for its role in relieving the feeling of heaviness in the lower pelvis.

Trace elements usually come from the diet, which should be varied and of high quality. In cases of deficiency, they can be given as a medicinal supplement.

Dietary sources of copper

This element is found in small quantities in almost all foods, except in milk which contains almost none. The highest concentrations of copper come from (calf and sheep's) liver ++, seaweed, shellfish such as scallops and oysters, lobster, fish roe, almonds, avocados, cocoa, cereals (whole wheat and whole-grain rice), mushrooms, dried fruits, green vegetables, walnuts, plums, soya beans, and tea.

Dietary sources of magnesium

Magnesium is found in almost all foods, but principally in calorie-rich ones, unfortunately. The best sources are citrus fruits, bananas, whole-grain cereals (oat flakes or bran), cocoa and chocolate, shellfish (winkles, shrimps, oysters, and clams) and oily fish, snails, figs, hard cheese, nuts (almonds, peanuts, hazelnuts, and walnuts), vegetables such as spinach, green and dried beans, maize, split peas, and soya beans, as well as whole-grain bread.

Natural healing

• Copper and magnesium treatments: these are available in various brands and formats, such as Organic Minerals (Colloidals) which contains 70+ trace minerals:
– Available in 946ml bottles
– Take 1–3 caps just before breakfast and/or evening meal
– Children 1 teaspoon daily for each 20lbs of body weight
Or Maximol (Ionised colloidals):
– Available in 500ml bottles
– Take ½ capful once or twice daily on an empty stomach

Homeopathy

Cantharis, Formica rufa
– Four 5c tablets of each of these remedies to be sucked slowly every ten minutes, reducing the frequency once the symptoms improve.

Cantharis

– Animal origin: the whole green blister beetle or Spanish fly is used
– The homeopathic remedy for any burning pain
– Also a remedy for conditions with itching, burning vesicles or blisters (rashes or shingles, for example)
The blister beetle or Spanish fly secretes an irritating, toxic substance used in the past for 'love potions' as an aphrodisiac.

Formica rufa

– Animal origin: the red ant
– The homeopathic remedy for cloudy, foul-smelling urine

• You could also try Lehning® Juniperus Complex 6, whose ingredients include Belladonna 3x and Cantharis 8x:
– Sold in 30ml bottles of oral drops
– Fifteen drops to be taken in a little water, three times a day

In order to ward off further occurrences of the infection, Colibacillinum (a treatment made from a sterilized, diluted E. *coli* culture) is often prescribed.
– Six 7c tablets to be taken once a week for several months

• It is also essential to determine the constitutional remedy that will get at the root of the problem, but this requires an in-depth consultation with a professional homeopath and is not a matter for self-treatment

Herbal Remedies

Wild lime sapwood, which helps pain and inflammation.

Blueberry is effective against the E. *coli* bacterium.

– Either drink a cup of herbal tea (tisane) or a decoction of lime sapwood twice a day, or ask your herbalist to make up a 30ml bottle of mother tincture of blueberry, and take 40 drops of this in a little water twice a day for a fortnight

Lime sapwood

Lime sapwood comes principally from the Roussillon area of the south of France. Sapwood is the trunk's second, living, layer of bark, below the outer bark. It contains many active principles, which make it a useful remedy, particularly for its draining action.

Blueberry

Whilst the fresh berries are a laxative, the dried fruits have a more constipating and anti-infective effect, and the leaves are good for cystitis.

You could also try Solgar® Blueberry Leaf Extract; each capsule provides 100mg of standardized Blueberry Leaf extract:
– Available in containers of 60 vegicaps
– One or two vegicaps daily with meals

Plant essential oils

Oregano and **mountain savory**
Add one drop of essential oil of Spanish oregano and one drop of essential oil of mountain savory to an infusion of thyme mixed with one spoonful of honey. Take after lunch and dinner.

Oregano

Still sometimes called wild marjoram, this hardy mountain plant also acts to soothe the nervous system. The ancient Greeks and Romans used to place it or plant it near tombs in order to bring peace to departed souls.

Kidney stones (renal colic)

Urine's function is to eliminate water and micro-crystals that have come from natural wastes, and it circulates within narrow ducts (called ureters) only a hairsbreadth in diameter. If the urine flow should diminish due to dehydration (from excess heat or insufficient liquid), or if the quantity of waste material increases, these crystals may clump together to form a stone (a process called lithiasis). In 80 per cent of cases, this occurs in someone who consumes a lot of milk and chocolate, and the stone is made of calcium oxalate, is small, fairly hard, and spiny like a sea urchin. In 20 per cent of cases, the sufferer is someone who enjoys rich food, including a lot of meat. In these cases, the stone is larger, harder, more rounded, and made of uric acid. In very rare cases, the stone is formed of phosphates, ammonia, or magnesium.

The onset of intense, continuous pain in the abdomen or lower back, radiating down to the pubis, usually indicates kidney stones. No position brings any relief from the pain, which may be accompanied by a state of extreme agitation. A few drops of blood may be passed in the urine. A previous history of kidney stones, or perhaps a recent trip to a hot country, will also help confirm the diagnosis.

Renal colic can normally be treated at home, except in four situations in which you need to go to hospital:

– in cases of doubt as to the diagnosis,

which could become a surgical emergency
– the presence of a high temperature (above 38.5° C), since a simple case of renal colic never involves a fever
– unbearable pain
– the cessation of urination altogether (known as anuria)

Extreme discomfort may justify the prescription of powerful antispasmodic medicines, along with complementary therapies.

Important general advice

The last thing you must do during an attack of renal colic is to drink large quantities of water, since that will only increase the amount of blocked urine, and thus increase the pain. Limit yourself to half a litre per day. When the crisis abates, two litres a day is the recommended quantity of water.

• If you have a calcium-containing stone, cut down on your consumption of dairy products, tea, coffee, and chocolate

• If you have a uric acid stone, limit your intake of game meat, offal, smoked or cured meats, tinned meats, fish (such as anchovies, herring, or sardines), and shellfish. Vegetables are safe, except for mushrooms, but chocolate may also bring on an attack. Taking the waters at a spa may be sufficient to dissolve a uric acid stone in about ten days

The various medicines we have at our disposal nowadays may tempt patients to think that diet is of secondary importance. In fact, diet is crucial, since any excess, particularly of fats, sugars, and alcohol, has an immediate impact on the metabolism of uric acid.

Homeopathy

Belladonna and **Calcarea carbonica**

– Four 5c tablets of both these remedies to be sucked slowly every ten minutes, reducing the frequency as the symptoms improve

Belladonna

– Vegetable origin: the deadly nightshade plant
– The homeopathic remedy for intense, paroxysmal pain, such as migraine or renal colic
– A specific indication: the sudden, violent onset of the pain

Calcarea carbonica

– Mineral origin: oyster-shell calcium
– The homeopathic remedy for infectious conditions, skin complaints – and kidney stones. It is the logical treatment, since most kidney stones are calcium-based
– A specific indication: an extreme sensitivity to cold

You can also try Plantago-Homaccord® (Heel) which contains Belladonna, Plantago major and Ignatia in various potencies:
– Available in drop bottles of 30 and 100ml
– In general, 10 drops 3 times daily. In

acute disorders, initially 10 drops every 15 minutes

- It is also essential to determine the constitutional remedy that will get at the root of the problem. A professional homeopath is likely to prescribe Calcarea carbonica, Lycopodium or Sulfur It is worth noting that Calcarea carbonica can be used both as a short-term remedy for acute episodes and as a constitutional remedy – only the modalities will vary.

Herbal Remedies

Parietaria

– This is available mainly as a herbal tea (tisane), two or three cups to be drunk daily. You can improve its unpleasant, insipid taste by adding one drop of essential oil of orange

Parietaria

Parietaria, or pellitory-of-the-wall, is a member of the nettle family. It has a long treatment history as a urine 'softener' (or emollient).

Prostate problems

The prostate, the male sex gland, is roughly the shape and size of a chestnut and weighs about three-quarters of an ounce in a 30-year-old man. It is normally elastic and flexible, easily allowing the neck of the bladder to open for urination purposes. However, over time, the prostate grows larger, loses its elasticity and begins to obstruct the bladder, which marks the beginning of the urinary difficulties.

Adenoma (or benign hypertrophy) is almost inevitable in the older male, affecting 80 per cent of men. A longer life expectancy, and the ageing of the population in general, are transforming this condition into a public health problem, particularly as cancer of the prostate is the second most common form of cancer among men.

The prostate's secretions, a milky, slightly acidic fluid due to the presence of citrates, form the first approximately 30 per cent of the ejaculate.

The role of the prostate

The prostate has numerous functions:
– it plays a part in the production of sperm by improving its quality, and therefore its fertility
– it acts on the viability and the motility of the sperm cells
– it supplies a liquid environment for the sperm, providing immune protection
– it allows the bladder to empty by relaxing its muscular area, something it does less and less well over time
– prostate fluid also seems to provide some protection against infection, perhaps due to its zinc content

There is a marked contrast between the diminished function of the prostate after the age of 60, and the increased risk of disease in the organ.

Symptoms

Although the symptoms vary from one patient to the next, the normal progression of the adenoma takes place in stages, starting generally after the age of 50:

– the first phase is marked by the frequent need to urinate (pollakiuria), especially at night, a need that may become urgent and cause considerable inconvenience

– this is followed by difficulties with micturition itself: trouble with the first stage of urination, with the need to push or strain, a diminished urine stream, requiring more time to finish emptying the bladder, with occasional signs of a few drops of post-urination incontinence

– a slow, but steady worsening of these symptoms

– the possible occurrence of acute episodes of urinary retention, requiring hospital treatment

These clinical symptoms are likely due to hormonal influences, since men who have been castrated before puberty (fortunately, there are very few nowadays) do not develop adenoma.

Monitoring

This is done by means of questions, a clinical exam, and ultrasound and biological indications.

• The types of questions the doctor asks are a reflection of the difficulties you may be having: Do you feel you have to strain when you urinate? Is there a delay before the urine starts to flow? Do you feel any burning sensation as you pass urine? Does your urine stream seem weaker than in the past? Does it take longer to urinate now? Do you feel your bladder is completely emptied when you finish? How many times do you have to get up in the night to go? Do you ever feel the need to urinate when you cannot hold it in? In what circumstances?

• The three standard tests for the monitoring and diagnosis of prostate problems are a rectal examination, a PSA (prostatic specific antigen) blood test, and an ultrasound scan

• Medical treatment is enough in most cases, over a number of years. If the discomfort the prostate causes becomes too severe, the possibility of surgery may be discussed

A few tips

• Keep up moderate physical activity

• Avoid fizzy drinks, alcohol, or other liquids in the evening

• Cut out spicy food so as to help limit prostate enlargement

Homeopathy

Sabal serrulata is the standard remedy, which you can take for life.

– Four 5c tablets to be sucked slowly like sweets twice a day for months

You could also try Lehning ® 6 Juniperus ComplexJ, whose ingredients include Sabal 2x, Thuja 3x and Belladonna 3x:

– Available in 30ml bottles of oral drops
– Twenty drops to be taken in a little water, three times a day

Or you can take Sabal-Homaccord® (Heel) which contains tincture and potencies of Sabal serrulatum as well as Hepar sulfur in various potencies:
– Available in drop bottles containing 30 and 100ml
– In general, 10 drops 3 times daily. In acute disorders, initially 10 drops every 15 minutes

Sabal or saw palmetto

The hazelnut-scented berries of this small North American palm tree are said to have some hormonal effects that increase prostatic health, cleanse the urine and stimulate the libido.

Herbal remedies

Onion, nettle, and **saw palmetto**

Onion

The onion bulbs from our kitchen gardens contain anti-infective agents, and have been used for this purpose since Greek and Roman times. During the Middle Ages, onions were hung beside cloves of garlic in the doorway of the house to ward off the plague. The onion's decongestive, diuretic, and anti-inflammatory properties recommend it for prostatitis.

Nettle

The roots of the stinging nettle were used in country remedies to cure bed-wetting in children. In adults, nettle can help prostatitis and revive sexuality. The young shoots can be eaten like vegetables or in soups for their nutritional, depurative (blood purifying) and tonic value.

POSSIBLE PRESCRIPTION: Ask your herbalist to prepare a 125ml bottle of nettle in a whole fresh-plant suspension. Take half a teaspoonful in a little water morning and night.

You could also try Nature's Plus Pygeum, which contains 100mg of pygeum, an African plant:
– Available in containers of 30 softgels
– One softgel to be taken daily

• Alternatively you could take Prostanol® (Bional) which is a combination of vitamin E, magnesium, zinc, pumpkin seeds, saw palmetto and extract of nettle:
– Available in containers of 40 capsules
– Take 1 capsule 3 times daily for a month, then 1 capsule daily as maintenance

Pygeum africanum

The wood from this African plum tree is extremely hard, and is used for making carts. The bark is the source of the extract that is helpful in prostate conditions.

Oligotherapy

Magnesium

This trace element usually comes from the diet, which should be varied and of high quality. In cases of deficiency, which often occurs with magnesium, it can be given as a medicinal supplement.

Magnesium treatment: this is available in various brands and formats, such asOrganic Minerals (Colloidals) which contains 70+ trace minerals:
– Available in 946ml bottles
– Take 1–3 caps just before breakfast and/or evening meal
– Children 1 teaspoon daily for each 20lbs of body weight
Or Maximol (Ionized colloidals):
– Available in 500ml bottles
– Take ½ capful once or twice daily on an empty stomach

Skin troubles

The skin is not simply an envelope for the body, but is an organ in its own right, with several functions: the protection of the body from outside attack, the maintaining of body temperature, the elimination of toxins through sweat and sebum, as well as a fundamental sensing role via its millions of nerve endings. Our skin reflects our general state of health, looking radiant when we are well, and unhealthy when we are ill or under stress. It is an organ visible to others, and may in certain cases (such as acne or psoriasis) be accompanied by relationship problems that only compound the underlying anxiety. The skin is also an outward sign of social status, as the importance of a tan will testify. We will try any number of beauty products and medical and surgical treatments to try to mask the skin's tell-tale signs of ageing, as we try to hold back the idea of our own mortality.

Acne – Eczema – Psoriasis – Cold sores (herpes simplex) – Warts and verrucas – Burns – Shingles – Heavy perspiration – Hair problems – Nail problems

Acne

This skin condition may be quite a harmless and minor ailment, but it does not seem that way to the 80 per cent of all teenagers who have it. It is in many ways a rite of passage destined to blight some part of our adolescent years. The various unsightly combinations of red spots, pustules, blackheads, and cysts appear mainly on the face and back. While hormonal in origin, it is also linked to the sebaceous glands (source of the sebum that covers and protects the skin), which become infected. Acne most often diminishes or cures itself spontaneously by the age of 18 or 20. The rarer, more severe forms (four per cent of cases) may require treatment with antibiotics or vitamin A (Roaccutane®)

What causes acne?

– Just before the onset of puberty, the sebaceous glands on the face, shoulders, and chest begin producing an excess of sebum

– This glandular hypersecretion, which is linked with the production of male hormones (in girls as well as in boys), combines with an increase in dead cells that block up the pilo-sebaceous gland. The sebum then accumulates beneath the skin, forming micro-cysts and blackheads

– The skin's bacteria find a favourable growing environment in the oily sebum, which only exacerbates the symptoms

Some tips on cleanliness

These are important to follow:

• Do not use household soap on your face, very good though it may be for laundry, for this will dry out your skin. Similarly, avoid antibacterial solutions (liquid soaps), which are too harsh

• Instead, use facial cleansing bars, moisturizing soaps, and mild cleansing gels, which cut down on the production of sebum without harming the skin

• Do not scrub your face with a flannel, still less with a massage glove, for this will eliminate the skin's protective film and promote irritation

• Be careful in the sun, because although sunlight improves the skin in the short term, there may be a further outbreak of spots when the holidays are over

Dietary advice

• Avoid sweetened foods as much as possible

• Do not eat too much bread or starchy foods (such as pizza or quiche), fats (dishes with sauces, cream, mayonnaise), or chocolate

• Limit your intake of dairy products, especially of whole, unskimmed milk

• Stay away from smoked or cured meats, ready meals, and hamburgers

• Tinned foods should be avoided if possible

• Eat plenty of fruit, vegetables, and cereals +++

• Take one tablespoonful of olive oil or borage (Starflower) oil per day

• Cigarettes and alcohol will not improve your skin

• Treat any constipation through simple, natural nutritional means (see the section on 'Digestive disorders', p. 163)

The natural food for the skin

Brewer's yeast

ORIGIN: A living substance specially prepared as a supplement, from a minute fungus that serves as a ferment in the preparation of beer. It is not the same as baker's yeast, and is better tolerated by the digestive system.

COMPOSITION AND PROPERTIES: Yeast is packed with B vitamins, minerals (such as chromium, phosphorus, potassium, and selenium) and essential amino acids. It reinforces the immune system, helps fight infections, and restores the balance of intestinal flora. It boosts the health of the skin, nails, and hair.

METHOD OF USE: It is obtainable from health food shops and pharmacies in the form of tablets, capsules, and flakes for sprinkling on food.

Oligotherapy

Zinc

Trace elements are usually found in the diet, which should be varied and of high quality. In cases of deficiency, zinc can be given as a medicinal supplement.

Dietary sources of zinc

Zinc is most plentiful in seafood, oysters ++, fish, and shellfish, but it is also found in cereals, some vegetables (broccoli, mushrooms, spinach, and beans), brewer's yeast, walnuts, wholemeal bread, egg yolks, and meat.

• Zinc treatment: this is available in various brands and forms – such as Organic Minerals (Colloidals) which contains 70+ trace minerals:
– Available in 946ml bottles
– Take 1–3 caps just before breakfast and/or evening meal
– Children 1 teaspoon daily for each 20lbs of body weight
Or Maximol (Ionized colloidals):
– Available in 500ml bottles
– Take ½ capful once or twice daily on an empty stomach

• You could also try trace-element combinations such as Premtis® (Lamberts), which includes iron, magnesium, calcium, folic acid, copper, zinc, vitamins B12, B6 and others:
– Available in containers of 120 tablets
– 2 tablets to be taken daily

• You could also try Lamberts® Zinc/Copper, which contains a blend of zinc(15mg per tablet), and copper (1mg per tablet):
– Sold in containers of 90 tablets

– Take 1 tablet daily on an empty stomach

Vitamins

Principally vitamins A, B, C, and E:
– Vitamin A preserves the skin's elasticity,

promotes healing, and helps the skin resist infections
– the B vitamins play an important role in the health of the skin, helping to combat seborrhoea and blackheads
– Vitamin C contains anti-infective properties
– Vitamin E speeds up the healing process and helps prevent skin ageing

• You could also try Megavit® (Lamberts), which combines vitamins A, B, C, and E, and zinc, selenium and the bioflavonoids:
– Sold in containers of 60 and 180 tablets
– 1 to 2 tablets daily

A mineral treatment: clay

This substance cleans the skin deep down by absorbing all the impurities like blotting paper, tightening the dilated pores of the skin as it dries.

PREPARATION: You can buy it as a loose powder from a speciality shop or from some pharmacies. Prepare it by adding it to water (and not the other way round) in order to avoid lumps, and stir. Leave the mixture for at least an hour before applying it to the affected areas twice a day.

Homeopathy

Kalium bromatum and **Selenium**
– Four 5c tablets of one or both of these remedies to be sucked slowly between meals, twice a day for several weeks

Kalium bromatum

– Chemical origin: potassium bromide
– The specific homeopathic remedy for hardened pustules in oily skin

Selenium

– Mineral origin: metallic selenium
– The homeopathic remedy for oily skin with blackheads
– A specific indication: marked fatigue

• You could also try Psorinoheel® (Heel), a type of homeopathic skin purifier which contains Sulfur D6, Psorinum D10, Medorrhinum D12
– Available in drop bottles of 30 and 100ml
– Take 10 drops 3 times daily

• It is also important that you combine these treatments with a constitutional remedy, to be chosen after consultation with a professional homeopath. Some likely choices are Natrum muriaticum, Sepia, or Sulfur

Sulfur

– Mineral origin: sulphur
– The constitutional homeopathic remedy for skin problems
– Two specific indications: the skin condition is made worse by water, and improved by cold

Herbal remedies

Burdock and **heartsease**
POSSIBLE PRESCRIPTION: Ask your herbalist to make up a 30ml bottle of mother tincture of one of these two plants. Take

25 drops in a little water three times a day for several weeks.

Burdock

This plant has long been used for making poultices, but is also very effective against skin infections, and helpful for most skin conditions generally. It also acts as a depurative (or blood-purifying agent), which makes it a useful treatment for bouts of fever or rheumatism.

Heartsease

Also known as wild pansy, this plant is a member of the violet family, and has always been used to treat skin ailments. Its aerial parts have a detoxifying effect which helps treat itching, acne, or eczema.

- You could also try Herba Naturelle Heartsease:
  - Available in bottles of 50ml and 100ml
  - 20 drops 3 times daily in a little water

Ask your herbalist to make up a 60ml bottle of burdock in a whole fresh-plant suspension (this formulation's cold stabilization process restores the full natural therapeutic effect of the plant). Take half a teaspoonful in a glass of water twice a day. This is not to be taken by children under 15 years of age.

Calendula

POSSIBLE PRESCRIPTION: Obtain a 30ml bottle of mother tincture of calendula (or marigold) from your herbalist. Sprinkle a few drops on a compress and apply it two or three times daily to the affected areas.

Calendula

The petals of the marigold flower possess healing and antiseptic properties that make this a most useful plant for minor skin wounds that have developed a secondary infection, and it is a principal ingredient in most soothing creams. This herb also promotes purification and drainage, which means that it is helpful in eliminating toxins.

Nettle

- You could try Nature's Plus Nettle, which contains 250mg of extract of nettle:
  - Available in containers of 30 capsules
  - Take 1 capsule daily

Nettle

Nettle has always been widely used for its medicinal properties, despite its painful, stinging hairs. These contain histamines and formic acid, which produce the itching, painful rash. But the plant itself has depurative, tonic, and remineralizing properties, and is also helpful for skin complaints. The young shoots can be eaten as a vegetable (cooked in soup) for their fortifying virtues, and the aerial parts are used in the preparation of herbal remedies. Nettle root has a diuretic effect.

Eczema

Eczema is a skin complaint characterized by patches of red, irritated, inflamed skin with small, itching blisters or scabs. It is likely that the illness is linked to some allergen. Although it can affect all ages, babies and small children are the most prone to eczema. It generally appears at about seven or eight months, and is usually cured by the age of three, but may occasionally persist into adulthood, remaining a chronic condition that flares up periodically. Eczema, like other skin problems, is difficult to live with on a day-to-day basis, both for the patient and for those close to him or her.

General advice

- It is important to try to identify any food allergy that may be triggering the condition, especially in children (see page 304 of the section on 'Allergies')
- Use moisturizing skin bars so as not to dry out the skin
- Take warm baths, avoiding water that is too hot or cold
- Take care not to let the skin dry out, by using moisturizing lotions and humidifiers
- Avoid wearing jewellery containing nickel, as this can often provoke contact dermatitis
- Wear cotton, not synthetic, underwear

Some tips on diet

- Avoid sweetened foods as much as possible
- Do not eat too much bread or starchy foods (such as pizza or quiche), fats (dishes with sauces, cream, mayonnaise), or chocolate
- Limit your intake of dairy products, especially of whole, unskimmed milk
- Stay away from smoked or cured meats, ready meals, and hamburgers
- Tinned foods should be avoided if possible
- Eat plenty of fruit, vegetables, and cereals +++
- Take one tablespoonful of olive oil or borage (starflower) oil per day
- Keep cigarettes and alcohol to a minimum, and treat any constipation through simple, natural nutritional means (see page 163 of the section on 'Digestive Problems')

The natural food for the skin

Brewer's yeast

ORIGIN: A living substance specially prepared as a supplement, from a minute fungus that serves as a ferment in the preparation of beer. It is not the same as baker's yeast, and is better tolerated by the digestive system.

COMPOSITION AND PROPERTIES: Yeast is packed with B vitamins, minerals (such as chromium, phosphorus, potassium, and selenium) and essential amino acids. It reinforces the immune system, helps fight infections, and restores the balance of intestinal flora. It boosts the health of the skin, nails, and hair.

METHOD OF USE: It is obtainable from health food shops and pharmacies in the form of tablets, capsules, and flakes for sprinkling on food.

Homeopathy

Graphites and **Petroleum**
– Four 5c tablets of one or both of these remedies to be sucked slowly, twice a day for several weeks

Graphites

– Mineral origin: black lead or graphite
– The homeopathic remedy for skin complaints with oozing, irritant discharge
– Two specific indications: the condition is improved by cool temperatures, and made worse by heat

Petroleum

– Mineral origin: unrefined oil
– The homeopathic remedy for skin irritations with blisters, cracked, or broken skin
– Two specific indications: the condition is improved by heat, and made worse by cool temperatures

• You could also try Graphites-Homaccord® (Heel), which includes Graphites and Calcium carbonicum in various potencies:
– Available in drop bottles containing 30 and 100ml
– In general, 10 drops 3 times daily. Long term administration (several months) should be supervised by a therapist

• It is also important that you combine these treatments with a constitutional remedy, to be chosen after consultation with a professional homeopath. Some likely choices are Calcarea carbonica, Lycopodium, or Sulfur

Calcarea carbonica

– Animal and mineral origin: calcium carbonate from the oyster shell
– One of the constitutional remedies for eczema of the scalp (or cradle cap)

Oligotherapy

Copper, selenium, and **zinc**
Trace elements are usually found in the diet, which should be varied and of high quality. In cases of deficiency, these minerals can be given as medicinal supplements.

Dietary sources of copper

This element is found in small quantities in almost all foods, except in milk which contains almost none. The highest concentrations of copper come from (calf and sheep's) liver ++, seaweed, shellfish such as scallops and oysters, lobster, fish roe, almonds and walnuts, some vegetables (such as avocados and mushrooms), cereals (whole wheat and whole-grain rice), cocoa, dried fruits, green vegetables, plums, and tea.

Natural healing

Dietary sources of selenium

Selenium comes principally from animal products, meat (liver, kidney), saltwater fish (herring and tuna), shellfish (such as oysters), and eggs. It is also present in whole-grain cereals, wheatgerm, brewer's yeast, brazil nuts, and certain vegetables (garlic, broccoli, carrots, and mushrooms).

Dietary sources of zinc

Zinc is most plentiful in seafood, oysters ++, fish, and shellfish, but it is also found in meat, egg yolks, cereals, wholemeal bread, brewer's yeast, walnuts, and some vegetables (broccoli, mushrooms, spinach, and beans).

• Copper and zinc treatments: these are available in various brands and forms, such as: Organic Minerals (Colloidals) which contains 70+ trace minerals:
– Available in 946ml bottles
– Take 1–3 caps just before breakfast and/or evening meal
– Children 1 teaspoon daily for each 20lbs of body weight
Or Maximol (Ionized colloidals):
– Available in 500ml bottles
– Take ½ capful once or twice daily on an empty stomach

• You could also try Lamberts® Zinc/Copper, which contains a blend of zinc (15mg per tablet), and copper (1mg per tablet):
– Sold in containers of 90 tablets
– Take 1 tablet daily on an empty stomach

• For a topical solution, you could also try Weleda Copper ointment:
– Available in tubes of 25 g
– To be applied twice daily with a thin layer

• Selenium treatment. You could try Lamberts® Selenium 200µg plus A+C+E, which contains selenium plus vitamins A, C, and E:
– Available in containers of 100 tablets
– One tablet to be taken daily

Vitamins

Primarily A, B, C, and **E**
– Vitamin A preserves the skin's elasticity, promotes healing, and helps the skin resist infections
– the B vitamins play an important role in the health of the skin, helping to combat seborrhoea and blackheads
– Vitamin C contains anti-infective properties
– Vitamin E speeds up the healing process and helps prevent skin ageing

• You could also try Megavit® (Lamberts), which combines vitamins A, B, C, and E, and zinc, selenium and the bioflavonoids:
– Sold in containers of 60 and 180 tablets
– 1 to 2 tablets daily

Herbal remedies

• Ask your herbalist to make up a 60ml bottle of burdock in a whole fresh-plant suspension (this formulation's cold stabilization process restores the full natural therapeutic effect of the plant). Take half a teaspoonful in a glass of water twice a day. This is not to be taken by children under 15 years of age

Burdock, heartsease, and calendula

Burdock, long used in poultices, is very effective against skin infections; heartsease (or wild pansy) also has a long history as a herbal remedy for skin troubles; and calendula (or marigold), much used for healing wounds, is the principal ingredient in many soothing skin creams.

• You could also try Herba Naturelle Heartsease:
– Available in bottles of 50ml and 100ml
– 20 drops 3 times daily in a little water

Borage
The seeds of the plant are used for the extraction of cold-pressed oil for therapeutic purposes. It is available most commonly in the form of capsules obtainable from your herbalist.

ORAL TREATMENT: One capsule to be taken twice a day for several days, for skin and infectious ailments.

TOPICAL APPLICATION: One capsule, opened up and applied to the skin, may reinforce the oral treatment.

Borage

Borage, a pretty, herbaceous plant originally from southern Spain and Morocco, is primarily grown for the oil extracted from its seeds. Its effectiveness in treating skin complaints is greater than that of oil of evening primrose. Both of these plants have been increasingly used in medicine, ever since researchers discovered a particular substance in their composition, one of the 'good' essential polyunsaturated fatty acids, essential for overall good health, and especially for the skin.

Lavender water is beneficial for morning cleansing of oily skin, whilst sage is more appropriate for dry skin.

Lavender

This fragrant plant has been cultivated for centuries and is known for multiple benefits: it perfumes, soothes, cleanses, disinfects, stimulates, and regulates. Its essential oil has powerful antiseptic and antibacterial properties, as well as soothing pain and calming the nerves.

• You can make your own, home-made soothing skin lotion, by placing two teaspoons of rose petals in a cup of cold water and leaving them to steep overnight

The rose bush

This shrub with the thorny stems comes originally from Iran. It has been grown since ancient times not only for the beauty of its flowers, but also for its medicinal properties. Rose water was first brought to Europe from Damascus by the Crusaders. It was long considered a cure-all, and Avicenna believed it to be the specific cure for consumption. Nowadays, however, it is used only for cosmetic purposes, for its tonic effect on the skin, and for its perfume.

Psoriasis

We do not know at this point what causes psoriasis, although it may well have a genetic origin. Psoriasis appears as well-defined red patches of scaly, dead skin. It does not cause pain or itching, but comes and goes in bouts, affecting mainly the scalp and ears, the elbows, cuticles, and knees.

The average age of onset for psoriasis symptoms is about 25, with most sufferers aged between 16 and 22 – but it can appear at any stage in life. It affects men and women equally, but many either do not know they have it, or are indifferent to it, as psoriasis does not cause great inconvenience much of the time.

The first episode of psoriasis is often triggered by a particular incident or condition:
– a course of medical treatment: lithium, beta-blockers, or the end of a course of cortisone, are some examples
– an infectious illness, especially in children
– some sort of mechanical friction, such as a wound or area of skin dried out by sunburn
– physical or emotional stress (such as bereavement or the ending of a relationship)
– smoking or alcohol consumption
– the period after giving birth (although psoriasis tends to improve during pregnancy)
– a weight gain
– the change of seasons

Once psoriasis has made an appearance, it is likely to return, eventually becoming a chronic condition. Episodes are likely to be triggered by emotional stress or by infectious illnesses. While psoriasis is certainly not a life-threatening condition, many patients do not want to live with it, and it is difficult to treat. The various traditional medical treatments are not well tolerated by the body, and may pose a risk of toxicity in the long term. They can also only treat the symptoms, reducing the lesions until the patient feels they are not so noticeable.

Oligotherapy

Sulphur

This trace element is usually found in the diet, which should be varied and of high quality. In cases of deficiency, sulphur can be given as a medicinal supplement.

Dietary sources of sulphur

Sulphur is found primarily in sulphurated amino acids, and thus mostly in protein. It is plentiful in eggs (165mg of sulphur per 100g of egg yolk), meat, fish, and seafood, as well as in garlic, onions, broccoli, cabbage, and dried beans.

• Sulphur treatment: this is available in various brands and forms – such as Organic Minerals (Colloidals) which contains 70+ trace minerals:
– Available in 946ml bottles
– Take 1–3 caps just before breakfast and/or evening meal

– Children 1 teaspoon daily for each 20lbs of body weight
Or Maximol (Ionized colloidals):
– Available in 500ml bottles
– Take ½ capful once or twice daily on an empty stomach

Homeopathy

Arsenicum album and **Arsenicum iodatum**
– Four 7c tablets of one or both of these remedies to be sucked slowly between meals, twice a day for several weeks

Arsenicum album

– Chemical origin: arsenic oxide or white arsenic
– The homeopathic remedy for dry skin covered with large patches of dead scales (squamae)
– Two characteristic indications: the alternate appearance and disappearance, and the periodicity, of the symptoms

Arsenicum iodatum

– Chemical origin: arsenic iodide
– The homeopathic remedy for dry skin with smaller scaly patches than in the case of the previous remedy

• You could also try Lehning® Sulphur Complex 12 , whose ingredients include Arsenicum album 4x and Sulfur 3x:
– Available in boxes of 80 tablets
– One tablet to be sucked twice a day

• It is also essential that you combine these treatments with a constitutional remedy, to be chosen after consultation with a professional homeopath. Some likely choices are Calcarea carbonica, Psorinum, or Sulfur

Vitamins

Primarily A, B, C, and E
– Vitamin A preserves the skin's elasticity, promotes healing, and helps the skin resist infections
– the B vitamins play an important role in the health of the skin, helping to combat seborrhea and blackheads
– Vitamin C contains anti-infective properties
– Vitamin E speeds up the healing process and helps prevent skin ageing

• You could also try 'Health from the Sun' EFA Derma-Skin Formula, which contains borage and flaxseed oils beneficial to the skin, as well as vitamins A, C, D, E, zinc and extracts of burdock root and yellowdock:
– Available in containers of 60 capsules
– Take 2 capsules once daily

Herbal remedies

Cadewood

Oil of cade

The oil comes from a process of dry distillation of the cadewood, which is a species related to juniper.

Borage
– Borage oil capsules can be obtained from your herbalist. Take one capsule twice a day for several weeks

TOPICAL APPLICATION: One capsule, opened up and applied to the skin, may reinforce the oral treatment.

Borage

This pretty, herbaceous plant originally from southern Spain and Morocco is, like evening primrose, mostly grown for the oil extracted from its seeds. The oils from both these plants have been shown to be important in numerous chemical reactions essential to good health. Borage oil appears to be the more effective treatment for skin conditions.

• You could also try 'Nature's Plus' Borage oil:
– Available in containers of 30 softgels
– Take 1 softgel daily

• Alternatively you could take 'Health from the Sun' Borage oil; each capsule contains 300mg of borage oil:
– Available in containers of 30 capsules
– Take 1 capsule daily

Acupuncture

This treatment is worth trying – but patience will be the order of the day.

TREATMENT SCHEDULE: Several sessions will be needed, spread out over the course of several months, in combination with other therapies.

Water cures

Several spa towns in France specialize in the treatment of psoriasis: Aix-les-Bains, Avène-les-Bains, La Bourboule, Castera-Verduzan, Les Fumades, Lons-le-Saunier, Molitg-les-Bains, Neyrac-les-Bains, Rochefort-sur-Mer, La Roche-Posay, Salins-les-Bains, Saint-Christau, Saint-Gervais-les-Bains, Salies-de-Béarn, Salies-du-Salat, Salins-les-Bains, Tercis-les-Bains, and Uriage-les-Bains…

PUVA phototherapy

This consists of treatment with ultraviolet light, and has been in use since 1974. Unlike the other therapies recommended in this book, this one cannot be qualified as gentle or risk-free, due to its contraindications and its numerous short-, medium-, and long-term side effects. What it does do is whiten psoriasis lesions in 80 per cent of cases – but it could be dangerous. It can only be performed by dermatologists who have specialized facilities.

Cold sores (herpes simplex)

Cold sores are a harmless, but chronic and recurring infection caused by the herpes virus (a relative of the chickenpox and shingles viruses). Cold sores are extremely common, affecting millions of people per year. The condition is benign, except for women in the later stages of pregnancy, as there is a risk that the virus will be passed on to the newborn baby during delivery.

Cold sores are likely to reappear during an infectious illness or at menstruation, or may come back to spoil one's first few days out in the sun. They are infectious, and are most contagious when the blisters are newly formed, as they are full of the virus.

You may experience a few warning tingling sensations, a redness, a burning or itching feeling; then about two or three hours later, a sore appears on the lips, buttocks, or in the genital area. It consists of small, fluid-filled blisters that sting or burn. The fluid is clear at first, but eventually it clouds and thickens to form a scab, which falls off in eight or ten days, leaving no scar.

Treatment will be both general and topical, and has three main objectives: to shorten the duration of the outbreak, to reduce discomfort, and to strengthen the patient's terrain in order to try to prevent further outbreaks. At the current time, there is no definitive cure for cold sores that would eliminate them once and for all.

Preventive measures

It is vital to:

- Protect yourself from the sun's rays by using an effective sunblock, especially when you are in the mountains or by the sea
- Reapply the sunscreen every two hours
- Rinse your face and lips with fresh water after a bath, because dry, cold conditions on dry lips only encourage the return of herpes

Dietary advice

These tips are essential:

- Eliminate all heavy, fatty foods, especially dairy products, fried foods, and sauce dishes
- Avoid salted peanuts
- Drink large quantities of water
- Eat plenty of foods rich in vitamins B and C, and in copper
- Increase your consumption of onion and garlic
- Garnish your food frequently and consistently with condiments such as thyme, cinnamon, and oregano, herbs recognized for their ability to combat infection

Foods rich in vitamin C

Citrus fruits (lemons, oranges, and grapefruit), green vegetables (celery, green cabbage ++, watercress, spinach, sorrel, parsley, and horseradish), fruits (such as pineapple, blackcurrants ++, guava, and kiwi fruit ++), red berries (strawberries, raspberries, and redcurrants), potatoes, peppers, and tomatoes.

Homeopathy

Vaccinotoxicum to be taken early and systematically.
– Six 7c tablets to be sucked slowly between meals, once a day for one week

Vaccinotoxicum

– Animal origin: nosode made from the herpes vaccine
– The specific homeopathic remedy for herpes and shingles

Nosodes are homeopathic remedies prepared from microbial materials, animal or vegetable tissues, secretions or excretions taken from patients suffering from certain diseases. This is the case with the smallpox virus.

Rhus toxicodendron
– Four 5c tablets to be sucked slowly like sweets, three times a day as soon as the first symptoms appear. Reduce the frequency once there are signs of improvement, stop the treatment when cured

Rhus toxicodendron

– Vegetable origin: the fresh leaves of the sumach or poison ivy plant
– The homeopathic remedy for blistered skin
– A specific indication: the condition improves with heat

• You could also try Mezereum-homaccord® (Heel), which contains mezereum and Acidum arsenicosum in various potencies:
– Available in drop bottles containing 30 and 100ml
– In general, 10 drops 3 times daily. In acute disorders, initially 10 drops every 15 minutes

Oligotherapy

Copper or a combination of **copper, silver, and gold**

Copper is usually found in the diet, which should be varied and of high quality. In cases of deficiency, copper can be given as a medicinal supplement.

Foods rich in copper

Seaweed, almonds, avocados, cocoa, cereals (especially whole wheat and whole-grain rice), mushrooms, shellfish, oysters, calf and sheep's liver ++, dried fruit, green vegetables, walnuts, fish roe, plums, and tea.

• Copper treatment: this is available in various brands and forms – such as Organic Minerals (Colloidals) which contains 70+ trace minerals:
– Available in 946ml bottles
– Take 1–3 caps just before breakfast and/or evening meal
– Children 1 teaspoon daily for each 20lbs of body weight
Or Maximol (Ionized colloidals):
– Available in 500ml bottles
– Take ½ capful once or twice daily on an empty stomach

• You could also try Lamberts® Zinc/Copper, which contains a blend of zinc (15mg per tablet), and copper (1mg per tablet):
– Sold in containers of 90 tablets
– Take 1 tablet daily on an empty stomach

Vitamin C
This vitamin is to be taken systematically at a dose of 1,000mg per day for adults, 500mg daily for children.

Vitamin C-based supplements

*Synergisti-C (Thorne) which contains 650mg ascorbic acid, 400mg Echinacea angustifolia, 100mg Baptisia tinctoria and 100mg hesperidin:
– Available in containers of 60 capsules
– Take one to two capsules twice daily

Biocare vitamin C (citrus free) 500mg containing magnesium ascorbate and bilberry:
– Available in containers of 180 vegetarian capsules
– Take one to two capsules daily

Lamberts®. Rutin+C+bioflavonoids (containing vitamin C 500mg, citrus bioflavonoids 100mg, rutin 50mg and hesperidin complex 30mg):
– Available in containers of 90 capsules
– Take one to two capsules daily

You can take natural vitamin C in chewable form – Lamberts® vitamin C 100mg:
– Sold in containers of 90 tablets
– One to three tablets daily

Or you can take chewable Redoxon® which contains vitamin C (500mg) and Zinc (5mg):
– Available in containers of 30 tablets
– Adults up to 2 tablets per day. Children (6–12 years) ½ tablet per day

Herbal remedies

Echinacea for fighting infection.

Ginseng as a tonic.

POSSIBLE PRESCRIPTION: Ask your herbalist to make up a 30ml bottle of mother tincture of each of these plants. Take 25 drops of echinacea solution in a little water three times a day; 25 drops of ginseng solution twice a day.

• You can use Echinaforce (Bioforce), a tincture of Echinacea purpurea:
– Available in 50ml and 100ml bottles of oral drops
– Fifteen drops to be taken in a little water, three times a day by adults, seven drops three times a day by children (6–12 years old)

– You can also use Red Kooga, a mixture of ginseng and multivitamins and minerals:
– Sold in boxes of 32 tablets
– Adults (over 12 years old): one tablet to be taken each day

Plant essential oils

Spanish oregano, mountain savory, or **common thyme**
HERBAL PRESCRIPTION: Ask your herbalist to make up a 1ml bottle of essential oil of one of these plants. Take two drops in a little honey, twice a day.

The essential oils of oregano and thyme have anti-inflammatory, antiseptic, and expectorant effects, but their concentration depends largely on their geographical origin. Savory's properties are also very similar.

• You could also try Gouttes aux essences® (Lehning), whose ingredients include essential oils of cinnamon, lavender, and thyme:

– Sold in 45ml bottles of oral solution
– Twenty drops to be taken in a little water, three times a day. For children over the age of 30 months: five drops to be taken in a little water, four times a day

Topical applications

It may be useful to apply mother tincture of calendula, essential oil of lemon, or camomile lotion, two or three times a day for a few minutes. They can be used alone or in combination with acyclovir cream, Zovirax®. To my mind, it is perfectly justifiable to use a classical medical treatment in this way if it is effective and well tolerated, which is the case with Zovirax.

Warts and verrucas

These small outgrowths of flesh, of varying consistency, may appear anywhere on the body, but by far the most common locations are the hands and feet. They are caused by a virus that thrives in damp, confined spaces, such as in sports shoes, swimming pools, showers, or on judo mats.

Warts can be passed on from one person to another, but their degree of infectiousness is, fortunately, highly variable.

They may disappear on their own, but their unsightliness and the embarrassment they cause make it understandable that most people want them quickly treated.

Preventive measures

• Do not walk barefoot in damp places, as these are where the virus is most likely to be contracted

• Wear plastic sandals or flip-flops when you go to a swimming pool

• Wash your sports shoes each time you wear them

• Make sure the shoes are dry before putting them on again

Oligotherapy

Magnesium

This trace element usually comes from the diet, which should be varied and of high quality. In cases of deficiency, which often occurs with magnesium, it can be given as a medicinal supplement.

Dietary sources of magnesium

Present in almost all foods, but mostly in the calorie-rich ones, unfortunately. The best sources of magnesium are: citrus fruits, bananas, whole-grain cereals (oat or bran flakes), cocoa and chocolate, shellfish (winkles, shrimps, oysters, and clams) and oily fish, figs, hard cheeses, nuts (almonds, peanuts, hazelnuts and walnuts), vegetables (spinach, dried and green beans, maize, split peas and soya beans), and wholemeal bread.

• Magnesium treatment: this is available in various brands and forms, such as Organic Minerals (Colloidals) which contains 70+ trace minerals:
– Available in 946ml bottles
– Take 1–3 caps just before breakfast and/or evening meal
– Children 1 teaspoon daily for each 20lbs of body weight

• Or Maximol (Ionized colloidals):
– Available in 500ml bottles
– Take ½ capful once or twice daily on an empty stomach

The foods rich in magnesium are also rich in calories, but it is worth noting that four ounces of plain chocolate (which is a generous portion, since it is the equivalent of almost half a bar) contain fewer calories than an average eight-ounce portion of chips (fries).

• In serious cases, you could try a higher-dose magnesium supplement, such as Magasorb® (Lamberts) containing 150mg of magnesium (as citrate):
– Available in containers of 60 and 180 tablets
– One to three tablets daily

Mineral water brands containing the most magnesium

– Hépar: contains 110mg of magnesium per litre
– Badoit: contains 92mg of magnesium per litre
– Contrex: contains 84mg of magnesium per litre
– Volvic contains 80mg of magnesium per litre
– Evian contains 24mg of magnesium per litre
– Vittel contains 20mg of magnesium per litre
– Pellegrino contains 54mg of magnesium per litre

Homeopathy

Antimonium crudum and **Nitricum acidum**
– Four 5c tablets of one or both of these remedies, to be sucked slowly twice a day for several weeks

Antimonium crudum

– Chemical origin: black sulphide of antimony
– The homeopathic remedy for hard, callused warts
– A specific indication: the child who is apt to be greedy, who cannot help wolfing down his or her food and then feels ill afterwards

Nitricum acidum

– Chemical origin: nitric acid
– The homeopathic remedy for warts with irregular edges, that are cracked, inclined to bleed, located mostly on the soles of the feet
– A specific indication: the yellowish colour of the wart

• You could also try Galium-Heel® (Heel), which contains Nitricum acidum D6, Thuja D3, Galium aparine D3, Echinacea angustifolia D5:
– Available in drop bottles containing 30 and 100ml
– Ten drops, to be taken three times daily

• Another possibility is to ask your herbalist to make up a small bottle of a blend of 3g of mother tincture of thuja and 30g of collodion. Apply a few drops of this solution to the wart; a thin film will form as the solution dries. Reapply a few drops as the film starts to peel away, until the warts have been removed

• It is also important that you combine these treatments with a constitutional remedy, to be chosen after consultation with a professional homeopath. Some likely choices are Calcarea carbonica, Lycopodium, or Thuja

Thuja occidentalis

– Vegetable origin: a conifer tree, the white cedar
– The homeopathic remedy for excrescences of the skin, vesicles, or papules
– Two specific indications: the skin appears grimy and oily

Herbal remedies

Greater celandine (chelidonium)

Herbal prescription: If celandines grow in your garden, you can apply the fresh sap locally to the warts, two or three times a day. If not, ask your herbalist to make up a 30ml bottle of mother tincture, and apply several drops of that.

Celandine

Celandines from the woods are a traditional remedy for warts and corns, for the fresh sap applied directly is one of the surest methods of curing them. Be careful when taking this plant internally, however, as it very quickly becomes toxic, and you need a herbalist's knowledge before you ingest it.

• You could also try Bioforce Chelidonium (a tincture for external use)
– Apply once or twice daily to the wart

Plant essential oils

Mountain savory

Possible prescription: Obtain a 2g bottle of essential oil of mountain savory from your herbalist. Apply one drop of the oil to the warts, morning and evening, for a few weeks until they disappear

Mountain savory

This sun-loving plant is much used in cooking and, like thyme, eucalyptus, oregano, also contains active principles that make it most effective against various skin infections.

A depurative

You could use a depurative, as the first homeopaths often did, to detoxify the body. One possible brand is Nutri Cleanse which contains psyllium, bentonite clay, slippery elm, barberry, oregon grape, rhubarb root, burdock root, cloves and fennel seed:
– Available in containers of 120 capsules

– Take 2 to 4 capsules daily

A depurative is a 'purifying' or cleansing remedy that eliminates poisons and toxins. We should not forget that the traditional concept of illness was based on the idea of a poisoning of the body, and that treatment consisted of banishing the 'evil humours', hence the recourse to blood-letting, enemas, and depuratives.

Burns

The vast majority of burns involve minor injuries that are most often treated at home. This section will deal only with these first-degree burns, affecting a limited area of the uppermost layer of skin. Fortunately, serious burns constitute no more than about five per cent of the total. Fifty per cent of the injuries affect the hands, and thirty per cent involve the neck and face. Three-quarters of burn incidents are caused either by hot substances (water or oil) or by corrosive materials (such as bleach or caustic soda).

Essential advice

- Cold water is the best emergency treatment for a burn, and should be applied immediately, as it soothes the burning feeling and limits the extent of the burn. You can continue cooling down the burned area for as long as ten minutes, by running cold water over it (the water should be between 8 and 25° C)

- Do not apply oil or any creamy substance, and especially not butter

- Do not apply ice cubes directly to skin

- Do not disinfect the burn with alcohol or hydrogen peroxide, for both of these will add to the discomfort

- Do not apply any ointment, unless on professional advice

- Do not use an antiseptic that stains the skin, such as Mercurochrome®, as this makes it more difficult to assess the seriousness of the burn, and increases the inflammation

- Do not dress the wound with cotton wool, as once this dries it becomes difficult to remove from the skin

Homeopathy

Apis mellifica, Belladonna, and **Rhus toxicodendron**

– Four 5c tablets of one or all of these remedies to be sucked slowly two or three times in succession, reducing the frequency as the symptoms improve

Apis mellifica

– Animal origin: the whole bee, steeped in alcohol
– The specific homeopathic remedy for swellings
– Two specific indications: the pain is improved by cold, and made worse by heat

Belladonna

– Vegetable origin: the leaves and fresh flowers of the deadly nightshade plant

Natural healing

– The homeopathic remedy for red, swollen blotches
– A characteristic indication: the sudden, violent onset of the symptoms

Rhus toxicodendron

– Vegetable origin: the sumach or poison ivy
– The specific homeopathic remedy for blisters or vesicles

The name 'Belladonna' (beautiful woman) comes from the historical use of the plant by Italian women to dilate their pupils, making them more attractive.

• You could also try Traumeel® (Heel), which includes Belladonna D4, Calendula D2, Arnica D2

– Available in drops, tablets and ointment
– Drops: in general, 10 drops 3 times daily. Tablets: 1 tablet to be dissolved under the tongue 3 times daily

Herbal remedies

Calendula and **tepezcohuite**

POSSIBLE PRESCRIPTION: You can apply compresses soaked in boiled water with ten drops of mother tincture of calendula (marigold), three or four times daily, to the burn.

Calendula (marigold)/tepezcohuite

The common marigold is considered to be one of the best plants for healing. Tepezcohuite, a Mexican plant related

A natural remedy for sunburn

Mix a tablespoonful of brewer's yeast with a little sweet almond oil. Coat the burned area with this mixture and leave it on for 15 minutes.

The sun is both your friend and one of your worst enemies:
– it allows the skin to synthesize vitamin D3, vital to children, pregnant women, and the elderly
– it helps heal eczema and psoriasis
– it acts as an antidepressant by stimulating the brain's neurotransmitters

But... it can also lead to:
– burns of varying degrees (sunburn)
– premature ageing of the skin
– and above all, skin cancers, which are constantly on the rise

I can only advise against the use of sun-beds and tanning sessions, as the short-term benefits to the appearance are outweighed by the long-term harm (premature skin ageing and increased risk of cancer).

to mimosa, has been widely used to treat burns since the days of the Mayans.

- You could also try Calendula-Salbe-Heel S, which includes tincture of calendula:
  - Sold in 50g tubes of ointment
  - To be applied once or twice daily
- If you have nothing else to hand, you can apply slices of raw potato or cucumber to the burned area, to cool and moisten it

Plant Essential oils

Lavender

POSSIBLE PRESCRIPTION: A few drops of a blend of five drops of essential oil of lavender and 10ml of St. John's wort oil, to be applied directly to the burn two or three times in succession, at intervals of a few minutes. Then re-apply twice daily for two or three days.

Lavender

This plant scents, soothes, cleans, disinfects, stimulates, and regulates – all thanks largely to the essential oil contained within it.

St. John's wort

Although this plant is currently sought after for its effects on mood (depression), it has traditionally been used for its benefits to the skin.

Shingles

This distinctive and painful skin condition is caused by a virus related to herpes and chicken-pox, although less contagious. Shingles begins with a bout of pains that follow a nerve pathway, whether along the trunk, the limbs, or even from the eye. The pain is soon followed by the appearance in the same location of blisters that itch, burn, or throb, sometimes unbearably. These blisters then dry into scabs which last somewhat longer, and which may leave small but permanent scars.

In most cases, shingles is a painful, but benign condition, which usually resolves in three weeks. However, horribly painful after-effects do sometimes recur and may persist, particularly among the elderly. It becomes a serious, possibly an emergency, condition if it appears all over the body, if it affects the eyes, or if it occurs in an immuno-deficient patient.

Treatment

A powerful course of treatment should be used from the outset. Both topical and general, the treatment aims to shorten the duration of the condition, limit its seriousness, and above all, prevent the painful post-herpetic neuralgia.

Acupuncture

This treatment is almost essential for its effectiveness against acute pain. It is a good idea to start acupuncture treatments without delay, as soon as the first symptoms appear.

TREATMENT SCHEDULE: The frequency of the sessions may be quite intensive, ranging from one a day to three or four times a week, for the first two weeks.

Oligotherapy

Copper alone or in a **copper, gold, and silver** combination.

Magnesium and **zinc**
Trace elements are usually found in the diet, which should be varied and of high quality. In cases of deficiency, they can be given as medicinal supplements.

Dietary sources of copper

This element is found in small quantities in almost all foods. The highest concentrations of copper come from (calf and sheep's) liver ++, seaweed, shellfish such as scallops and oysters, lobster, fish roe, almonds and walnuts, some vegetables (such as avocados and mushrooms), cereals (whole wheat, whole-grain rice and soya), dried fruits, green vegetables, plums, cocoa, and tea.

Dietary sources of magnesium

Magnesium can be found in almost all foods, but comes mainly from citrus fruits, bananas, whole-grain cereals (oat- or bran flakes), cocoa and chocolate, shellfish (winkles, shrimps, oysters, and clams) and oily fish, figs, hard cheeses, nuts (such as almonds, peanuts, hazelnuts, and walnuts), vegetables (spinach, dried and green beans, maize, split peas, and soya beans), and wholemeal bread.

Dietary sources of zinc

Zinc is most plentiful in seafood, fish, oysters ++ and other shellfish. It is also found in meat, egg yolk, cereals, wholemeal bread, brewer's yeast, hazelnuts, and some vegetables (broccoli, mushrooms, spinach, and beans).

• Copper-magnesium-zinc treatments: each of these three trace elements can be taken in various forms, such as Organic Minerals (Colloidals) which contains 70+ trace minerals:
– Available in 946ml bottles
– Take 1–3 caps just before breakfast and/or evening meal

– Children 1 teaspoon daily for each 20lbs of body weight
Or Maximol (Ionized colloidals):
– Available in 500ml bottles
– Take ½ capful once or twice daily on an empty stomach

Vitamins

Vitamin C is vital for building up the immune system.

The **B vitamins** are needed to help regenerate the nerve cells.

Foods rich in vitamin C

Citrus fruits (lemons, oranges, and grapefruit), green vegetables (celery, green cabbage ++, watercress, spinach, sorrel, parsley, and horseradish), fruits (such as pineapple, blackcurrants ++, guava, and kiwi fruit ++), red berries (strawberries, raspberries, and redcurrants), potatoes, peppers, and tomatoes.

• You can find a vitamin supplement in Berocca®, a blend of calcium, magnesium, B vitamins, and 1,000mg of vitamin C:
– Sold in boxes of 10 or 20 effervescent tablets
– One tablet to be taken in the morning

• You could also try Megavit® (Lamberts), which combines vitamins A, B, C, and E, and zinc, selenium and the bioflavonoids:
– Sold in containers of 60 and 180 tablets
– 1 to 2 tablets daily

Brewer's yeast

ORIGIN: A living substance specially prepared as a supplement, from a minute fungus that serves as a ferment in the preparation of beer. It is not the same as baker's yeast, and is better tolerated by the digestive system.

COMPOSITION AND PROPERTIES: Yeast is packed with B vitamins, minerals (such as chromium, phosphorus, potassium, and selenium) and essential amino acids. It reinforces the immune system, helps fight infections, and restores the balance of intestinal flora. It boosts the health of the skin, nails, and hair.

METHOD OF USE: It is obtainable from health food shops and pharmacies in the form of tablets, capsules, and flakes for sprinkling on food.

Homeopathy

Vaccinotoxicum is systematically prescribed.
– Six 7c tablets to be sucked slowly between meals, once a day for four or five days

Vaccinotoxicum

– Animal origin: made from the smallpox vaccine
– The homeopathic remedy for blister-type rashes (herpes, chicken-pox, and shingles)

Also **Mezereum** and **Ranunculus bulbosus**

– Four 5c tablets of one or both of these remedies to be sucked slowly between meals, three times a day for several days

Mezereum

– Vegetable origin: a shrub, the Daphne mezereum tree
– One of the homeopathic remedies for rashes with itching blisters and scabs
– A specific indication: the condition is made worse by the heat of the bed

Ranunculus bulbosus

– Vegetable origin: the bulb of the buttercup plant
– The homeopathic remedy for acute, burning, stinging pain, with blood-filled blisters or blisters that itch until they bleed
– Two characteristic indications: the condition is made worse by being touched, or by the slightest movement

• You could also try Lehning® Euphorbium Complex 88, whose ingredients include Mezereum 4x, Rhus toxicodendron 4x, and Sulfur 4x:
– Sold in 30ml bottles of oral drops
– Fifteen drops to be taken in a little water, three times a day

• Another remedy would be Ranunculus-Homaccord® (Heel), which contains Ranunculus bulbosis and Asclepias tuberosa in various potencies:
– Available in drop bottles containing 30 and 100ml
– In general, 10 drops 3 times daily. In acute disorders, initially 10 drops every 15 minutes

Herbal remedies

Echinacea for fighting infection.

Eleutherococcus or **Siberian ginseng**, which strengthens the patient's terrain.

POSSIBLE PRESCRIPTION: Ask your herbalist to make up 30 capsules of a blend of dried extracts of all three plants, 100mg of each plant for each No.2 capsule (the size of the capsule that the herbalist will use for the ingredients). Take one capsule three times a day for ten days.

Siberian Ginseng / Echinacea

Siberian ginseng, or Eleutherococcus, belongs to the ginseng or ivy family, but comes from the plains of Siberia where it grows in abundance. It gained some notoriety after athletes from the former Soviet Union and Eastern bloc countries used it to increase their resistance to physical and mental fatigue. Echinacea (purple coneflower) comes from North America, where it was much used by native tribes to combat infections.

• You can use Echinaforce (Bioforce), a tincture of Echinacea purpurea:
– Available in 50ml and 100ml bottles of oral drops
– Fifteen drops to be taken in a little water, three times a day by adults, seven drops three times a day by children (6–12 years old)

• And Lamberts® Korean ginseng 600mg:
– Sold in containers of 60 capsules
– Take one to two capsules daily

• As a topical treatment, you could try applying cold compresses, two or three times daily, soaked in a few drops of a mother tincture of calendula (marigold), together with the usual daubing of the skin with soluble eosin, which dries out the blisters

Calendula

The common marigold, with its deep orange petals rich in active principles, possesses antiseptic, antibacterial, and antiviral properties, and helps heal many skin conditions.

Plant essential oils

Spanish oregano, for its effectiveness against infection.

True **Lavender**.

– Two drops of essential oil of Spanish

oregano to be taken in a little honey, twice a day for several days; two drops of essential oil of lavender to be applied to the affected area two or three times a day

Spanish oregano

Oregano has been in use since Greek and Roman times, and not only as a garnish for pizza. Like eucalyptus, savory, and thyme, it contains an essential oil with powerful infection-fighting properties.

Lavender

Lavender is one of the oldest plants to be cultivated for herbal treatments, and one of the most popular for minor wounds and bruises. Its aromatic and therapeutic properties come from the plant's essential oil.

• You could also try Gouttes aux essences®(Lehning), whose ingredients include essential oils of cinnamon, lavender, and thyme:
– Sold in 45ml bottles of oral solution
– Twenty drops to be taken in a little water, three times a day. For children over the age of 30 months: five drops to be taken in a little water, four times a day

Heavy perspiration

Perspiration is a natural function of the body, vital not only for the elimination of toxins produced by the body but particularly for maintaining the body's internal temperature at a steady 37° C, regardless of the outside conditions.

The body sweats little in cold temperatures, but production increases in the summer, or when the body produces its own heat after physical exertion, during a fever, or as a result of emotion.

Perspiration is made up of 99 per cent water, with a little salt, a few traces of oil and urea, and waste matter from muscle cells. Our bodies are equipped for this elimination with three million sweat glands, known as eccrine glands on the body's hairless surfaces. Apocrine glands are located in the armpits and pubic area. The consumption of meat, cheese, coffee, tobacco, alcohol, and spices increases the activity of the sweat glands.

Sweat has little or no odour when it is first produced, but takes on an unpleasant smell as a result of its chemical degradation upon contact with the skin's bacteria.

Any treatments whose aim is to stop perspiration are considered 'dangerous' by homeopaths, but this does not rule out the offer of some advice to patients.

Useful tips

• Some clothing materials cause more perspiration than others, for they prevent the moisture from evaporating:

A tennis match

When the outside temperature is 35° C, a two-hour tennis match will cause the body to lose about three litres of water. It is therefore essential to drink some water before the game, regular small amounts during the match, and large quantities afterwards.

In point of fact, the stomach cannot, for purely physiological reasons, process more than about half a litre (perhaps 600ml) of liquid per hour. It is therefore pointless to overload it with any more than that. Drinking more water during physical exertion will not help hydrate the body, as the excess only 'sits on the stomach' and impedes physical activity without helping your performance in any way – quite the contrary.

So, during this two-hour tennis match, it makes no sense to drink more than a litre and a half in total. You must be prepared to come off the tennis court in a dehydrated state, in need of approximately two litres of water, a loss that you then make up over the following three hours. It is best to drink cool, but not ice-cold, water.

A four-hour match played in intense heat at a major tennis tournament can leave the players in need of four litres of water, possibly more. Such a liquid deficit would require about five hours' steady water consumption to make up. Some players resort to an intravenous drip to reduce this recovery time.

some examples are synthetic fabrics (nylon, polyester, or acrylic) or artificial fibres, such as viscose. Cotton and linen, which are made of plant fibres, are much more absorbent

• It is advisable to remove the hair under the arms in cases of heavy perspiration, as hair traps odours and maintains a warm, humid environment that encourages the development of odour-producing bacteria

• Antibacterial deodorants pose no risk to your health

• Antiperspirants most often contain aluminium compounds, and act by reducing the secretion of perspiration. They have an astringent effect on the pores and should not be used more than two or three times per week

A substance is said to be an astringent when it brings about a contraction of the tissues, thus reducing bodily secretions or bleeding, for example

Oligotherapy

Magnesium reduces the stress that can sometimes be placed on the body by fluid loss from very heavy sweating.

This trace element usually comes from the diet, which should be varied and of high quality. In cases of deficiency, which often occurs with magnesium, it can be given as a medicinal supplement.

Dietary sources of magnesium

Present in almost all foods, but mostly in the calorie-rich ones, unfortunately. The best sources of magnesium are: citrus fruits, bananas, whole-grain cereals (oat or bran flakes), cocoa and chocolate, shellfish (winkles, shrimps, oysters, and clams) and oily fish, snails, figs, hard cheeses, nuts (almonds, peanuts, hazelnuts and walnuts), vegetables (spinach, dried and green beans, maize, split peas and soya beans), and wholemeal bread.

• Magnesium treatment: this is available in various brands and forms, such as Organic Minerals (Colloidals) which contains 70+ trace minerals:
– Available in 946ml bottles
– Take 1–3 caps just before breakfast and/or evening meal
– Children 1 teaspoon daily for each 20lbs of body weight
Or Maximol (Ionized colloidals):
– Available in 500ml bottles
– Take ½ capful once or twice daily on an empty stomach

• You could also try a Stress formula such as Lamberts® B-100 complex, a mixture of vitamins B1, B2, B3, B5, B6, B12, folic acid, biotin, choline, inositol and PABA:
– Available in containers of 60 and 200 tablets
– One tablet to be taken each day

Homeopathy

Calcarea carbonica and **Thuja**
– Four 5c tablets to be sucked slowly like sweets twice a day, as needed or as a long-term treatment

Calcarea carbonica

– Animal and mineral origin: calcium from oyster-shells
– The homeopathic remedy for acid perspiration on the head and feet
– A specific indication: the condition is made worse by cold

Thuja occidentalis

– Vegetable origin: the white cedar tree
– The homeopathic remedy for unpleasant-smelling perspiration
– A specific indication: oily, shiny skin

• You could also try Psorinoheel® (Heel), which includes Thuja D6, Psorinum D10, Sulfur D6...
– Available in drop bottles of 30ml and 100ml
– 10 drops 3 times daily

Herbal remedies

Sage
POSSIBLE PRESCRIPTION: Ask your herbalist to prepare a 30ml bottle of mother tincture of sage. Take 25 drops in a little water, twice a day.

Sage

Its name comes from the Latin, *salvare*, to save, which gives an indication of its importance among the various plant remedies. It acts as an antiseptic, a tonic, a regulator of hormones... and of perspiration. The Chinese, convinced of its value, were willing to give the English two cases of tea in exchange for one case of sage. Its essential oil contains phyto-oestrogens, which make it very useful in treating gynaecological problems, particularly the menopause.

• You could also try Menosan (Bioforce) Sage drops:
– Available in tincture form in bottles of 50ml
– 15 to 20 drops in a little water, 3 times daily before meals

Hair problems

The desire for beautiful hair has long been a part of human culture, as it is a symbol of strength and seductiveness – and so we are distressed when it looks lifeless, and feel devastated when we begin to lose it.

Our hair is a living substance, and consequently each hair has its own life cycle of birth, growth, decline, and fall.

– We have on average 200,000 hairs, a quantity that is regulated by the influence of male hormones

– We lose approximately 50 hairs per day, which is perfectly normal, although of course this loss must be replaced by an equal regrowth

– If the lost hair is not replaced, we develop baldness, a condition that affects, to a greater or lesser degree, forty per cent of men and eight per cent of women

– In order to avoid or at least delay the onset of baldness, hair roots must receive a good supply of blood, nutrients, and oxygen

– A scalp that is too oily will stifle the hair and weaken it

– A dry scalp means that the hair receives too little sebum, making it lifeless and liable to break

Important tips

• Contrary to popular belief, even fine hair needs to be washed often – but only with gentle, low-foaming shampoo (even baby shampoo is not necessarily gentle on the hair, although it does not sting if it gets in your eyes)

• Try not to use a large quantity of shampoo, or rub it into your scalp. Rinse thoroughly as soon as possible

• Avoid using very hot water, which damages the hair

• Try to leave your hair to dry naturally whenever possible. If you need to use a hairdryer, hold it six inches away from your head

• Avoid brushing your hair too vigorously, as this encourages dandruff. Your brush should be made of silk fibres and should be neither too inflexible nor too hard

• If you swim in the sea, rinse your hair

Dandruff

Half the population of the Western world, particularly men, complain of these flakes of dead skin that come from the outer layer of the scalp and shed in profusion all over their jacket collars.

Dandruff is brought on by the frequent use of harsh shampoos, fatigue, stress, and poor diet, not to mention the role played by male hormones and a genetic predisposition.

Dandruff may also be accompanied by the overgrowth of a fungus which is normally present on the scalp, and which can be treated. Anti-dandruff shampoos contain fungicides for this purpose, or products like tar that control the flaking of the skin.

afterwards in water to which vinegar or lemon juice has been added

Dietary advice for healthy hair

• Be careful not to eat too much sugar in any form

• Limit your intake of dairy products, especially of whole, unskimmed milk

• Stay away from smoked or cured meats and fast food

• Tinned foods should be avoided if possible

• Eat plenty of fruit, vegetables, and cereals +++

• Take one tablespoonful of olive oil or borage oil per day

Vitamins for your hair

The best vitamins for healthy hair are **vitamins B5** and **H**, which are mostly to be found in cereals, royal jelly, wheatgerm, green vegetables, fruit, brewer's yeast, milk, wholemeal bread, and meat (especially offal).

• You could also try Maxi-Hair® (Lamberts), which contains vitamins A, C, D, E and all the B group as well as trace elements:
– Sold in containers of 60 tablets
– One tablet to be taken daily

• Alternatively you could take Cheveux Plus (Arkopharma) which contains a combination of vitamins B2, B3, B5, B6, biotin, zinc, nettle, cysteine and methionine to help support hair growth:
– Available in containers of 75 capsules
– Take 3 capsules per day for 15 days, then 2 capsules per day as maintenance. Do for 3 months

There is no particular advantage in taking these vitamins via intramuscular injection, as this works no better than taking the tablets.

Oligotherapy

Silica and **sulphur**

Natural healing

These trace elements are usually found in the diet, which should be varied and of high quality. In cases of deficiency, they can be given as medicinal supplements.

Dietary sources of silica

Plants in general are rich in silica, but modern eating habits mean that we are not getting as much of it as we used to. It is most plentiful in the outer layers of vegetables and cereals (except for maize and rye), citrus fruits, beer, mushrooms, olives, radishes, and bran ++.

Dietary sources of sulphur

Sulphur is found primarily in sulphurated amino acids, and thus mostly in protein. It is plentiful in eggs (165mg of sulphur per 100g of egg yolk), meat, fish, and seafood, as well as in garlic, onions, broccoli, cabbage, and dried beans.

Sulphur and silica treatment: these are available in various brands and forms – such as: Organic Minerals (Colloidals) which contains 70+ trace minerals:
– Available in 946ml bottles
– Take 1–3 caps just before breakfast and/or evening meal
– Children 1 teaspoon daily for each 20lbs of body weight
Or Maximol (Ionized colloidals):
– Available in 500ml bottles
– Take ½ capful once or twice daily on an empty stomach

Sulphurated amino acids

These slow down the rate of hair loss, and contribute to more beautiful hair.

• You could try Solgar® Skin, Nails and Hair formula, which contains MSM, vitamin C, lysine and silicon:
– Available in containers of 60 tablets
– Two tablets, to be taken daily with meals

Homeopathy

It is important to select the constitutional remedy appropriate for you, in consultation with a professional homeopath. Some likely choices are Arsenicum album, Sulfur, or Thuja.

Herbal remedies

Burdock and **henna** – which is widely used in Africa to colour the hair, prevent it from becoming too oily, and give it volume.

– Obtain a 30ml bottle of mother tincture of burdock from your herbalist. Take twenty-five drops in a little water, twice a day for several days

• Ask your herbalist to make up a 60ml bottle of burdock in a whole fresh-plant suspension (this formulation's cold stabilization process restores the full natural therapeutic effect of the plant). Take half a teaspoonful in a little water twice a day. This treatment is not for children under 15 years of age

Borage oil is very beneficial for the skin and hair.
– You can buy this remedy in capsule form from your herbalist. Take two capsules per day for several weeks

Topical application: one capsule

Health formula for your hair

– One multivitamin tablet every day
– A B-complex vitamin tablet or a dose of brewer's yeast
– Wheatgerm
– 1,000mg of vitamin C
– Olive and borage oil
– Cysteine
– Silica
– A decoction of panama bark (15g per litre of water), to be used as a shampoo

You can ask your herbalist to make up a blend of essential oils or lotions of sage, rosemary, wild thyme, and mountain savory. Place a few drops in your hair and rub in gently for about a minute each day, for several days.

opened up and applied directly to the scalp may reinforce the oral treatment

• You could also try 'Health from the Sun' Borage oil; containing 300mg of borage oil:
– Available in containers of 30 capsules
– Take 1 capsule daily

• Alternatively you can take Lamberts® High GLA which contains 220mg of gamma-linoleic acid, derived from 1,000mg of borage oil:
– Available in containers of 90 capsules
– Take 1 capsule daily

Nail problems

This is a very common complaint, as three out of five women say their nails are too soft or dry, or are liable to split or break. This horn-like substance that grows from the ends of our hands and feet is often a reflection of our general state of health, and the slightest illness has an almost immediate impact on the condition of our nails.

Nails grow approximately one millimetre per week, faster in summer than in winter, more rapidly during the day than overnight, and more quickly in children than in adults. Much to women's chagrin, they also grow faster in men, who pay no attention to them. It takes six months to replace a fingernail, and one year for a completely new toenail.

Important advice

• Make sure you keep your hands and fingers scrupulously clean with soap and a nail brush

• Keeping your nails trimmed will prevent the development of bacteria underneath them that could spread, and damage them

• Wear gloves to protect your hands from repeated contact with harsh cleaning or household repair products

Oligotherapy

Silica and **zinc**

These trace elements are usually found in the diet, which should be varied and of high quality. In cases of deficiency, they can be given as medicinal supplements.

Keratin

This protein, essential for the building of hair and nails, is synthesized by the body from cysteine. Zinc is not only essential for this synthesizing process to take place, it also helps protect cysteine. Silica reinforces all these chemical processes.

Zinc and silica treatment: these are available in various brands and forms, such as Organic Minerals (Colloidals) which contains 70+ trace minerals:
– Available in 946ml bottles
– Take 1–3 caps just before breakfast and/or evening meal
– Children 1 teaspoon daily for each 20lbs of body weight
Or Maximol (Ionized colloidals):
– Available in 500ml bottles
– Take ½ capful once or twice daily on an empty stomach

Health food for the nails

Brewer's yeast

ORIGIN: A living substance specially prepared as a supplement, from a minute fungus that serves as a ferment in the preparation of beer. It is not the same as baker's yeast, and is better tolerated by the digestive system.

COMPOSITION AND PROPERTIES: Yeast is packed with B vitamins, minerals (such as chromium, phosphorus, potassium, and selenium) and essential amino acids. It reinforces the immune system, helps fight infections, and restores the balance of intestinal flora. It boosts the health of the skin, nails, and hair.

METHOD OF USE: it is obtainable from health food shops and pharmacies in the form of tablets, capsules, and flakes for sprinkling on food.

Sulphurated amino acids

These improve the quality of the nail and encourage its growth.

• You can find cysteine as one of the ingredients in several commercially prepared remedies, by taking, for example, Solgar® L-Cysteine, which contains 500mg of cysteine i:
– Available in bottles of 30 vegicaps
– Take 1 vegicap daily with a little juice or water between meals

Homeopathy

Antimonium crudum and **Graphites**

– Four 5c tablets of one or both of these remedies to be sucked slowly twice a day for several weeks

Antimonium crudum

– Chemical origin: black sulphide of antimony
– The homeopathic remedy for thickened, hard, cracked nails

– A specific indication: the nail is broken along its length

Graphites

– Mineral origin: the black lead used in pencils
– One of the homeopathic remedies for brittle or misshapen nails
– Two specific indications: the skin is dry and thick

• You could try Lehning® Silica Complex 11, whose ingredients include Antimonium crudum 3x and Arsenicum album 5x:
– Sold in 30ml bottles of oral solution
– Twenty drops to be taken in a little water, three times a day

• These treatments should be used in combination with a constitutional remedy, to be chosen after consultation with a professional homeopath. Some likely choices are Natrum muriaticum, Silica, or Thuja

Herbal remedies

Alfalfa and **Horsetail** are both effective for replacing lost minerals.

POSSIBLE PRESCRIPTION: Obtain from your herbalist a 30ml bottle of mother tincture of alfalfa, and an equal quantity of mother tincture of horsetail. Take 25 drops of the alfalfa solution in the morning in a little water, and 25 drops of the horsetail solution in the evening. This treatment should be continued for several weeks.

Alfalfa/horsetail

Alfalfa, a very common plant in temperate regions, is known to be rich in minerals and to have a marked revitalizing effect. When combined with horsetail, which contains high levels of silica, the two treatments complement one another very well.

• You can obtain horsetail from your herbalist, as a whole fresh-plant suspension (this formulation's cold stabilization process restores the full natural therapeutic effect of the plant). Take half a teaspoonful in a little water twice a day. This is not to be taken by children under 15 years of age

Borage oil is very beneficial for the skin, hair, and nails.
– You can buy this remedy in capsule form from your herbalist. Take two capsules per day for several weeks

TOPICAL APPLICATION: one capsule opened up and applied directly to the nails may reinforce the oral treatment

• You could also try 'Health from the Sun' EFA Derma-Skin Formula, which contains borage and flaxseed oils beneficial to the skin, as well as vitamins A, C, D, E, zinc and extracts of burdock root and yellowdock:
– Available in containers of 60 capsules
– Take 2 capsules once daily

Cardiovascular problems

There is no question that progress has been made in the diagnosis of heart disease, as well as in our understanding of the risk factors and the treatment of cardiovascular problems. Yet this area still remains one of medicine's main concerns, as heart disease is one of the primary causes of death, along with cancer. Complementary therapies, through their interest in the patient's 'terrain' and in the question of diet, have an enormous contribution to make in the management of these serious illnesses.

Heart and blood vessels

Tinnitus (ringing in the ears)

This has been variously described as resembling the humming of a ventilator or fan, a buzzing sound, a steady roar like a waterfall, or the hissing of a pressure cooker. This sound is perceived intermittently or permanently in one or both ears, or in some other part of the head, when there is no external sound source. External noises may, however, either worsen or temporarily drown out the sounds in the head.

Tinnitus is unpleasant and difficult to cope with, although it is almost always a benign condition. While a medical consultation may sometimes be able to trace the cause of the sounds, treatment is most often a difficult process.

Osteopathy and chiropractic

Small muscles in the neck can sometimes block and pinch certain networks of nerves. The most common symptom produced is pain, but various nerve troubles can also result, including dizziness and tinnitus. Once a medical examination has localized the source of the muscle spasm, manipulation of the spine eliminates the troublesome symptoms almost immediately. Some patients who have already had their symptoms treated in this way soon come to recognize the signs of a cervical blockage, see their practitioner without delay, and know they will soon obtain relief from a simple adjustment.

TREATMENT SCHEDULE: As few as two sessions, ten days apart, may bring signs of improvement.

Acupuncture and mesotherapy

These two therapies are both worth trying, as they soothe nerves, help relax muscle spasms, and relieve pain generally.

TREATMENT SCHEDULE: Five or six sessions, one week apart, of acupuncture or mesotherapy, or a combination of the two, are sometimes enough to bring relief when everything else has failed.

I have placed mesotherapy among the non-medicinal therapies, as it uses only tiny injectable doses of traditional medicines or homeopathic blends, and it strikes me as being similar to acupuncture, both in its areas of application and in its results. It is still classified as one of the reflex therapies. This therapy is more common in France and is rarely used in Britain. Those who do use it are GPs who have trained in homeopathic medicine.

Electro-Acupuncture

This is sometimes used to reinforce the effects of traditional acupuncture. A weak electric current is delivered by a nerve stimulator through needles or carbon electrodes. It is primarily used for chronic pain, but some practitioners advocate it for stubborn cases of tinnitus.

Transcutaneous Electrical Nerve Stimulation (TENS)

This is a neurophysiological technique, derived from numerous scientific studies undertaken in an effort to understand how acupuncture works. It has become more practical in recent years through the miniaturization of the TENS equipment, and is now used mainly in pain-management centres for the treatment of such conditions as the after-effects of amputations, or shingles. But some acupuncturists also use it for tinnitus.

Acupressure and shiatsu

These two therapies, of Chinese and Japanese origin respectively, are based on the massage, rubbing, and stretching of acupuncture points, or of points that examination reveals to be painful. They may well be of use in tinnitus, as they both seek to restore the circulation of energies that may have been disrupted. Sessions usually last half an hour or one hour, and are repeated weekly.

In very resistant cases of tinnitus, a condition for which there are not many therapeutic solutions available, it is important to be both open to new ideas, and very patient. Before deciding that a particular treatment has done no good, you should be willing to try several sessions, as these are often necessary before even the beginnings of an improvement can be seen.

Homeopathy

Aurum and **Glonoinum**

Four 5c tablets of one or both of these remedies to be sucked slowly between meals, twice a day for several weeks.

Aurum metallicum

– Mineral origin: the metal gold
– The homeopathic remedy for vascular congestion in the head
– The symptoms appear most readily among the elderly and those prone to depression

Glonoinum

– Chemical origin: nitroglycerine, usually used for chest pains (angina)
– The homeopathic remedy for circulatory problems with a rush of blood to the head
– A specific indication: the condition is made worse by heat

• You could also try Lehning® Aurum Complex 38, whose ingredients include Aurum muriaticum 8x:
– Available in boxes of 80 tablets
– One tablet, sucked three times a day

• It is also important that you combine these treatments with a constitutional remedy, to be chosen after consultation with a professional homeopath. Some likely choices are Aurum, Baryta carbonica, or Sulfur

Oligotherapy

Manganese and **cobalt**

Trace elements are usually found in a varied and high-quality diet. In cases of deficiency they can be given as medicinal supplements.

Natural healing

Dietary sources of manganese

This is primarily to be found in plants, especially whole-grain cereals, chocolate, oil-producing nuts (such as almonds, walnuts, and hazelnuts), wheatgerm, some herbs and spices (cloves, ginger, and thyme), vegetables (carrots, beetroot, chestnuts, beans, peas, and soya beans), coffee, and tea. It is pretty much nonexistent in animal products (meat, fish, or eggs) or fruits.

Dietary sources of cobalt

This mineral cannot be synthesized by the body, and comes essentially from animal products: meat, milk, and shellfish (crayfish). Plant and vegetable matter contains only a form of cobalt that our bodies cannot use.

• Manganese-cobalt treatment: this combination is available in various brands and forms, such as Organic Minerals (Colloidals) which contains 70+ trace minerals:
– Available in 946ml bottles
– Take 1–3 caps just before breakfast and/or evening meal
– Children 1 teaspoon daily for each 20lbs of body weight
Or Maximol (Ionized colloidals):
– Available in 500ml bottles
– Take ½ capful once or twice daily on an empty stomach

Herbal remedies

Garlic, ginkgo biloba, and **melilot** for their effects on circulation.

Angelica, hawthorn, and **black horehound** for their soothing action.

These two groups of plants can be taken singly or in combination.

Angelica

Angelica promotes blood circulation, as well as having antispasmodic effects that make it useful for colicky pains and aerophagia (nervous swallowing of air, producing abdominal wind). Angelica is widely used in cakes and pastries, in confectionery, and is one of the ingredients in Benedictine liqueur.

POSSIBLE PRESCRIPTION: Ask your herbalist to make up 60ml bottle of mother tincture of ginkgo biloba. Take 25 drops in a little water, three times a day.

• You could also ask your herbalist to prepare a 60ml bottle of melilot or hawthorn in a whole fresh-plant suspension (this formulation's cold stabilization process restores the full natural therapeutic effect of the plant). Take half a teaspoonful in a little water morning and evening

Melilot

This fodder plant, which thrives on fallow land and in limestone areas, contains natural blood-thinners that are very beneficial for circulatory problems. Melilot also has calming, antispasmodic properties, which have recommended it for use in mild problems of the autonomic nervous system.

High blood pressure (hypertension)

Blood circulates through the arteries at a certain pressure in order for it to reach the organs. Normal blood pressure ranges between 70 and 130mm of mercury) for the first number (systolic pressure). The second figure, often neglected by patients who focus only the first, is still important: this diastolic pressure should not be higher than 100mm of mercury.

The measuring of blood pressure by means of an inflatable cuff is an Italian invention that has now been in use for a hundred years.

When these figures are too high, a diagnosis of high blood pressure, or hypertension, is made. However, at least two different readings should be taken, at rest, and one month apart – if both readings show high numbers, the diagnosis can be confirmed. Medical management of the condition may possibly continue for the rest of the patient's life, but should not be undertaken without repeated confirmation that the high readings are accurate and consistent. Cardiologists are debating the necessity of treating so-called 'borderline' hypertension, in which the first number may range up to140–160, and the second number may vary between 85 and 95.

Hypertension affects millions of people in the Western world. It may be manifested as pain or throbbing in the head, dizziness, ringing in the ears, tiredness, or sometimes a very sudden or recurring nosebleed. This disease may develop quietly and insidiously, and should be taken seriously. By reducing the calibre of the blood vessels, it poses a threat to the heart, brain, and kidneys, increasing the burden on these organs to their detriment. High blood pressure is directly responsible for heart attacks (cardiac infarction), and strokes that may lead to paralysis on one side of the body (hemiplegia).

Four important points

– In most cases of hypertension, no identifiable cause for the condition is found

– In half of all cases, there is a family history of high blood pressure

– Hypertension is not exclusively linked to stress, although stress certainly is a factor

– Salt added to food has played a large part in the widespread development of this condition. We are all born with different levels of tolerance, even for salt itself, but diets are less strict now when it comes to salt intake than in the past, as diuretics are so effective at eliminating the excess. Most fruits and vegetables are rich in potassium and low in sodium, which makes them ideal for low-salt or salt-free diets

Natural healing

Five useful tips

These tips are in many ways the logical conclusion of what has just been said, but following them may be enough to save you taking medicines that are all too easy to prescribe, that may have unwanted side-effects, and that are never completely harmless:
– lose any excess weight you may have gained
– get some sort of regular, moderate exercise, for about 45 minutes, two or three times per week
– cut down on your salt intake
– stop smoking
– try to reduce your stress levels!

Homeopathy

Its role will depend on the nature of the case. It may be used as a constitutional remedy for those who are predisposed to hypertension, or as a 'back-up treatment' in more serious cases.

Aconite and **Aurum**

– Four 5c tablets of one or both of these remedies to be sucked slowly between meals, twice a day

Aconitum napellus

– Vegetable origin: the monk's-hood plant, also known as wolf's-bane (traditionally used by hunters as an arrow poison against the animal)
– The homeopathic remedy for illnesses that come on very suddenly
– Two specific indications: the sudden onset of the symptoms, and intense anxiety

Aurum metallicum

– Mineral origin: the metal gold
– The homeopathic remedy for arterial congestion in the head
– The symptoms are likely to appear in angry, intolerant personalities, or in those prone to depression

• You could also try Lehning® Aurum Complex 38, whose ingredients include Aurum 8x:
– Sold in boxes of 80 tablets
– One tablet to be sucked, three times a day

Oligotherapy

Magnesium

This trace element usually comes from the diet, which should be varied and of high quality. In cases of deficiency, which often occurs with magnesium, it can be given as a medicinal supplement.

Dietary sources of magnesium

Present in almost all foods, but mostly in the calorie-rich ones, unfortunately. The best sources of magnesium are: citrus fruits, bananas, whole-grain cereals (oat or bran flakes), cocoa and chocolate, shellfish (winkles, shrimps, oysters, and clams) and oily fish, snails, figs, hard cheeses, nuts (almonds, peanuts, hazelnuts and walnuts), vegetables (spinach, dried and green beans, maize, split peas, and soya beans), and wholemeal bread.

• Magnesium treatment: this is available in various brands and forms, such as Organic Minerals (Colloidals) which contains 70+ trace minerals:
– Available in 946ml bottles
– Take 1–3 caps just before breakfast and/or evening meal
– Children 1 teaspoon daily for each 20lbs of body weight
Or Maximol (Ionized colloidals):
– Available in 500ml bottles
– Take ½ capful once or twice daily on an empty stomach

• You can also take higher doses of magnesium by using remedies such as Magasorb® (Lamberts) containing 150mg of magnesium (as citrate):
– Available in containers of 60 and 180 tablets
– One to three tablets daily

Herbal remedies

Garlic, birch, and **olive tree** for their effectiveness in lowering blood pressure.

Cypress, ginkgo, and **common periwinkle**, which protect the arteries and capillaries.

POSSIBLE PRESCRIPTION: Ask your herbalist to prepare a blend of dried extracts of garlic, cypress, and olive, 100mg of each plant for each No.2 capsule (the size of the capsule that the herbalist will use for the ingredients). Take one capsule three times a day for two or three weeks.

• You could also try Pure-Gar (Lamberts); each capsule contains 500mg of garlic powder:
– Available in containers of 90 capsules
– 1 to 3 capsules daily

Garlic

As well as its legendary use for warding off vampires, garlic is a medicinal plant with many virtues. It fights off infection in the ears, nose, and throat, and was widely used for this purpose before the discovery of antibiotics. It can bring remarkable benefits to circulatory problems (thinning the blood, bringing down high cholesterol and blood pressure readings). It also works as a hypoglycaemic, and can be a valuable adjunct to the diabetic diet.

Birch

The leaves of this tree with the slender trunk and silvery bark have always been used for their ability to promote elimination by the gall bladder and kidneys. Its sap acts as a diuretic, and its essential oil is very effective against skin troubles such as eczema and psoriasis. It is one of the best depuratives and detoxifiers.

Olive

The olive tree has played an important role since the days of the Greeks and Romans, both for its medicinal properties and for its symbolic aspect. Its leaves reduce tension, improve circulation, encourage the elimination of urine – as well as serving to symbolize peace.

Its oil was an important element in the culture of ancient Crete, and is now considered an essential part of a healthy diet.

• You can take Olive-X (Thorne), which contains Olive leaf extract (500mg):
– Available in containers of 60 capsules
– 1 capsule 3 times daily

Palpitations

Palpitations are the exaggerated, and unpleasant, feeling of the heart beating, or racing, when normally it is not felt at all. The 'turn' may last only a few seconds, a few minutes, or even several hours, and it may come and go or become a permanent condition. The subject may also experience an oppressive feeling, that only hinders his or her activity somewhat, or a stronger sensation of sickness or faintness that brings any activities to an end.

If you experience palpitations, it is worth consulting a cardiologist, especially if they are persistent or recurring. They usually turn out to be a benign and minor nuisance, but the specialist can determine the cause and the seriousness of the condition. The episodes may disappear if you follow such simple advice as eliminating stimulants (like tea or coffee) from your diet – but it is occasionally necessary to prescribe a mild sedative.

If there is one organ that symbolizes all our emotions, it is, of course, the heart. I do not need to remind you of the obvious links between the heart and the mind.

Homeopathy

Cactus and **Nux vomica**
– Four 5c tablets of one or both of these remedies to be sucked slowly like sweets, three or four times in succession

Cactus grandiflorus

– Vegetable origin: the young stems of the night-blooming cereus plant
– The homeopathic remedy for tight chest pains
– A specific indication: the symptoms improve when out in fresh air

Nux vomica

– Vegetable origin: the fruit of the Strychnos nux-vomica tree, also known as poison nut
– The specific homeopathic remedy for symptoms resulting from too much alcohol or coffee
– A specific indication: the symptoms improve after a nap

Warning: it is essential to consult your doctor if this pain is intense or long-lasting, if it recurs, or if it spreads towards the jaw or left arm.

• You could also try Bioforce Hawthorn-Garlic Complex:
– Available in containers of 150 capsules

– Take 1 to 2 capsules twice daily with a little water

Oligotherapy

Magnesium

Trace elements usually come from the diet, which should be varied and of high quality. In cases of deficiency, which often occurs with magnesium, it can be given as a medicinal supplement.

Dietary sources of magnesium

Present in almost all foods, but mostly in the calorie-rich ones, unfortunately. The best sources of magnesium are: citrus fruits, bananas, whole-grain cereals (oat or bran flakes), cocoa and chocolate, shellfish (winkles, shrimps, oysters, and clams) and oily fish, snails, figs, hard cheeses, nuts (almonds, peanuts, hazelnuts and walnuts), vegetables (spinach, dried and green beans, maize, split peas, and soya beans), and wholemeal bread.

• Magnesium treatment: this is available in various brands and forms, such as Organic Minerals (Colloidals) which contains 70+ trace minerals:
– Available in 946ml bottles
– Take 1–3 caps just before breakfast and/or evening meal
– Children 1 teaspoon daily for each 20lbs of body weight
Or Maximol (Ionized colloidals):
– Available in 500ml bottles
– Take ½ capful once or twice daily on an empty stomach

• You can also take higher doses of magnesium by using remedies such as Magasorb® (Lamberts) containing 150mg of magnesium (as citrate):
– Available in containers of 60 and 180 tablets
– one to three tablets daily

The herb for palpitations

Hawthorn

Hawthorn

This tree has been in use since ancient times, and for a variety of purposes, whether for dissolving gall bladder or kidney stones, or for making the executioner's block. It was only in the 19th century, however, that it gained recognition when its cardiosedative benefits were discovered. Hawthorn can slow down a racing heart, reduce or eliminate palpitations, act as a heart tonic and a vasodilator for those who have suffered a heart attack, thus improving their heart function. It also brings down high blood pressure, and calms anxiety, both in children and adults, without inducing drowsiness or memory lapses. It has the added advantage of being nontoxic.

Possible prescriptions:

– Mother tincture, the most common therapeutic form of hawthorn: ask your herbalist to prepare a 30ml bottle. Take 25 drops two or three times a day, for nervous or heart conditions

– Dried extracts: you can ask your herbalist to make up 20 capsules containing 200mg of dried extract for each No.2 capsule (the size of the capsule that the herbalist will use for the ingredients). Take one capsule 2 or 3 times a day, depending on the symptoms

– Whole fresh-plant suspension: this formulation's cold stabilization process restores the full natural therapeutic effect of the plant. Obtain a 60ml bottle of hawthorn in a whole fresh-plant suspension from your herbalist. Take half a teaspoonful in a little water twice a day

– Herbal tea: one dessertspoonful of hawthorn blossoms for each cup of boiling water. Allow the blossoms to steep for ten minutes before drinking the tea

– Decoction: hawthorn branches can be used in a herbal decoction for circulatory problems

• You could also try Lamberts® Hawthorn; each tablet contains 2,500mg of powdered hawthorn:
– Available in containers of 60 tablets
– One tablet daily for a minimum of 6 weeks

• Another alternative is Bio-Health's Hawthorn Berry, which contains 450mg of hawthorn:
– Available in containers of 120 capsules
– Take 1 capsule twice daily with water

Nosebleeds

The mucous membrane inside the nose is fed by many blood vessels, and it is not surprising that it bleeds from time to time. This may simply be a spontaneous event, or could be the result of repeated childhood or adolescent picking, and is now most often precipitated by high blood pressure in the adult. Nine times out of ten, nosebleeds are not serious, and cause more shock than anything else.

How can you help?

These measures should be taken immediately:

• Sit the patient down in a chair

• Explain the situation calmly, without over-dramatizing things – the aim is to reassure the patient

• Get the subject to blow his or her nose very gently, so as to get rid of all the blood clots

• The patient should lean forward rather than back, as any blood that runs down into the back of the throat is liable to set off a coughing fit, and may get into the bronchial tubes

• Pinch the subject's nostrils gently between your thumb and forefinger for several minutes, and ask the person to breathe through his or her mouth

• Avoid any hasty or needless intervention that could make the situation worse, especially as most nosebleeds end of their own accord anyway

• Do not put any cotton wool in the nose, as it is very difficult to remove once it has dried

Homeopathy

Arnica and **China**
– Four 5c tablets of one or both of these remedies to be sucked slowly like sweets, three or four times in succession

Arnica montana

– Vegetable origin: the whole of the leopard's-bane plant is used
– The specific homeopathic remedy for traumatic injuries and bruises
– Be careful, arnica is a poisonous plant; it is not for internal use, and should not be applied to broken skin

China

– Vegetable origin: the bark of the cinchona tree, source of quinine
– The specific homeopathic remedy for the after-effects of haemorrhaging

• You could also try Lehning® Arnica Complex 1, whose ingredients include Arnica 3x and China 3x:
– Sold in 30ml bottles of oral drops
– Fifteen drops to be taken three to four times in succession by adults; children should take five drops, three to four times

Herbal remedies

Nettle
– How to use it: a soup or herbal tea made from nettle leaves, which taste a little like spinach, can halt a nosebleed, and even reduce menstrual flow

Nettle

Though feared for its stinging leaves, nettle is a medicinal plant with many properties: it is a depurative, a tonic, a mild diuretic, an astringent, and reduces allergic symptoms.

• You could also ask your herbalist to make up a 30ml bottle of nettle in a whole fresh-plant suspension (this formulation's cold stabilization process restores the full natural therapeutic effect of the plant). Take half a teaspoonful in a little water twice a day

Cypress, ginkgo, and **common periwinkle** for their benefits in protecting the arteries and capillaries.

– Ask your herbalist to prepare a 30ml bottle of mother tincture of one of these three plants. Take 25 drops in a little water, three or four times a day

Cypress

This conifer tree from the East has always held an important place in poetry, as well as in medicine for its power to reduce bleeding. In the past, its seeds were ground up and used to treat wounds. Cypress acts on the veins much as witch hazel does.

Ginkgo biloba

The ginkgo is an ornamental tree from China and Japan, with a legendary and mythical past. It acts a vasodilator, while also reducing the blood's viscosity. This capillary regulation results in improved circulation.

Common periwinkle

The common periwinkle, or *Vinca minor*, has astringent and haemostatic properties, which allow it to reduce menstrual blood flow or stop nosebleeds. It also improves blood flow to the brain, and has lent its name to a class of medicines used for that purpose, the vincamines.

• You could also try Ginkgo biloba 2000mg (Lamberts): each tablet contains 40mg of a 50:1 extract of Ginkgo biloba:
– Available in containers of 60 tablets
– 1–3 tablets daily.

Vertigo

Patients with this condition most often describe a fleeting feeling of instability or faintness, with light-headedness and loss of balance, sometimes accompanied by nausea, vomiting, and headache. Dizzy spells are a very frequent symptom, and are the third most common reason people go to the doctor, after fever and pain. Although these symptoms can be frightening and unpleasant, they are almost always harmless. In most cases, in fact, the cause is never found, and any tests carried out show normal results. The only exception is cervical osteoarthritis, but although this often appears on X-rays, it is rarely responsible for the dizzy symptoms.

Maintaining our balance is no simple matter, as we constantly readjust our body's position in space through a delicate system of receptors located in the inner ear. If certain pathological conditions are responsible, these mechanisms can fail or become scrambled, like radar, thus causing a sensation of dizziness.

General advice

If you are feeling dizzy:

• Do not get behind the wheel of your car

• Get some rest by lying down in a quiet place, away from bright light

• Stay away from high or windy areas, stay on your usual diet, and avoid stimulants

Osteopathy and chiropractic

Small muscles in the neck can sometimes block and pinch certain networks of nerves. The most common symptom produced is pain, but various nerve troubles can also result, including dizziness and sometimes tinnitus. Once a medical examination has localized the source of the muscle spasm, manipulation of the spine eliminates the troublesome symptoms almost immediately.

Some cases of dizziness, which only appear in a reclining position when the subject turns his or her head, are caused by the displacement of sensory cells in the inner ear. The diagnosis is confirmed by a test that goes by the barbaric name of an electronystagmogram. The treatment is a simple matter in comparison, involving a specific mobilizing adjustment that rapidly improves the debilitating clinical symptoms, sometimes permanently.

Acupuncture and mesotherapy

These two therapies are both worth trying, as they soothe nerves, help relax muscle spasms, and relieve pain generally.

TREATMENT SCHEDULE: Two or three sessions of acupuncture or mesotherapy, or a combination of the two, are often enough to bring the first signs of improvement, or even a cure.

I have placed mesotherapy among the non-medicinal therapies, as it uses only tiny injectable doses of traditional medicines or homeopathic blends, and it strikes me as being similar to acupuncture, both in its areas of application and in its results.

Homeopathy

Conium and **Phosphorus**

– Four 5c tablets of one or both of these remedies to be sucked slowly between meals, two or three times a day

Conium maculatum

– Vegetable origin: the giant hemlock plant
– The homeopathic remedy for dizzy spells with visual disturbance
– A specific indication: the condition is made worse by sexual continence

Phosphorus

– Mineral origin: white phosphorus
– The homeopathic remedy for dizziness following loss of blood
– A specific indication: the condition is made worse by storms

• You could also try Lehning® Conium Complex 36, whose ingredients include Conium 4x and Arsenicum album 4x:
– Sold in 30ml bottles of oral drops
– Fifteen drops to be taken in a little water, three times a day

• For dizziness caused by circulatory problems in the elderly, you could try Vertigoheel® (Heel), which contains Cocculus D4, Conium D3, Ambra D6 and Petroleum D8:
– Available in drop bottles containing 30 and 100ml and tablets (packs of 50 and 250)
– In general, 10 drops or 3 tablets to be dissolved under the tongue 3 times daily. In sporadic dizziness and nausea, initially 10 drops or 1 tablet every 15 minutes

• It is also vital that you combine these treatments with a constitutional remedy, to be chosen after consultation with a professional homeopath. Some likely choices are Aurum, Phosphorus, or Sulfur

Aurum metallicum

– Mineral origin: the metal gold
– The homeopathic remedy for vascular congestion in the head
– The symptoms appear most readily among the elderly and those prone to depression

Oligotherapy

Manganese and **cobalt**
Trace elements are usually found in a varied and high-quality diet. In cases of deficiency, which is unlikely with these two minerals, they can be given as medicinal supplements.

• Manganese-cobalt treatment: this combination is available in various brands and forms, such as Organic Minerals (Colloidals) which contains 70+ trace minerals:
– Available in 946ml bottles
– Take 1–3 caps just before breakfast and/or evening meal
– Children 1 teaspoon daily for each 20lbs of body weight
Or Maximol (Ionized colloidals):
– Available in 500ml bottles
– Take ½ capful once or twice daily on an empty stomach

Herbal remedies

Garlic, ginkgo biloba, and **melilot** for their effects on circulation.

Angelica, hawthorn, and **black horehound** for their soothing action.

These two groups of plants can be taken singly or in combination.

POSSIBLE PRESCRIPTIONS: Ask your herbalist to prepare a 60ml bottle of mother tincture of ginkgo. Take 30 drops in a little water, twice a day.

• You could also ask your herbalist to make up 30 capsules of a blend of dried extracts of angelica, hawthorn, and melilot, 100mg of each plant for each No.2 capsule (the size of the capsule that the herbalist would use for the ingredients). Take one capsule two or three times a day for about ten days.

Ginkgo biloba

This ornamental tree from China and Japan is venerated for its legendary and mythical associations. It is one of the oldest and hardiest trees on the planet, as it survived both the last ice age and the atomic bombing of Hiroshima. It has also sometimes been dubbed the 'tree of forty gold crowns', because of its high price in times gone by, and because its yellow or green fan-shaped leaves fall to the ground in a golden carpet.

• You could ask your herbalist for a 60ml bottle of hawthorn or melilot in a whole fresh-plant suspension (this formulation's cold stabilization process restores the full natural therapeutic effect of the plant). Take half a teaspoonful in a little water twice a day

Hawthorn

This is the plant for the heart: it promotes heart function, regulates its rhythm, re-establishes normal blood pressure, and even helps blood circulation to the brain.

Melilot

This plant is capable of producing some of the most wide-ranging benefits to the circulation. It is effective in treating both haemorrhoids and varicose veins, and also helps reduce the risk of phlebitis, thanks to its anti-coagulant properties.

• You could also try Pure-Gar (Lamberts); each capsule contains 500mg of garlic powder:
– Available in containers of 90 capsules
– 1 to 3 capsules daily

Garlic

This the oldest and most remarkable of the medicinal herbs, and was used by the labourers who built the pyramids. For several centuries it was considered a cure-all, powerful enough to prevent and cure the plague, as well as to keep vampires away. It has potent infection-fighting properties, as well as bringing marked benefits to the circulation. There is no doubt that it should be part of the diet of every heart patient. It has only one drawback, its devastating effects on the breath.

Limbs and extremities

Restless legs

If your legs won't stay still, by day or – especially – night, you have restless legs syndrome. The symptoms include stinging, burning, or tingling sensations, or outright pain.

Fifteen per cent of the population suffers from the condition to some degree. It is most often benign, but quite often runs in families, affecting more women than men. It may be made worse by the consumption of alcohol, coffee, or cigarettes.

Homeopathy

Zincum
– Four 5c tablets to be sucked slowly between meals, twice a day

Zincum metallicum

– Mineral origin: the metal zinc
– The specific homeopathic remedy for restless legs

• You could try Lehning® Tarentula Complex 71, whose ingredients include Tarentula 6x and Zincum valerianum 6x:
– Available in 30ml bottles of oral drops
– Fifteen drops to be taken in a little water, three times a day

• Another alternative is Spascupreel® (Heel), which contains Magnesium phosphoricum D6, Colocynthis D4, Gelsemium D6
– Available in packs of 50 and 250 tablets

Natural healing

– In general, one tablet to be sucked three times daily. In acute disorders, one tablet every 15 minutes.

Oligotherapy

Zinc

Trace elements usually come from the diet, which should be varied and of high quality. In cases of deficiency, zinc can be given as a medicinal supplement.

Dietary sources of zinc

Zinc is most plentiful in seafood, fish, oysters ++, and shellfish, as well as in cereals, some vegetables (broccoli, mushrooms, spinach, and beans), brewer's yeast, walnuts, wholemeal bread, egg yolk, and meat.

Zinc treatment: this is available in various forms, such as Organic Minerals (Colloidals) which contains 70+ trace minerals:
– Available in 946ml bottles
– Take 1–3 caps just before breakfast and/or evening meal
– Children 1 teaspoon daily for each 20lbs of body weight
Or Maximol (Ionized colloidals):
– Available in 500ml bottles
– Take ½ capful once or twice daily on an empty stomach

• You could also try Pic-Mins (Thorne), a trace mineral combination (in picolinate form) which includes a blend of selenium, vanadium, manganese, chromium, boron, molybdenum and zinc:
– Sold in containers of 90 capsules
– 1 capsule 3 times daily.

Raynaud's disease

This condition is not only inconvenient, but downright unpleasant, and occasionally painful. It leaves the fingers white, numb, and cold, while for some reason, the thumbs remain untouched.

The condition, which usually starts between the ages of 20 and 30, and affects more women than men, involves a vasospasm that temporarily cuts off the circulation of the blood. It is usually triggered by cold, but the emotions may also play a role – although it has not been confirmed, it seems likely that there is a psychological element to it.

Some medicines (such as migraine treatments derived from rye ergot, beta-blockers, or diuretics) and nicotine can also impair the micro-circulation, promoting Raynaud's disease.

Homeopathy

Agaricus and **Pulsatilla**

– Four 5c tablets of one or both of these remedies to be sucked slowly, two or three times a day

Agaricus muscarius

– Vegetable origin: a fungus, the fly agaric

– The homeopathic remedy for red, itching skin, that feels as though pierced by ice needles
– A very specific indication: cold makes the condition worse

Pulsatilla

– Vegetable origin: the meadow anemone or windflower
– The homeopathic remedy for blotched or marbled skin
– A specific indication: the desire for fresh air even when feeling chilled

• You could also try Abropernol® (Heel), which contains Pulsatilla D4, Hamamelis D4, Agaricus D5...
– Available in packs of 50 and 250 tablets.
– 1 tablet dissolved under the tongue 3 times daily

Oligotherapy

Magnesium

Trace elements usually come from the diet, which should be varied and of high quality. In cases of deficiency, which often occurs with magnesium, it can be given as a medicinal supplement.

Dietary sources of magnesium

Present in almost all foods, but mostly in the calorie-rich ones, unfortunately. The best sources of magnesium are: citrus fruits, bananas, whole-grain cereals (oat or bran flakes), cocoa and chocolate, shellfish (winkles, shrimps, oysters, and clams) and oily fish, snails, figs, hard cheeses, nuts (almonds, peanuts, hazelnuts, and walnuts), vegetables (spinach, dried and green beans, maize, split peas, and soya beans), and wholemeal bread.

• Magnesium treatment: this is available in various brands and forms, such as Organic Minerals (Colloidals) which contains 70+ trace minerals:
– Available in 946ml bottles
– Take 1–3 caps just before breakfast and/or evening meal
– Children 1 teaspoon daily for each 20lbs of body weight
Or Maximol (Ionized colloidals):
– Available in 500ml bottles
– Take ½ capful once or twice daily on an empty stomach

• You can also take higher doses of magnesium by using remedies such as Magasorb® (Lamberts) containing 150mg of magnesium (as citrate):
– Available in containers of 60 and 180 tablets
– one to three tablets daily

Herbal remedies

Melilot and **white willow**

POSSIBLE PRESCRIPTION: Ask your herbalist to prepare 20 capsules of a blend of dried extracts of melilot and white willow, 150mg of each plant for each No.2 capsule (the size of the capsule that the herbalist would use for the ingredients). Take one capsule twice a day for several days.

Melilot

This plant offers a wide range of benefits

to the circulation. It is effective in treating both haemorrhoids and varicose veins, and also helps reduce the risk of phlebitis, thanks to its anti-coagulant properties.

White Willow

The bark of this tree is the source of salicylic acid, from which aspirin is derived. It has long been used to bring down fever, and remains one of the current treatments for rheumatic pains.

• You can ask your herbalist to prepare a 60ml bottle of melilot in a whole fresh-plant suspension (this formulation's cold stabilization process restores the full natural therapeutic effect of the plant). Take half a teaspoonful in a little water twice a day

The Mediterranean or Cretan diet

• This diet is currently a model in terms of its benefits to the heart. It consists of cereals, pasta, fruits and vegetables, and olive oil. It is an enjoyable regimen to follow, for although it does not allow for excess, it does not impose deprivation either. It appears to be a passport to a long life with a healthy heart

• The emphasis on cereals, and especially on pasta, provides a healthy portion of slow sugars (starches). The pasta is often served with garlic, onions, herbs, spices, and tomatoes. These ingredients form the basis of the diet, and constitute the main dish in most meals

• Fruits and green or dried vegetables are served at each meal

• Walnuts and almonds are frequent accompaniments

• Any fat is almost always of vegetable origin, in the form of olive oil. No butter or cream is used

• Priority is given to poultry and fish, with eggs served from time to time – rather than red meat (beef, mutton, or pork), which is rarely eaten

• Sugar and sweets are not part of the Mediterranean diet

• Wine is served regularly, but in moderate quantities

Vasomotor problems (acrocyanosis)

These very inconvenient symptoms are often encountered among those suffering from neurosis (see page 71 of the section on 'Nervous problems'): the fingers go numb and turn white or blue as soon as they are exposed to the cold.

Homeopathy

Lachesis and **Pulsatilla**

– Four 5c tablets of one or both of these remedies to be sucked slowly, two or three times a day

Lachesis mutus

– Animal origin: the venom from the bushmaster snake
– The homeopathic remedy for swollen, blue, or purplish skin
– One character trait: alternation between excitable moods and depression

Pulsatilla

– Vegetable origin: the meadow anemone or windflower
– The homeopathic remedy for swollen veins with blotched or marbled skin
– A specific indication: the desire for fresh air even when feeling chilled

• You could also try Hamamelis-Homaccord® (Heel), a homeopathic witch hazel compound containing Hamamelis and Carduus marianus in various potencies
– Available in drop bottles of 30 and 100ml
– In general, 10 drops 3 times daily. In acute disorders, initially 10 drops every 15 minutes

Oligotherapy

Magnesium

Trace elements usually come from the diet, which should be varied and of high quality. In cases of deficiency, which often occurs with magnesium, it can be given as a medicinal supplement.

Magnesium deficiency is very common in the West, and causes one of the most rich and varied symptomatologies we know.

Dietary sources of magnesium

It is to be found in almost all foods, but mostly in the calorie-rich ones, unfortunately. The best sources of magnesium are: citrus fruits, bananas, whole-grain cereals (oat or bran flakes), cocoa and chocolate, shellfish (winkles, shrimps, oysters, and clams) and oily fish, snails, figs, hard cheeses, nuts (almonds, peanuts, hazelnuts, and walnuts), vegetables (spinach, dried and green beans, maize, split peas, and soya beans), and wholemeal bread.

The main source of magnesium in the Western diet is cereals, followed by dairy products, vegetables, and meat.

• Magnesium treatment: this is available in various brands and forms, such as Organic Minerals (Colloidals) which contains 70+ trace minerals:
– Available in 946ml bottles
– Take 1–3 caps just before breakfast and/or evening meal
– Children 1 teaspoon daily for each 20lbs of body weight
Or Maximol (Ionized colloidals):
– Available in 500ml bottles
– Take ½ capful once or twice daily on an empty stomach

• You can also take higher doses of magnesium by using remedies such as Magasorb® (Lamberts) containing 150mg of magnesium (as citrate):
– Available in containers of 60 and 180 tablets
– One to three tablets daily

• Another alternative is a Stress formula such as Lamberts® B-100 complex, a mixture of vitamins B1, B2, B3, B5, B6, B12, folic acid, biotin, choline, inositol and PABA:
– Available in containers of 60 and 200 tablets
– One tablet to be taken each day

Herbal remedies

Melilot

POSSIBLE PRESCRIPTION: Ask your herbalist to prepare 20 capsules of dried extract of melilot, 300mg for each No.2 capsule (the size of the capsule that the herbalist would use for the ingredients). Take one capsule twice a day for ten days.

Melilot

This herbaceous plant with yellow flowers has a beneficial effect on most circulatory problems. It also acts as a mild sedative and is helpful against intestinal cramps, and so it was traditionally used as a remedy for colic.

• You could ask your herbalist to prepare a 60ml bottle of melilot in a whole fresh-plant suspension (this formulation's cold stabilization process restores the full natural therapeutic effect of the plant). Take half a teaspoonful in a little water twice a day

Veins

Vein trouble and varicose veins

Venous conditions affect a large proportion of the population in the West, particularly women – there are four times as many female sufferers as male, commonly ranging in age from 35 to 50. Vein problems include a wide range of leg symptoms, such as heaviness, swelling, unpleasant tightness, pain, restless legs, or burning or tingling sensations – most of which are worsened by heat or fatigue at the end of the day.

The contributing causes most often cited are:
– work that involves prolonged standing or sitting
– floor heating
– exposure to the sun or to heat
– how many pregnancies a woman has had
– hormonal factors
– being on the pill
– being overweight, especially if this goes with an excessively rich, spicy, or unbalanced diet, or heavy drinking or smoking

A detailed clinical examination, supplemented with haemodynamic tests (such as a Doppler or ultrasound), is essential in order to arrive at an accurate diagnosis, to choose the most appropriate treatment, and to ensure the best monitoring possible.

Vein problems are linked to one unavoidable factor, and that is heredity, which is beyond our control at the moment. But there are other factors that can trigger or aggravate the condition, and these should be acted upon.

Our evolution from quadrupedal to bipedal status put a significant strain on the venous system. The stagnation of blood flow, and the resulting increased pressure, have led to unsightly, sometimes painful, dilation of the veins and to varices.

General advice

These tips are both important and effective in the improvement or slowdown of the condition. You should:

- Avoid heat in all its forms: sunbathing, saunas, Turkish baths, hair removal using hot wax, floor heating, or tanning sessions with UVA rays
- Take cool showers, rather than hot baths
- Help promote good venous return by wearing heels that are neither too high nor too flat, by avoiding tight clothing, socks, shoes, or boots, and by remembering to put your feet up whenever possible
- Lose any excess weight, which only puts extra strain on the legs
- Give preference to physical activities that promote venous drainage, such as walking, gentle jogging, cross-country skiing, swimming, and cycling – rather than weightlifting, basketball, fencing, volleyball, tennis, or squash, which tend to dilate the veins

Oxygen-bearing blood leaves the heart and travels round the body through the arteries. It returns, carrying waste products, through the veins a process doctors call 'venous return'.

Dietary advice

Your diet should be:

- High in vitamin C, which comes primarily from citrus fruits (lemons, oranges, grapefruit), spinach, parsley, and tomatoes
- High in vitamin E, which is most abundant in whole-grain cereals, wheatgerm, soya beans, lettuce, spinach, asparagus, and cold-pressed vegetable oils such as olive or sunflower oils
- High in selenium, which comes principally from pineapple, cereals, and fish

Mechanical measures

– Elastic support for the legs is now available as fine compression stockings or tights, which still show off the shape of the legs while preventing dilation of the veins

– Lymph drainage, through massage, the application of gentle pressure, or the use of specialized equipment, improves the circulation of lymph fluid (the liquid in which our cells are bathed) and thus improves the symptoms

Homeopathy

Aesculus and **Vipera**

– Four 5c tablets of one or both of these remedies to be sucked slowly, twice a day between meals

Aesculus hippocastanum

– Vegetable origin: the horse chestnut
– The homeopathic remedy for swollen veins
– One specific sensation: the feeling of heaviness

Vipera redii

– Animal origin: the venom from the poison asp
– The homeopathic remedy for inflammation and dilation of the veins

• You could also try Aesculus-Heel® (Heel), which contains Aesculus D2:
– Available in drop bottles of 30 and 100ml
– In general 10 drops 3 times daily

• It is also important that you combine these treatments with a constitutional remedy, to be chosen after consultation with a professional homeopath. Some likely choices are Calcarea fluorica, Pulsatilla, or Sepia

Calcarea fluorica

– Mineral origin: calcium fluoride
– The homeopathic remedy for slackened tissues (such as prolapsed organs, sprains, and varicose veins)

Oligotherapy

Manganese and **cobalt**

Trace elements are usually found in a varied and high-quality diet. In cases of deficiency, which is unlikely with these two minerals, they can be given as medicinal supplements.

Dietary sources of cobalt

Cobalt is most plentiful in mushrooms, white cabbage, shellfish (crayfish), onions, radishes, and meat (especially liver).

Dietary sources of manganese

The best sources of manganese are beetroot, blackcurrants, cereals, chestnuts, chocolate, nuts (such as almonds, hazelnuts, and walnuts), wheatgerm, ginger, cloves, green vegetables, soya beans, egg yolk, and tea.

• Manganese-cobalt treatment: this combination is available in various brands and forms, such as Organic Minerals (Colloidals) which contains 70+ trace minerals:
– Available in 946ml bottles

– Take 1–3 caps just before breakfast and/or evening meal
– Children 1 teaspoon daily for each 20lbs of body weight
Or Maximol (Ionized colloidals):
– Available in 500ml bottles
– Take ½ capful once or twice daily on an empty stomach

Herbal remedies

Blackcurrant, chestnut, and red vine leaf all have an elective action on venous circulation.

POSSIBLE PRESCRIPTION: Ask your herbalist to

make up 60ml bottle of mother tincture of red vine leaf. Take 25 drops in a little water, three times a day for several weeks.

• You could also try 'Health from the Sun' Blackcurrant:
– Available in containers of 50 capsules containing 500mg of Blackcurrant
– 2 to 3 capsules to be taken daily

Red vine leaf

This shrub possesses a wealth of benefits to human health. We all know the virtues of red wine: a grape treatment purifies the body (although watch out for the calories), while the vinegar soothes the skin. The leaves and fruit promote circulation in the veins and help strengthen fragile capillaries.

• You could try a topical treatment such as vitamin k Crème Plus (Jason) which contains horse chestnut, calendula and bioflavonoids:
– Available in 60g tubes
– Rub in the cream twice a day

Plant essential oils

Mint

– You can massage your legs gently with a few drops of essential oil of mint, alone or diluted in virgin olive oil. You could also soak your feet in lukewarm water to which a few drops of essential oil of mint have been added.

Mint

Fifteen different mint species are used throughout the world for their digestive and refreshing properties. Peppermint is the most sought-after for its delicacy and its effectiveness, both of which are related to the quality and concentration of its essential oil.

Haemorrhoids

These sacs of venous blood act as shock-absorbers, swelling up and deflating when we pass a stool. When they are painful, burn, swell, bleed, or when they protrude from the anus, they become the painful 'piles' that afflict so many people. They are most common among people between the ages of 30 and 50, and in fact they are highly unusual in children and rare among the elderly.

The main cause of haemorrhoids is constipation, which should be treated or prevented. Other irritants are alcohol, spices, and prolonged physical effort, which also cause swelling and may trigger a bout. There is no connection between haemorrhoids and varicose veins, as the two involve completely different venous systems. Haemorrhoidal thrombosis, which is a fairly frequent complication after childbirth, involves the development of a small blood clot that blocks the vein. It is treated with medicines or by making a small incision under local anaesthetic.

Natural healing

Bleeding

Any bleeding from the anus, even if it is only a minute quantity, or occurs only once, should be medically examined in order to confirm that it is a haemorrhoid and to localize it. There are three anatomical types of haemorrhoids:
– external haemorrhoids are more likely to turn into thromboses
– internal haemorrhoids require a particular kind of examination, an anuscopy, in order to examine them. This type may involve moderate pain, itching, bleeding, oozing of serous fluid, and occasional prolapse with protrusion of the dilated veins
– Mixed types of haemorrhoids are, by definition, both internal and external

General advice

• Do not sit on the toilet for too long, as straining dilates the veins and encourages the development of painful haemorrhoids

• Treat any constipation you may be suffering from (see page 164 of the section on 'Digestive disorders').

Topical remedies

• Be gentle when you use toilet paper after a bowel movement

• Wash the area with a moist toilet tissue such as Germoloids® (Bayer), available in boxes of 10 sachets

• Have sitz baths in cool water to which a few drops of mother tincture of calendula have been added

Dietary advice

• During painful bouts, avoid too much alcohol, spicy meals, and condiments

• Give preference to food that is:
– high in vitamin C, which is most plentiful in citrus fruits (lemons, oranges, and grapefruit), spinach, parsley, and tomatoes
– high in vitamin E, primarily in wholegrain cereals, wheatgerm, soya beans, asparagus, spinach, lettuce, and cold-pressed vegetable oils, such as olive or sunflower oils
– high in vitamin B3, whose highest concentrations are found in blackcurrants, redcurrants, brewer's yeast, blackberries, and blueberries
– high in selenium, mostly to be found in pineapples, cereals, and fish

Homeopathy

Aesculus hippocastanum and **Hamamelis**
– Four 5c tablets of one or both of these remedies to be sucked slowly, four or five times a day between meals

Aesculus hippocastanum

– Vegetable origin: the horse chestnut
– The homeopathic remedy for stretched, swollen haemorrhoids
– One characteristic indication: the symptoms improve with cold

Hamamelis virginiana

– Vegetable origin: the dried bark of the American witch hazel tree
– The homeopathic remedy for swollen,

heavy haemorrhoids that are painful to the touch
– Two characteristic indications: bleeding, and worsening of the symptoms with the slightest touch

• You could also try Lehning® Aesculus Complex 103, whose ingredients include mother tinctures of Aesculus and of Hamamelis, as well as Nux vomica 3x:
– Sold in 30ml bottles of oral drops
– Twenty drops to be taken in a little water, three times a day between meals

• Another alternative is Aesculus composition (Heel), which contains Aesculus D1, Hamamelis D4, Arnica D3...
– Sold in drop bottles of 30 and 100ml
– In general, 10 drops 3 times daily. In acute disorders initially 10 drops every 15 minutes

• It is also vital that you combine these treatments with a constitutional remedy, to be chosen after consultation with a professional homeopath. Some likely choices are Calcarea fluorica, Sepia, or Sulfur

Oligotherapy

Manganese and **cobalt**
Trace elements are usually found in a varied and high-quality diet. In cases of deficiency, which is unlikely with these two minerals, they can be given as medicinal supplements.

• Manganese-cobalt treatment: this combination is available in various brands and forms, such as Organic Minerals (Colloidals) which contains 70+ trace minerals:
– Available in 946ml bottles
– Take 1–3 caps just before breakfast and/or evening meal
– Children 1 teaspoon daily for each 20lbs of body weight
Or Maximol (Ionized colloidals):
– Available in 500ml bottles
– Take ½ capful once or twice daily on an empty stomach

Herbal remedies

Witch hazel, horse chestnut, and **red vine leaf** for their action on venous circulation.
POSSIBLE PRESCRIPTION: Ask your herbalist to prepare a 60ml bottle of mother tincture of witch hazel. Take 25 drops in a little water, two or three times a day for several weeks.

• Externally, you could use Nelsons Haemorrhoidal cream which contains Calendula and Hamamelis
– Available in 30g tubes
– Apply after going to the toilet.

Witch hazel

This small tree from the woods of North America resembles the hazelnut tree. Native people believed it had magic powers, hence its common name. It improves venous circulation and strengthens the resistance of the blood vessels.

Natural healing

Horse chestnut

The seeds of the horse chestnut tree, which originally came from the Balkans, benefit the veins in three different ways: they strengthen the walls of the blood vessels, prevent the dilation responsible for varicose veins and haemorrhoids, and combat the water retention that causes swollen legs.

Red vine leaf

This climbing shrub, whose products we already enjoy every day, is also one of the best plants for the circulation – it helps both vessel walls and venous return. One glass of wine with a meal is a good preventive measure to take against the risk of heart disease.

Allergies

Under normal circumstances, a healthy body quietly neutralizes the numerous foreign substances it encounters on a daily basis. But in millions of cases, the body overreacts to these irritants, producing great discomfort and sometimes life-threatening symptoms – these people are allergic, suffering from asthma, eczema, rhinitis, hay fever, or rashes. Some occasionally suffer from a more dramatic swelling of the mouth and throat, which requires urgent hospital treatment, possibly even a stay in the intensive care unit. Two ideas are important when it comes to allergies: a predisposition to allergies often runs in families, and a family history of the condition can regularly be discovered through questioning of the patient; and although psychological factors may worsen the symptoms, they are certainly not the cause of them. Cases of respiratory allergies have doubled over the last 20 years, most likely because of changes in lifestyle, and the overwhelming influence of environmental factors, such as atmospheric pollution, and greater exposure to recirculated air and food additives. But by following some of the complementary therapies I propose in this chapter, the great majority of allergy sufferers should be able to lead almost normal lives.

Dust and dust mite allergies

These two particular allergies are extremely common: dust is pretty much inescapable, while dust mites have found ideal living conditions in our houses and multiply happily in our quilts and duvets, mattresses, woollen blankets and carpets, and fabric wall coverings. This would be a matter of purely academic interest, if it were not for the fact that these cousins of the spider, which live on dead, shed skin cells, are responsible for various allergic reactions, such as rhinitis, spasmodic coughs, and possibly asthma attacks.

Medical management

This consists first of all of eliminating contact with the allergen, then of acting on the patient's 'terrain' in order to modify and reinforce it.

Allergy tests are a useful procedure, even for a professional homeopath – not so as to be able to give desensitizing treatments, but to be able to tell the patient what to avoid. It is a waste of time trying to prescribe any sort of treatment without trying to eliminate the cause of the allergy.

Once the allergen has been pinpointed, every effort should be made to avoid contact with it. In the case of dust mites, no treatment is as effective as getting rid of the creatures, as far as one can.

Essential measures

It is vital to try to remove dust mites, especially from the bedroom. You should:

– air the bed thoroughly, as dust mites hate cool, dry air

– avoid having fitted carpets and fabric wall coverings in your room

– wrap your mattress in a plastic cover

– be careful to keep the dust under control at all times

– use synthetic blankets on your bed, and wash them frequently

– spray against dust mites in your bedroom. Two treatments, six weeks apart, should be enough

Homeopathy

Homeopathy's approach is akin to that of a desensitizing programme, but without its drawbacks – it uses what is known as isotherapy.

Once the allergen (the substance that causes the allergic reaction) has been accurately identified, it is collected and brought in to the homeopath, who then prepares the isotherapeutic remedy. There are two types:

– Self-isotherapeutic remedies were prepared from secretions supplied by the patient, taken from the nose or throat, or from a urine sample. Current legislation no longer permits their preparation in France. However, in

Britain, there is no such regulation and homeopaths often prescribe on this basis. Most usually the preparation will is made from a sample of the patient's urine or from small skin scrapings

– Hetero-isotherapeutic remedies, on the other hand, are still made up and distributed to patients. The remedy is derived from house dust, mould, or pollen, and given to the patient in the form of granules or tablets

• The specific homeopathic remedy derived from generic house dust or taken from the bedroom

SAMPLE PRESCRIPTION: Ask your homeopath for two tubes of isotherapeutic remedy made of house dust at a dilution of 5c. Take four tablets twice a day for several weeks.

• It is also essential that you combine this treatment with a constitutional remedy, to be chosen after consultation with a professional homeopath. Some likely choices are Arsenicum album, Nux vomica, or Sulfur

Sulfur

– Mineral origin: sulphur
– The main constitutional homeopathic remedy for allergies
– Three specific indications: the symptoms are made worse by heat and water, and improve in cool temperatures

Self-isotherapeutic remedies were banned without any concrete scientific evidence against them, but purely as a precautionary measure. In Britain (where no such regulation exists), homeopaths rarely take blood samples, preferring urine or skin to create the remedy. I would simply point out that homeopathy's detractors also criticize the discipline for the complete absence of active principles once a certain dilution has been reached – which would make the transmission of any disease a highly unlikely possibility.

Oligotherapy

Manganese and **cobalt**
Trace elements are usually found in a varied and high-quality diet. In cases of deficiency, which is unlikely with these two minerals, they can be given as medicinal supplements.

Dietary sources of manganese

This is primarily to be found in plants, especially whole-grain cereals, chocolate, nuts (such as almonds, walnuts, and hazelnuts), wheatgerm, some herbs and spices (cloves, ginger, and thyme), vegetables (beetroot, chestnuts, beans, peas, and soya beans), and tea.

Dietary sources of cobalt

This mineral comes essentially from meat and milk, and shellfish (crayfish). Vegetables offer very little cobalt, although it is found in mushrooms, white cabbage, onions, and radishes.

• Manganese-cobalt treatment: this combination is available in various brands and forms, such as Organic

Minerals (Colloidals) which contains 70+ trace minerals:
– Available in 946ml bottles
– Take 1–3 caps just before breakfast and/or evening meal
– Children 1 teaspoon daily for each 20lbs of body weight
Or Maximol (Ionized colloidals):
– Available in 500ml bottles
– Take ½ capful once or twice daily on an empty stomach

• You could also take a manganese-only supplement, such as Lamberts® Manganese (as Amino Acid Chelate), containing 5mg of manganese:
– Available in containers of 100 capsules
– 1 to 3 capsules daily

Acupuncture

Allergies are acupuncture's third great treatment area, after pain and autonomic nervous system problems. Its role here is primarily one of prevention, and it can be used in combination with the two preceding therapies.

TREATMENT SCHEDULE: Two sessions per month for several months.

An average of six sessions are needed in order to judge whether the treatment is working.

Food allergies

This sort of allergy usually causes stomach upsets, rashes, and more rarely, swelling of the mouth and throat (sometimes called Quincke's disease) or anaphylactic shock, both of which require emergency treatment.

In all cases of food allergy:
– be sure to institute an exclusion diet
– make cooked fruits and vegetables a priority in your diet

Swelling of the throat and mouth should be treated urgently, as this allergic reaction prevents air from reaching the lungs, and the patient may die of suffocation.

The best treatments consist of
– identifying the allergen responsible, which may well be no easy task
– then eliminating the food from your diet

Several categories of foods may be responsible for reactions such as rashes:
– Foods with a high histamine content: fermented foods and drinks (sauerkraut, Roquefort cheese, and beer), spinach, tomatoes, oily fish (such as anchovies, sardines, salmon, and tuna), shellfish, and sausages

– Foods that cause unusually high levels of histamines to be released: alcohol (especially brandy, gin, and liqueurs), fresh pineapple, white of egg, peanuts, chocolate, citrus fruits (lemons, clementines, oranges, grapefruit), shrimps, and strawberries

Different allergens responsible:

– before the age of six months: cow's milk (13 per cent of cases), eggs (30 per cent), fish (12.5 per cent), oranges, pork, and wheat

– between six months and two years of age: peanuts (20 per cent), celery, tomatoes, and peas

– from two years: almonds, chocolate, shrimps, strawberries, lentils, walnuts, cashews and hazelnuts, pistachios, apples, and soya

Histamine is a substance released during an allergic reaction, and antihistamines are prescribed in order to suppress this allergic response.

– Foods that contain tyramine: chocolate, cheeses (such as Brie, Camembert, Cheddar, Emmental, Gruyère, Mozzarella, Parmesan, and Roquefort), fish (caviar, herring, and tuna), meat ('high' game, salami, and fermented sausages), and grapes

– Preserving agents: mostly monosodium glutamate, which is added to a lot of Chinese food. This can cause headaches, burning in the chest and throat, and tingling all over the body. Although the symptoms may be rather dramatic and cause many people to ring for an ambulance, this is largely unnecessary as most cases are not serious and the symptoms disappear rapidly on their own

– Sulphites, mainly those numbered E 210, E 211, E 223, and E 250, are used to suppress the development of unpleasant odours in wine, to lighten or stabilize the colour of certain foods and drinks, and to prevent bacteria from multiplying

– Nitrates are powerful vasodilators, and may trigger an allergic response

– Certain colouring agents, such as E 102 (tartrazine), E 110 (sunset yellow), or E 123 (amaranth, prohibited for use except in caviar) may cause rashes or hives

– Other allergens, such as some exotic fruits (kiwi fruit ++), for example, are being identified more frequently

I am sure you now understand how difficult it is to identify one single food as a culprit, since different additives are now so widespread throughout the food industry. You could, of course, inspect every manufacturer's label with a magnifying glass, but you may have to come to a general conclusion about certain foods or particular brands: do they agree with you or not?

Homeopathy

Only a constitutional remedy, selected in consultation with your professional homeopath, can modify the terrain in the hope of long-term changes for the better. In the case of allergies, you must be patient, and not expect any 'miracle' cures within a few days.

Asthma

This illness manifests itself as wheezing and breathlessness, coughing, or breathing difficulties, symptoms that come and go in bouts. Asthma is linked to allergies, as well as to psychological and environmental factors, and affects millions of people in the west to some degree. Children are twice as likely to suffer from asthma as adults, and its incidence appears to be on the rise all over the world, despite all the medical treatments available to combat it.

Management of asthma

This comprises four important aims:

- Teaching patients to avoid or control those elements that trigger their asthma attacks
- Treating these attacks rapidly and effectively
- Evaluating and monitoring the seriousness of the asthma through regular, objective measurements of lung function
- Putting a long-term treatment plan into place, as the asthma attacks may diminish in frequency, or even disappear at some point

Asthma is very much influenced by the patient's state of mind, and no one can deny the role played by psychology in the onset of asthma attacks or in their disappearance. However, asthma remains very much a multifaceted disease that is also influenced by heredity, as well as by allergies triggered by dust mites, cat hairs (the most common household allergen), other allergens derived from pets' skin and claws, feathers, and pollen. Other factors that could contribute to asthma, but whose role has not yet been well defined, are smoking (whether passive or active), atmospheric pollution, and infections.

Animals trigger many allergic reactions: birds with their feathers, cats through the dried saliva that remains on their fur after grooming, rabbits, guinea pigs, and hamsters. Dogs, however, seem to cause fewer allergies.

Having asthma does not rule out keeping up physical exercise, especially endurance activities such as walking, jogging, swimming, cross-country skiing, or cycling. Any of these activities will bring benefit if performed two or three times a week, for about 45 minutes per session. Such physical activity will not actually treat the asthma, but can increase the body's stamina and lung capacity, thus reducing the asthmatic's breathlessness, and raising the threshold of the onset of an attack.

Acupuncture

Allergies in general, and asthma in particular, constitute acupuncture's third great forte, after pain and nervous disorders. Acupuncture is not an instantaneous remedy, and is therefore not suitable for treating acute asthmatic symptoms – however, it can, and should, be part of a long-term programme of prevention.

TREATMENT SCHEDULE: Several bimonthly sessions to be followed over the course of a few months.

Oligotherapy

Manganese and **cobalt**

Trace elements are usually found in a varied and high-quality diet. In cases of deficiency, which should not occur with these two minerals, they can be given as medicinal supplements.

Dietary sources of manganese

This is primarily to be found in plants, especially whole-grain cereals, chocolate, nuts (such as almonds, walnuts, and hazelnuts), wheatgerm, some herbs and spices (cloves, ginger, and thyme), vegetables (beetroot, chestnuts, beans, peas, and soya beans), and tea.

Dietary sources of cobalt

This mineral comes essentially from animal products: meat, milk, and shellfish (crayfish). Plant and vegetable matter contains very little cobalt in general, with the exception of mushrooms, white cabbage, onions, and radishes.

• Manganese-cobalt treatment: this combination is available in various brands and forms, such as Organic Minerals (Colloidals) which contains 70+ trace minerals:
– Available in 946ml bottles
– Take 1–3 caps just before breakfast and/or evening meal
– Children 1 teaspoon daily for each 20lbs of body weight
Or Maximol (Ionized colloidals):
– Available in 500ml bottles
– Take ½ capful once or twice daily on an empty stomach.

• You could also take a manganese-only supplement, such as Lamberts® Manganese (as Amino Acid Chelate), containing 5mg of manganese:
– Available in containers of 100 capsules
– 1 to 3 capsules daily

Homeopathy

Antimonium tartaricum and **Sambucus nigra**

– Four 5c tablets of one or both of these remedies to be sucked slowly between meals, two or three times in succession at the start of an asthma attack

Antimonium tartaricum

– Chemical origin: antimony potassium tartrate
– The homeopathic remedy for lung conditions with thick, copious secretions that are difficult to expel

Sambucus nigra

– Vegetable origin: elderflowers
– The specific homeopathic remedy for attacks of breathlessness (stridulous laryngitis)

• You could also try Tartephedreel® (Heel), which contains Lobelia inflata D4, Ephedra vulgaris D3,Tartarus stibiatus D4

– Available in drop bottles of 30 and 100ml
– In general, 10 drops 3 times daily; in acute disorders initially 10 drops every 15 minutes

• It is also vital that you combine these treatments with a constitutional remedy, to be chosen after consultation with a professional homeopath. Some likely choices are Arsenicum album or Sulfur

Herbal remedies

White horehound and **plantain**
Ask your herbalist to prepare a 30ml bottle of mother tincture of plantain. Take 25 drops in a little water three times a day.

• You could also try Herba Naturelle White Horehound:
– Available in bottles of 50ml and 100ml
– 20 drops in a little water 3 times daily

White horehound

This plant, which grows in the hot, dry landscape of Provence, has various beneficial properties for the airways: it helps coughs, loosens bronchial secretions, and dilates the bronchial tubes, all of which are helpful for asthma. It is one of herbalism's five traditional bitter herbs, as can be confirmed by its taste.

Plantain

Plantain's leaves soothe irritations and bladder infections, promote healing, and help stop bleeding. The lanceolate variety is the most effective against allergies and inflammation of the airways.

• You can take T. Asthmatica Plus® (Thorne), which contains extracts of Tylophora asthmatica, Boswellia serrata, Picorhiza kurroa, Piper longa and quercetin:
– Available in containers of 120 capsules
– 1 to 2 capsules two to three times daily

Hay fever

This is another common allergy, affecting ten to twenty percent of the population. It is hardly ever seen in children under the age of five, but usually appears after puberty. The incidence of hay fever diminishes rapidly in those aged over 35.

The symptoms of this seasonal allergy come on during the flowering season, and are characterized by itching in the roof of the mouth and in the nose, sneezing fits, copious, but clear nasal discharge, and red, watery, irritated eyes that sting or itch. Hay-fever sufferers wait impatiently both for rain, which temporarily damps down the pollen, and for the end of the flowering season, which will cure them… at least until next year.

Managing allergies

When faced with any allergy problem, you need to:

- Identify the culprit by means of skin tests performed by applying various common allergens to the skin and noting any possible reactions
- Eliminate the allergen from your surroundings through avoidance measures
- Treat the allergy with a desensitizing programme set up by your allergy specialist, or preferably with homeopathic remedies to strengthen your individual 'terrain'

Avoidance measures

It is essential, although certainly not always easy, to take these measures, as it is difficult to get a child (or even an adult) to agree to stay shut up at home for the several weeks of the flowering season.

It may help if you discourage the sufferer from going out on long walks in the woods during the height of the allergy season, especially in fine, windy weather, unless he or she has taken some sort of allergy remedy, possibly antihistamines. Thanks to pollen samples taken every day by specialized monitoring bodies, we now know that the atmospheric pollen count varies tremendously from one day to the next, and depends largely on weather conditions. A dry, windy day will thus cause more problems to allergy sufferers than rain or windless weather.

Be aware of allergy confusion – just as with trains, there may be another allergy coming along behind the most obvious one. We now know that some

Pollen calendar: three successive waves

From the end of winter to early spring:
– most commonly cypresses and white cedar pollen, especially in the Mediterranean areas of Europe, from the end of January to mid-March
– mostly birch, hornbeam, and hazelnut tree pollen, especially in the North and East, in March and April
– primarily plane trees in April
– mostly ash and olive trees in successive waves from January to June
– most commonly oak, all over France and Britain, in May and June

In spring and early summer:
– primarily grasses (the most common culprit) from May to July or August
– occasionally plantain and nettles

Late summer and autumn
– mostly weeds and ragweed

patients who are allergic to inhaled pollens are also sensitive to other, apparently quite different, substances. Thus, there are combined allergies to birch pollen and apples (and to fruits with stones), to latex and bananas, to mugwort and celery, to ragweed and melons. And this list of combinations continues to grow.

Acupuncture

Acupuncture should really be recommended in these cases, for allergies constitute one of this therapy's most successful areas, after pain and nervous disorders. Acupuncture can both prevent and cure, so it can bring rapid relief during acute periods.

TREATMENT SCHEDULE: One session every fortnight from January to April, then two sessions per week for two or three weeks at the beginning of the pollen season, when you notice, for example, that the roof of your mouth feels itchy and your eyes begin to sting.

Oligotherapy

Manganese and **cobalt**

Trace elements are usually found in a varied and high-quality diet. In cases of deficiency, which should not be the case with these two minerals, they can be given as medicinal supplements.

Dietary sources of manganese

This is primarily to be found in plants, especially whole-grain cereals, chocolate, nuts (such as almonds, walnuts, and hazelnuts), wheatgerm, some herbs and spices (cloves, ginger, and thyme), vegetables (beetroot, chestnuts, beans, peas, and soya beans), and tea.

Dietary sources of cobalt

This mineral comes essentially from animal products: meat, milk, and shellfish (crayfish). Plant and vegetable matter contains very little cobalt in general, with the exception of mushrooms, white cabbage, onions, and radishes.

• Manganese-cobalt treatment: this combination is available in various brands and forms, such as Organic Minerals (Colloidals) which contains 70+ trace minerals:
– Available in 946ml bottles
– Take 1–3 caps just before breakfast and/or evening meal
– Children 1 teaspoon daily for each 20lbs of body weight
Or Maximol (Ionized colloidals):
– Available in 500ml bottles
– Take ½ capful once or twice daily on an empty stomach

– One dose of manganese-cobalt treatment to be taken three times a week as an ongoing treatment from Easter onwards. Increase the frequency to two doses per day during the pollen season

Homeopathy

Allium cepa

– Four 5c tablets to be sucked slowly two or three times per day for several days

Allium cepa

– Vegetable origin: the common or garden onion
– The homeopathic remedy for irritant nasal discharge
– The patient's symptoms will resemble those brought on when a healthy person peels an onion: sneezing, running nose, and weeping eyes

• You could also try Nelsons Pollena, which includes Allium cepa 6c, Sabadilla 6c and Euphrasia 6c:
– Available in boxes of 72 tablets
– Two tablets to be sucked every 2 hours for the first 6 doses, then 2 tablets 3 times daily between meals

• Another alternative is QC Nasal Spray (Thorne) which contains Euphorbium 6x and Quercetin 2x:
– Available in 1 fluid ounce metered bottles
– 1 to2 metered sprays in each nostril as needed

• **Pollen** and **Lung histamine**
– Four 5c tablets of one or both of these remedies to be sucked slowly, two or three times per day for several days. (Contact your homeopath)

Pollen

– Vegetable origin: a blend of tree and flower pollens
– The specific homeopathic remedy for hay fever

Lung histamine

– Animal origin: the lung of a guinea pig sacrificed while undergoing anaphylactic shock
– The specific homeopathic remedy for allergies

When the allergen has been clearly identified, it can be harvested, and the homeopath can then prepare an isotherapeutic remedy.

–Self-isotherapeutic remedies were prepared from secretions supplied by the patient, taken from the nose or throat, or from a urine sample. Current legislation no longer permits their preparation in France. However, in Britain, there is no such regulation and homeopaths often prescribe on this basis

– Hetero-isotherapeutic remedies, on the other hand, are still made up and distributed to patients. The remedy is derived from house dust, mould, or pollen

Sabadilla if the roof of the mouth is itchy
– Four 5c tablets to be sucked slowly two or three times per day for several days

Sabadilla

– Vegetable origin: the seeds of the cevadilla plant
– The specific homeopathic remedy for an itching palate, which the patient feels the need to scrape at with the tongue

Euphrasia for irritated eyes
– Four 5c tablets to be sucked slowly

two or three times per day for several days

Euphrasia

– Vegetable origin: the eyebright plant
– The specific homeopathic remedy for conjunctivitis accompanied by irritant discharge

• It is essential that you combine this treatment with a constitutional remedy, to be chosen after consultation with a professional homeopath. Some likely choices are Arsenicum album or Sulfur, which the homeopath may say should be taken two or three times per week throughout winter and spring

Herbal remedies

Plantain

POSSIBLE PRESCRIPTION: Ask your herbalist to prepare a 60ml bottle of mother tincture of plantain. Take 25 drops in a little water three times a day for the duration of the pollen season.

Plantain is a contradictory herb. Its pollen is one of the known triggers of hay fever, yet the plant (*Plantago major*, or greater plantain) supplies one of the best anti-allergy remedies. Plantain was used in the past in order to stop bleeding, promote healing, and calm upset stomachs.

For greater well-being

For this last chapter, I have selected three subjects that may seem at first glance to be quite unrelated, but that have all helped bring complementary medicine to the fore in their different ways. These three common situations cause many people so much worry that they will seek any solution, no matter how far-fetched, if it appears to offer a glimmer of hope. How is one to lose weight easily? Is there a manageable way to give up smoking? Are there natural methods to boost one's sex life? These are all areas in which complementary therapies should definitely be tried.

Weight loss – Giving up smoking – Preventing or treating sexual dysfunction

Weight loss

Slimming – that magic word synonymous with grace, slenderness, and beauty, for which millions of people are ready to follow any approach, any gimmick, as long as it promises they will lose ten pounds or one inch from their thighs in one week. Yes, it may involve a little dieting – and sometimes it may promise no dieting is needed at all.

We are long past the age when matronly women ruled the social world, when curves denoted health or wealth, or provided inspiration for artists (from Rubens to Fellini). On the contrary, we live in a period in which slenderness, if not actual thinness, rules, and we are tyrannized by magazine covers showing a succession of skinny models. This makes women feel constantly guilty and leads them into a permanent battle with their weight, which may be unreasonable or even unjustified, but is certainly never easy.

Women patients want not only to lose weight, but to lose it from 'certain areas', fuelling the increasing demand for meal replacements, the ever-popular reducing creams, and the use of all possible topical treatments to try to lose the 'hateful' saddle bags. The capsule, tablet, or herb that will bring (or bring back) a slender, firm, or muscled body with no effort simply does not exist yet, any more than a 'miracle solution' to banish forever unsightly rolls of flesh on the stomach, buttocks, or thighs. What is required is a commonsense and gentle approach, a healthy, balanced diet, and some nonaggressive remedies to bring about long-term weight loss that also allow the weight to stay off. It is important to avoid 'yo-yo' dieting, which is not only discouraging, but also seems to become more unavoidable with each successive attempt to lose weight.

What is the ideal weight?
There is no mathematical formula – it is the weight at which you 'feel well' in both body and mind, and at which the doctor has no complaints.

Being overweight is a significant public health problem: the list of health complications stemming from being obese is so lengthy, it explains why doctors have for so long focused on this aspect of the condition. But obesity is also a real social handicap, both in its aesthetic aspects and simply in the everyday difficulties it adds to moving about, travelling, or getting dressed and undressed.

The body that is generally apple-shaped (the upper body is well-developed, the abdomen protuberant, and the lower body also tends to bulge) presents more risks to the heart than a pear-shaped body (slender upper body, heavy lower body). Moreover, overweight men are more prone to cancers of the prostate and colon, and overweight women to breast, ovarian, and uterine cancers.

An obesity update
"All men are not created equal... when it comes to the ability to eat anything, at any time, in any way..."

In fact, we are all very unequal when it comes to the question of weight. Some of us are more 'prone' than others to weight gain, whether for hereditary reasons (20 per cent of cases) or due to environmental factors, such as lifestyle, education, eating habits, and inclination (or not) to exercise. For some of us, dieting consists only of putting a little less jam on one's toast, or of eating cake only every other day. For the less fortunate, it means tightening one's belt in drastic fashion for the rest of one's life, or taking a whole week to lose a 'few' extra ounces gained after only one small lapse – "two seconds on the lips, a lifetime on the hips", as the saying goes.

Recent studies have reportedly shown that calories consumed in the evening 'count double' – so it is particularly important to try to curb dietary excesses after 5pm.

Energy expenditure
An individual's weight depends on the balance achieved between the calories consumed and the energy expended. This second factor is itself linked to three others:

– The basal metabolism regulates the body's functioning, which is what burns up the greatest number of calories. The metabolic rate is influenced by heredity, but is closely related to muscle mass. The metabolic rate may slow down when food is restricted, or under chronic stress – we all know people who actually gain weight when they go on a diet, simply because they are preoccupied

– The production of heat by the body, and consequently the expenditure of energy, depends very much not only on food eaten but also on the quality of the nutrition. Out of 100 calories from protein, 25 to 40 are used to produce heat. These figures are much lower for calories from sugars and very low for fats, which explains how these latter substances tend to be stored up rather than consumed, promoting weight gain

– Only 20 per cent of calories are burnt up in physical activity in a sedentary person. Exercise should be encouraged, but its role in the overall consumption of energy, and therefore in weight loss, is only partial

Why is it so hard to keep to a diet?
– Willy Pasini, the famous Italian psychiatrist, explains humorously that women are trapped in a hopeless dilemma because, "they are more attractive when they weigh two or three pounds less, but feel more sexual when they weigh two or three pounds more"

– Dr. Chiva, a professor at the University of Nanterre, explains mischievously why it is we are doomed to failure in advance: "The pleasures of the table are the first ones we are given, and the last ones left to us when all the others have abandoned us"

As if these two explanations were not already enough reason for patients to have doubts about following their diets, here are (unfortunately) a few more.

The dangers of weight-loss treatments
The risks of traditional medicines are well known. Four categories of medicines were used for a long time in slimming treatments, but are rarely used now:

– Thyroid extracts do bring about weight loss, but unfortunately it is only muscle mass, not fat, that vanishes. These medicines also cause not just nervous disorders involving palpitations, anxiety, and heightened emotionalism, but especially hormonal disruptions, thus lowering the basal energy expenditure, and causing the patient to gain weight as soon as he or she returns to a normal diet

– Diuretics do not cause fat to be lost from the body, only water and mineral salts (mainly potassium), which has never brought about long-term weight loss. The skin becomes wrinkled, and this is followed not long after by cramps, itchiness, and malaise of various kinds. Any water lost is, of course, immediately replaced, ounce for ounce, by drinking

– Appetite suppressants, while certainly effective, can sometimes be dangerous. They are now banned

– Tranquillizers may ease the early days of a diet, but often make the patient sleepy. They may also cause dependency, and reduce basal energy expenditure, all of which makes long-term success unlikely

Since conventional weight-loss medicines have now been largely abandoned by most doctors, patients are quite justifiably looking to complementary therapies for help.

Acupuncture, auriculotherapy, electricity, and mesotherapy

• Acupuncture's calming effects are helpful in the initial stages of the diet, and ease the later period of stabilization. Sessions may range from two per week to one every fortnight

• Auriculotherapy has the advantage of leaving small 'semi-permanent' needles in place for several days, which can help reduce the hunger pangs during the difficult first days of the diet

• Electrolipolysis, a combination of acupuncture and electrical stimulation, seems to be effective in stimulating local micro-circulation and in reducing cellulite on the abdomen and upper thighs

• Mesotherapy remains the leading beauty treatment in France. It consists of injecting small doses of remedies into areas affected by cellulite, in order to reduce the appearance of 'orange-peel skin'

Topical treatments
Lymph drainage, or massage to the areas of the body where lymph fluid circulates, is a gentle, effective, and pleasant treatment. It improves local circulation, and helps reduce swelling in the thighs.

- Caffeine applied topically has a direct effect on minor vein problems that may be causing cellulite, and thus helps reduce it

- 'Reducing' creams soften, smooth, and tone the skin, and may help reduce some of its orange-peel appearance – but, unfortunately, do not cause spectacular weight reduction. These products contain three active elements: substances that promote drainage and strengthen the veins, in order to improve micro-circulation; lipid-reducing molecules that help break up and disperse fats in the cells; and toning ingredients. They are easy to use, and are risk-free, but they require enormous patience because these are very, very long-term treatments. They do improve the skin's appearance, even if they are not ultimately that effective against cellulite

Homeopathy

Anacardium orientale
– Four 5c tablets to be sucked slowly like sweets, two or three times a day when you feel hunger pangs

Anacardium orientale

– Vegetable origin: the Malacca bean tree, originally from the American tropics, and grown in India for its nuts
– The homeopathic appetite suppressant

- You could also try Strumeel® (Heel), which include Fucus D4, Spongia D3, Acidum silicicum D4
– Available in packs containing 50 and 250 tablets
– 1 tablet to be dissolved under the tongue 3 times daily.

- It is also very important that you combine this treatment with a constitutional remedy, to be chosen after consultation with a professional homeopath. Some likely choices are Calcarea carbonica, Sulfur, or Thuja

There is no miracle homeopathic remedy that can make anyone lose seven pounds easily in a week or two. Anyone who tells you they have lost several pounds in no time, with almost no effort, has almost certainly not taken homeopathic remedies alone, whatever they might think or say.

Herbal remedies

Pink sage, hawkweed, and **dandelion** are diuretics.

Green tea eliminates water and fats.

Ispaghula and **konjac** swell up in the stomach and give a feeling of fullness.

Bladderwrack and **laminaria**, which are both rich in iodine, stimulate the metabolism.

POSSIBLE PRESCRIPTION: Ask your herbalist to prepare a 30ml bottle of mother tincture of pink sage or hawkweed. Add 75 drops to one litre of mineral water, which is to be drunk regularly throughout the day.

Pink sage

The leaves of the pink sage, or Java tea, are used in that region for their detoxifying and diuretic effect. They also help bring cholesterol down slightly, and stimulate bile secretion.

Hawkweed

This plant is also known as 'mouse-ear hawkweed' because of the white hairs that cover its leaves. In the past it was believed to strengthen vision and heal wounds because of its unquestionable infection-fighting properties. Nowadays, it is mostly used to encourage the elimination of water, salt, and urea.

• You could also ask your herbalist to make up a 60ml bottle of dandelion in a whole fresh-plant suspension (this formulation's cold stabilization process restores the full natural therapeutic effect of the plant). Take half a teaspoonful in a little water morning and evening

Dandelion

Dandelion leaves contain high levels of potassium, and also act as a diuretic. Use them in salads, along with spinach. Dandelion root is a powerful depurative that is as effective for the liver and gall bladder as for the kidneys.

Seaweed

Seaweed is very good for your health as long as it is not eaten too often or in large quantities. Bladderwrack contains high levels of iodine, which can very easily build up to toxic levels after only a few weeks. You should therefore limit your treatment to less than three weeks' duration, and to between 200 and 300mg per day.

• You could also try Bioforce Kelp:
– Available in containers of 240 tablets
– Two capsules to be taken twice daily before meals. Not to be taken before bed

• Another alternative is Konjac fibre (Health Plus), which contains 500mg per capsule of Konjac flour, in order to reduce your appetite:
– Available in boxes of 70 capsules
– Two capsules to be taken before breakfast, three capsules before lunch and five capsules before dinner. Make sure that you drink plenty of water throughout the day

Konjac

The flour derived from the konjac root, originally from Japan, consists of a dietary fibre (glucomannan) capable of absorbing 100 times its own volume of water, forming an indigestible, viscous gel that suppresses appetite.

Wild chicory acts as a depurative, a mild laxative, and a diuretic; it is a useful supplement to any reducing diet.

– You can prepare your own decoction by boiling three tablespoonsful of chopped, crushed chicory root in half a litre of water. Leave the mixture to steep for an hour, then drink one cup before each meal

Chicory

Chicory roots encourage the elimination of urine, as dandelion does, but they also act as a detoxifier and tonic.

Celery and **watercress** are also diuretics and depuratives.

• You could also try Watercress powder (Phyto):
– Available in 500g packs
A substance is said to be a depurative when it helps purify the body through the elimination of toxins and poisons.

Oligotherapy

Zinc, nickel, and **chromium** for their role in regulating the endocrine system.

These trace elements are usually found in a varied and high-quality diet. In cases of deficiency, they can be given as medicinal supplements.

Dietary sources of zinc, nickel, and chromium

These are mainly to be found in some vegetables (beetroot, broccoli, mushrooms, cabbage, spinach, beans, and lentils), whole-grain cereals, wheatgerm, brewer's yeast, meat (liver and kidneys), seafood, pepper, thyme, black tea, and parsley.

POSSIBLE PRESCRIPTION: one dose of zinc-nickel-cobalt treatment to be taken in the morning, and one dose of chromium treatment to be taken in the afternoon, for one month. This is designed to supplement your diet, not replace it!

You could take these trace elements in combination such as Organic Minerals (Colloidals) which contains 70+ trace minerals:
– Available in 946ml bottles
– Take 1–3 caps just before breakfast and/or evening meal
– Children 1 teaspoon daily for each 20lbs of body weight
Or Maximol (Ionized colloidals):
– Available in 500ml bottles
– Take ½ capful once or twice daily on an empty stomach

Psychological treatments

There are three different possible approaches to psychological management of weight loss:
– traditional psychotherapy for support
– relaxation methods, as these help to control the inevitable tension caused by dieting
– other, more recent behaviour modification approaches, such as 'neuro-linguistic programming' (NLP), which does not address the diet itself, but rather the mental image the patient has of his or her goal to lose weight

It is most important for the therapist to:
– identify the patient's real wishes and desires
– evaluate his or her level of motivation
– get the patient to identify, in his or her own words, the positive elements

or the arguments that from the outset allow him or her to justify failure
– identify anything that may undermine the patient's goal of keeping the weight off in the long term

Muriel Robin: "I've been on a diet for a fortnight now, and I've already lost... two whole weeks."

Giving up smoking

In 1561, Jean Nicot introduced Europe to a herb that very quickly became fashionable in aristocratic circles. Soon noblemen were regularly taking snuff and smoking pipes. This habit remained the privilege of the few until the 19th century, when cigars and cigarettes appeared on the scene – now it seems nothing can stop the spread of the habit worldwide. We now know beyond any doubt that smoking poses enormous health risks, since two-thirds of all deaths that occur in middle age can be attributed to smoking. Smoking 20 cigarettes per day reduces life expectancy by seven years, by increasing the risk of heart disease and cancer.

Giving up smoking will benefit your health, no matter how old you are – but nicotine causes such a powerful addiction that giving up can cause significant withdrawal symptoms. These may include mood and behavioural disorders, a lump in the throat, spasms, cramps, acute hunger pangs, and often a gain in weight. The intensity of these withdrawal symptoms is not necessarily in direct proportion to the amount smoked.

The role played by cigarettes is a complex one – we may smoke as a way of asserting ourselves, to rebel, or to fit in with our friends, to increase our alertness, or calm our nerves, or simply to enjoy the cigarette. There is, therefore, no one purely pharmacological reason, attributable only to the chemical ingredients of the smoke or the nicotine content of the cigarette, to explain why giving up smoking is so difficult. Behavioural and psychological elements enter into the equation, too, and unless they are clearly understood, they will help sabotage your efforts to give up.

Let us examine the most effective **support methods** available to try to cope with the very difficult challenge of giving up cigarettes without too much pain.

The most effective method for stopping smoking is willpower, but the factor essential to success is motivation. Here are some examples:
– perhaps you have met someone who does not smoke
– you may have decided to have a baby, or you may already be pregnant
– you might want to take up physical exercise again, or train for a competition;

– you find you have a persistent cough in the mornings
– someone close to you may be affected by a serious illness caused by smoking
– you want to save money

In 1998, 27 per cent of adults aged 16 and over smoked cigarettes in England; 28 per cent of men and 26 per cent of women. In the same year, 69 per cent of smokers wanted to give up smoking. In 1999, 9 per cent of children aged 11–15 smoked cigarettes regularly – 8 per cent of boys and 10 per cent of girls. In the UK in 1995,over 120,000 deaths were caused by smoking; that is, one in five of all deaths.

Why do we smoke?
There are two types of addiction:
– psychological addiction, which is the most prevalent. We light up a cigarette when we are with friends, to make a phone call, while we watch television, or to go with a cup of coffee
– physical addiction, which is less common, but which goes deeper, and is related to the ingredients in nicotine. Nicotine reaches the brain in less time than it takes a sprinter to run 100 metres (after one inhalation, less than seven seconds). Once in the brain, nicotine stimulates the production of psychotropic or tranquillizing substances

Smokers have a sort of counter in the brain, a 'nicostat' that orders them to light another cigarette as soon as the level of nicotine drops below a certain threshold. Light or ultra-light cigarettes are smoked differently: smokers draw on them more deeply, for longer, more often – precisely in order to keep up the nicotine levels in the blood. In such cases, smoking stops being a pleasure and becomes an obligation, as going without a cigarette leaves the smoker feeling ill, irritable, and unable to concentrate. For every one cigarette smoked with genuine pleasure, several are smoked from pure addiction.

Essential general advice

The list of these tips is somewhat long, but must be followed if you are to give yourself the best possible chance of success. As soon as you decide not to smoke:

- Choose an appropriate time to give up
- Try to stop abruptly and completely, not gradually
- Do not try 'cutting down' first
- Avoid the temporary use of light or ultra-light cigarettes, which do not change the fact that smoking is still part of your daily routine – this is an important factor in the inability to give up
- Do not light up even one more cigarette
- Avoid the circumstances in which you usually smoke more, such as long meals, banquets, dinners with friends, card games, nightclubs, and bars
- Make sure you have a healthy, light, well-balanced diet, and that you eat

regularly throughout the day. Be aware that you will most likely want to eat more during the first few days

- Watch out for the tendency to nibble constantly, which may cause you to replace 20 cigarettes with 20 sweets instead
- Eat plenty of cereals, nuts, brewer's yeast (for its vitamin B content), fresh fruit and green vegetables for their vitamin C
- Cut back on stimulants such as coffee and tea, that only increase the craving for a cigarette
- Get up from the table before coffee, because the smell of coffee often causes the smoker to feel an irresistible desire for a cigarette
- Drink plenty of water at regular intervals. This will fill the stomach and suppress the urge to eat
- Take up physical exercise without delay, as this will prevent or reduce weight gain, and above all allow you to see the objective benefits of not smoking for your fitness and breathing

Some consequences of giving up smoking

In order to measure the undesirable effects of nicotine deprivation on weight, 9,000 Americans were followed over a ten-year period. On average, they gained between seven and nine pounds, but 13 per cent of the women and almost 10 per cent of the men gained two stone or more. Men generally find it easier to go back to their original weight than women. This very common tendency to gain weight only adds to the difficulties involved in giving up smoking.

According to the experts, it takes several years for the risk of cancer in an ex-smoker to drop down to that of someone who has never smoked. This is another reason to stop sooner rather than later.

Some conventional therapies

- **Nicotine replacement** consists of delivering nicotine to the body in the form of gum or a patch applied to the skin, which maintains a steady supply. The main disadvantage is that these nicotine-replacement methods often cause side-effects, such as hiccups, nausea, stomach upset, and the risk of heart complications, including increased heart rhythm or high blood pressure. And while nicotine may well be one of the factors in cigarette addiction, it is far from being the only one. Nicotine replacement continues over a period of two or three months, with the dose of nicotine being gradually reduced
- **The Venturi Method** gradually weans the body off nicotine by means of a series of cigarette filters, changed every week, that gradually filter out more and more of the tar and nicotine. After a period of about four weeks, it should be much easier to stop smoking altogether

• **The Five-Day Plan**, which has been in existence for 30 years, is a classic stop-smoking method. It brings people together in groups, and raises their awareness about what cigarettes do to the body through films and presentations. This method addresses the smokers' psychological needs, teaching them to avoid the pitfalls of certain situations, offering them dietary advice (vitamin and mineral supplementation) and relaxation sessions, in an effort to eliminate the dependency, so that people are less likely to relapse. Those who have tried this method find it to be hard going, but effective

• **Mental strategies**, such as hypnosis, relaxation, sophrology, and neurolingistic programming, help the smoker to reduce, eliminate, or channel the effects of the stress brought on by going without cigarettes, as well as reinforcing his or her motivation. These approaches help the person avoid taking up some other compensatory habit, particularly overeating

Acupuncture

This is the most widely used method to help give up smoking. Acupuncture helps the would-be nonsmoker by calming and balancing the nervous system, reducing the desire to smoke by inducing an aversion to tobacco. It produces a feeling of satiety that is most needed in the first few days when people are likely to turn to food instead, and lessens the craving, making this phase generally much easier to bear.

TREATMENT SCHEDULE: Sessions should initially be set up on a biweekly basis for the first three weeks of nicotine withdrawal. After that, maintenance sessions should be arranged depending on the subject's needs and any possible difficulties he or she encounters.

Auriculotherapy

This is acupuncture's little sister, and is also regularly used to bring about a successful cure.

TECHNIQUE: Auriculotherapy consists of piercing the earlobe with tiny needles the size of a pinhead, and leaving them in place for up to a week or more at a time. They are generally removed by the acupuncturist to avoid any septic problems but they may fall out of their own accord at some point anywhere from two days to two weeks later.

REMARKS: These 'semi-permanent needles' establish a longer-term readjustment that seems to be more effective than a single session of acupuncture. It is worth noting that these small needles can hardly be seen, and that they always fall towards the outside, rather than inwards, so there is no risk to the eardrum. While the needle treatment to the ears is not exactly pleasant, it is by no means really painful, and this therapy is not dangerous at all.

Mesotherapy

• Mesotherapy helps soothe and readjust the nervous system, helps develop an aversion to cigarettes that is most helpful, and can also be used to treat weight gain in specific parts of the body. It is this last area of application that has helped make mesotherapy better known in France. It is rarely practised in Britain other than by some GPs who have trained in homeopathic medicine

– The therapy consists of minute intradermic or subcutaneous injections of dilute classic medicines, that are applied to the face or body

The so-called 'Versailles treatment' is often used by therapists who deal with smokers in the process of giving up. This consists of micro-injections of solutions based on trace minerals and vitamins, delivered to the ear and nose areas, to help patients through the critical period of cigarette withdrawal.

Homeopathy

Tabacum

– Four 5c tablets to be sucked slowly three or four times a day during the first two weeks, then as needed after that

Tabacum

– Vegetable origin: the leaves of the tobacco plant

– The homeopathic remedy for nicotine-withdrawal symptoms

There are also the three great 'nervous tension' remedies: **Ignatia, Nux vomica**, and **Staphysagria**.

• **Ignatia**: for when giving up cigarettes is felt to be an enormous imposition, even when it is the individual's choice

• **Nux vomica**: for the heavy smoker who gives up completely and is worried about the effects on his or her mood

• **Staphysagria**: when the withdrawal period brings feelings of frustration and deprivation

– Four 7c tablets of one, two, or all three of these remedies to be sucked slowly between meals, twice a day for a fortnight

• You could also try Arteria-Heel® (Heel), which contains Tabacum D8, Secale comutum D4, Phosphorus D8, Viscum album D4

– Available in drop bottles containing 30 and 100ml

– 10 drops 3 times daily

• In France, one original homeopathic prescription involves the use of 'isotherapy', consisting of a remedy tailored to the individual based on his or her favourite brand of cigarettes. In Britain, a general remedy such as tobacco smoke in 30 potency is usually given for a few weeks followed by constitutional prescribing. Additional remedies such as Plantago or Caladium seguinum are often used in support

Herbal remedies

Hawthorn and **passionflower** for their calming effect.

Bladderwrack, fennel, and **pink sage** can help in the struggle against weight gain.

These plants can be made up singly or

in combination, as fluid extracts, mother tinctures, powder capsules, or dried extracts, for example. Ask your herbalist to prepare and package them for you.

POSSIBLE PRESCRIPTION: Ask your herbalist to prepare a 60ml bottle of hawthorn in whole fresh-plant suspension (this formulation's cold stabilization process restores the full natural therapeutic effect of the plant). Take one teaspoonful in a little water two or three times a day.

Hawthorn

This tree has been in use since Greek and Roman times, and for a variety of purposes. It was only in the 19th century, however, that it gained recognition when its cardiosedative benefits were discovered. Hawthorn can slow down a racing heart, reduce or eliminate palpitations, act as a heart tonic, and a vasodilator for those who have suffered a heart attack, thus improving heart function. It also brings down high blood pressure, and calms anxiety, both in children and adults, without inducing drowsiness or memory lapses. It has the added advantage of being nontoxic.

Passionflower

This vine or liana originally came from Brazil and Mexico, and was used by the Aztecs for its calming properties. It was introduced to Europe in the 17th century, and has been shown to be very effective against anxiety, nervous symptoms, and sleep disturbances.

• You could also try a mild tranquillizing remedy such as Passiflora Complex (Bioforce), which is a combination of tinctures of passionflower and oats:
– Available in bottles of 50ml
– 20 drops twice daily in a little water

I could suggest various other methods and remedies, but while it is encouraging that such a choice exists, it also goes to show that no one method stands out from the others as a miracle treatment. The ultimate success of any treatment finally depends on whether the subject genuinely wishes to stop smoking, and that is often the heart of the matter.

Preventing or treating sexual dysfunction

Sexual desire is such a subtle, complex, and fragile chemical combination, as intense as it may be fleeting, that I think I can safely say every man has had or will have a 'little problem' at some point in life – hence the popularity of Viagra®.

The symptoms of dysfunction are a reduction or loss of desire, and an erection that lacks endurance or intensity, or that cannot be maintained. This can mostly be attributed to psychological reasons (the role of stress, or relationship difficulties with the partner) or physiological ones (a reduction of the secretion of the male hormone).

There is no need to hunt down every last rhinoceros for its horn, fly to Canton in order to buy dried Spanish fly at the market, or go to the Costa Rican coast for turtle eggs buried in the sand, when complementary medicines can offer safe, affordable, and effective solutions to what are very common and harmless difficulties.

"The effect of stress on sex is as predictable as bromide in the soldier's mess tin", as popular wisdom would have it.

• While it is difficult to establish rules or statistics when it comes to frequency of lovemaking, the Simon Report published in France a few years ago is still the standard work
– between the ages of 20 and 30, one third of couples make love every night/on a daily basis
– between 30 and 40 years of age, this drops down to two or three times a week
– between the ages of 40 and 50, this frequency has dropped down to two or three times a month.

In Britain, the statistics are similar across the age groups but with a little less frequency on average. One recent survey proclaimed that couples in the UK make love about 149 times per year compared with 167 times per year in France. This of course is an average for all age groups. In older age, tenderness, communication, and emotional happiness now take priority over sexual relations, without this being felt to be a problem – unless there is a new partner. So the 'average' couple makes love somewhere between three times a week and three times a month, with a gradual decline in frequency that is due to various factors. One of these is the role played by certain prescription medicines, especially sleeping tablets, tranquillizers and anti-depressants, and beta-blockers

Some factors responsible for diminished sexual activity

This comes down to the effects of certain medicines:

– anti-hypertensive medicines (such as beta-blockers, diuretics, or ACE (angiotensin-converting enzyme) inhibitors

– tranquillizers and antidepressants

– anti-ulcer treatments

– medicines that reduce cholesterol levels

General advice

It is important to follow these tips:

• Stay in good physical condition by taking regular, moderate exercise. Overdoing it will be likely to have the opposite effect

• Eat a varied and balanced diet that

includes plenty of fruit, vegetables, cereals, wheatgerm, and seafood

- Stay away from fried and sweetened foods, which help block the arteries

- Choose foods containing the trace minerals and vitamins that bring vitality

- Spice up your meals with pepper, nutmeg, mustard seeds, cinnamon, and ginger

- Follow the example of the French king Henry IV who consumed large quantities of garlic to reawaken his ardour

- Be aware of the effects of alcohol, which is not a sexual stimulant – quite the opposite

- Round off an intimate meal with mint-flavoured green tea, coffee, or plain chocolate, all of which stimulate desire and provide energy for lovemaking – though they will not have any real effect on 'performance'

Lettuce versus mint

Lettuce has such calming properties that it was systematically served for dinner in convents. Mint, on the other hand, was always discouraged for homeopathic treatments because its stimulating action was incompatible with the promotion of abstinence and calm that was so important in former times.

Aphrodisiacs

Pepper, nutmeg, onions, leeks, watercress, orchids, mustard seeds, seafood, raw eggs, mandrake root, shark fin, sparrow's brain, lizard broth, rhinoceros horn, elephant tusk, crushed reindeer antler, dried Spanish fly… This list contains only a fraction of the multiplicity of products reputed to stimulate sexuality (a reputation undeserved in most cases) since the dawn of time.

Acupuncture

This treatment is recommended, and can be effective, as it stimulates and restores balance. An acupuncture point located in the small of the back should be pierced or massaged at regular intervals in order to reawaken dormant energies.

TREATMENT SCHEDULE: Biweekly or weekly sessions should be helpful during difficult periods.

Trace elements and vitamins

Selenium and **zinc, vitamins C** and **E**

Dietary sources

These are mostly to be found in garlic, broccoli, citrus fruits, green vegetables, red fruits, whole-grain cereals, mushrooms, wheatgerm, fish and seafood, meat (liver and kidney), and brewer's yeast.

These trace elements and vitamins usually come from a varied, high-quality diet.

- In cases of deficiency, they can be given as medicinal supplements. Some examples are: Lamberts® Natural Form vitamin E 400iu; Lamberts® Selenium 200µg; Lamberts® Zinc 30mg and Lamberts® vitamin C 1000mg with Bioflavonoids:

– One dose of zinc and of vitamin C to be taken in the morning, one dose of selenium and of vitamin E to be taken in the afternoon, for several weeks

• You could also try Lamberts® vitamin E with Selenium, which contains vitamin E 400iu and selenium 100ug:
– Available in containers of 60 tablets
– One tablet to be taken every day

• Another alternative is a dose of arginine, an amino acid that forms the proteins involved in reproduction. While this may not actually be your goal, arginine may help promote blood flow to the male sex organ. Arginine (Solgar) contains 500mg of Arginine per vegicap. It is available in bottles of 50 vegicaps. One vegicap daily with a little juice or water between meals

Herbal remedies

Plants and herbs have always been used to make up love potions, and **ginseng** is usually at the top of the list.

Ginseng

This mythic plant with multiple benefits has been known and venerated in China for 4,000 years. Ginseng is reputed to strengthen and stimulate the natural defence system, to act as an aphrodisiac, to combat stress, and to be an antidepressant and a tonic. It is traditionally prescribed and used during periods of overwork or during convalescence after an illness. It is an excellent remedy for physical and mental fatigue, and is often used by athletes for this purpose. This tonic action is likely to be the reason for its benefits to the libido. Ginseng has always been known as the 'plant of life', capable of slowing down the ageing process.

• You could also try Lamberts® Korean (Panax) Ginseng 600mg:
– Available in containers of 60 capsules
– 1 to 2 capsules daily

• Ginseng is in such demand the world over that many crop growers in the American West have taken it up, having decided it is much more profitable to grow than their traditional maize. Be sure to buy Panax ginseng, as only this variety has any effect on sexuality

Oats, Siberian ginseng, ginkgo, cola nut, yerba maté, and **yohimbine**

Possible prescription: Ask your herbalist to prepare 30 capsules of a blend of dried extracts of Siberian ginseng, Panax ginseng, and cola nut, 100mg of each plant for each No.2 capsule (the size of the capsule that the herbalist would use for the ingredients). Take one capsule three times a day for ten days.

Oats/Siberian ginseng/ginkgo/cola nut/yerba maté

Oats (*Avena sativa*) are said to have very beneficial effects on the erection response, as well as on its quality and duration; Siberian ginseng stimulates both the mind and the body; ginkgo promotes blood circulation; cola nut is known in West Africa as the plant that brings couples together at night; and Yerba maté is a South American tree that symbolizes strength and vigour.

Yohimbine

Yohimbine, used in a classical medicine for sexual dysfunction, is based on the yohimbé tree's ingredients. It is said one can see the places along African roadsides where the trees' bark has been partially stripped away to supply the citizens with yohimbine's stimulating properties.

• You could try Yerba Maté (Rio Health):
– Available in boxes of 40 teabags
– Infuse one teabag in a cup of boiling water

Plant essential oils

Anise, oregano, and **rosemary** for their stimulating effects.

Savory used to enjoy a reputation in the past for stirring up the 'fires of desire', and its Latin name, **satureia**, makes a clear reference to the satyr.

– Two drops of essential oil of one of these plants to be taken in a little honey before lovemaking

Mountain savory

Apart from its mildly aphrodisiac properties, savory, the little aromatic plant often confused with thyme, also brings benefits to the entire digestive system, combating flatulence, soothing colic pains, and stimulating digestion.

Homeopathy

Agnus castus
– Four 5c tablets to be sucked slowly like sweets two or three times a day for several days

Chasteberry or Agnus castus

– Vegetable origin: the chasteberry, the fruit from the chaste tree
– The basic homeopathic remedy for sexual problems

Chasteberry or **Agnus castus**

The fruit of this pungent tree, originally from Central Asia, is sometimes known as 'monk's pepper', and was used in medieval monasteries to calm sexual urges. But if chasteberry mostly has a soothing effect, it can sometimes be a stimulant, and is for this reason also classified among the aphrodisiac plants. It is also worth mentioning that chasteberry belongs in the list of herbs (along with yarrow, lady's mantle, sarsaparilla, and wild yam) that benefit the prostate.

• You can also take Bioforce Agnus castus in tincture form:
– Available in drop bottles of 50ml
– Take 15 to 20 drops in a little water twice daily

List of homeopathic remedies

Index

List of plants and herbs

List of trace elements, vitamins, and dietary supplements

List of illnesses and conditions

Natural healing